# Anti-Aging Therapeutics
## Volume VI
### 2003 Conference Year

*Editors*

Dr. Ronald Klatz

and

Dr. Robert Goldman

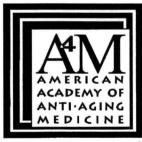 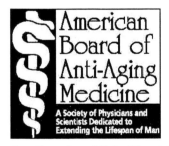 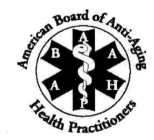

**An official educational work published by A4M Publications**
1510 West Montana Street
Chicago, IL 60614 USA
TEL: (773) 528-4333; FAX: (773) 528-5390; E-MAIL: a4m@worldhealth.net
WEBSITE: www.worldhealth.net

Visit
**The World Health Network,** at www.**worldhealth.net**, the Internet's leading anti-aging portal;
And
**The A4M's Special Information Center,** at www.**a4minfo.net**, the A4M's Publishing and Media Showcase

## IMPORTANT – PLEASE READ

The content presented in the *Anti-Aging Therapeutics, volume 6* is for educational purposes only and is specifically designed for those with a health, medical, or biotechnological education or professional experience. *Anti-Aging Therapeutics, volume 6* does not prevent, diagnose, treat or cure disease or illness.

While potentially therapeutic pharmaceuticals, nutraceuticals (dietary supplementation) and interventive therapies are described in the A4M's *Anti-Aging Therapeutics, volume 6*, this work serves the sole purpose of functioning as an informational resource. Under no circumstances is the reader to construe endorsement by A4M of any specific companies or products. Quite to the contrary, *Caveat Emptor*. It is the reader's responsibility to investigate the product, the vendor, and the product information.

Dosing of nutraceuticals can be highly variable. Proper dosing is based on parameters including sex, age, and whether the patient is well or ill (and, if ill, whether it is a chronic or acute situation). Additionally, efficiency of absorption of a particular type of product and the quality of its individual ingredients are two major considerations for choosing appropriate specific agents for an individual's medical situation.

Furthermore, anyone with malignancy should consult their physician or oncologist prior to beginning, or continuing, any hormone therapy program.

Finally, please be mindful that just because a product is natural doesn't mean it's safe for everyone. A small portion of the general population may react adversely to components in nutraceuticals (especially herbal products). A complete inventory of interventions utilized by a patient should be maintained by physicians and health practitioners dispensing anti-aging medical care.

*Anti-Aging Therapeutics, volume 6* is, again, designed for those with a health, medical, or biotechnological education or professional experience. It is not intended to provide medical advice, and is not to be used as a substitute for advice from a physician or health practitioner. If you are a consumer interested in any of the approaches discussed in these chapters, it is absolutely essential that you have a thorough discussion with your physician to understand all benefits and risks.

For those individuals interested in the diagnostics and/or therapies described by chapter authors of *Anti-Aging Therapeutics, volume 6*, A4M, A4M urges that you consult a knowledgeable physician or health practitioner, preferably one who has been Board Certified in Anti-Aging Medicine. You may find one by utilizing the Online Physician/Practitioner Locator at the A4M's educational website, www.worldhealth.net, or you may call our international headquarters in Chicago, IL USA at (773) 528-4333.

© Copyright 2004. American Academy of Anti-Aging Medicine.
1510 West Montana Street; Chicago IL 60614 USA.
All rights reserved.

**ISBN** 0-9668937-5-1 (print & CD-ROM)

Electronic and/or print reproduction, storage in an electronic and/or physical retrieval system, or transmission by any means (electronic, mechanical, photocopying, microfilming, recording, or otherwise) requires the advance written consent by the publisher.

Printed in the United States of America.

# TABLE OF CONTENTS

| | | |
|---|---|---|
| 1 | Anti-Aging Medicine at Eleven Years (2004): Reflections and Projections as a New Era Begins<br>*Dr. Robert Goldman and Dr. Ronald Klatz* | 1 |
| 2 | Putting It All Together: A Look at the Best Combination of Planning, Testing, Supplements, and Follow-Up For the Anti-Aging Clinician<br>*Eric Braverman, M.D.* | 7 |
| 3 | Is Growth Hormone Replacement for Normal Aging Safe?: Analysis of Current Medical Literature<br>*Ronald Rothenberg, M.D.* | 17 |
| 4 | "Fire in the Heart": New Developments in Diagnosis, Prevention & Treatment of Cardiovascular Disease<br>*Stephen Sinatra, M.D. and Graham Simpson, M.D.* | 27 |
| 5 | Integrated Anti-Aging: from Medical to Surgical Interventions<br>*Stephen M Pratt, M.D.* | 47 |
| 6 | Extreme Sports and Anti-Aging Medicine<br>*Bradley C. Grant, M.D., M.P.H.* | 53 |
| 7 | Testosterone, The Male Hormone Connection: Treating Diabetes and Heart Disease<br>*Michael Klentze, M.D., Ph.D.* | 59 |
| 8 | Current Status of Estrogen Therapy<br>*Seung-Yup Ku, M.D., Ph.D.; and Seok Hyun Kim, M.D., Ph.D.* | 73 |
| 9 | Hypercholesterolemia Treatment: A New Hypothesis or Just an Accident<br>*Sergey A Dzugan M.D., Ph.D.* | 89 |
| 10 | Eye Floaters: Causes and Alternative Treatment<br>*Scott Geller M.D.* | 99 |
| 11 | Plastic Surgery and Anti-Aging: A Natural Combination<br>*Robert L Peterson, M.D.* | 105 |
| 12 | The Impact of Nuclear Energy in Degenerative Disease<br>*Burton Goldberg, Hon Doctor of Humanities* | 113 |
| 13 | Implications for Medicine: New Energy Biophysics Discoveries<br>*Eugene Mallove Sc.D.* | 115 |
| 14 | Towards a Better Vaccine for Alzheimer's Disease<br>*Dr. Kevin A. Da Silva and Dr. Joanne McLaurin* | 121 |
| 15 | Fine-Tuning Mitochondria to Lose Weight: The Role of CIDE Proteins in the Development of Obesity and Diabetes<br>*Dr. Peng Li* | 137 |
| 16 | Anti-Aging Medicine: The Next Generation of Sports Medicine, Present and Future Challenges<br>*Robert Goldman, M.D., D.O., Ph.D.* | 143 |
| 17 | The Science Behind Growth Hormone<br>*Dr. Peter E. Lobie* | 149 |
| 18 | Update on Nutrient Supplements and Other Types of Treatment for Age Related Macular Degeneration<br>*Dr. Gerard Chuah* | 159 |
| 19 | Cartilage Repair with Autologous Chondrocytes and Stem Cells<br>*Dr. Eng Hin Lee* | 167 |
| 20 | Modern Management of Diseases of Neurological Deficits<br>*Dr. Ho King Lee* | 171 |

| | | |
|---|---|---|
| 21 | Free Radicals and Antioxidants: Where Are We Now?<br>*Dr. Barry Halliwell* | 179 |
| 22 | Growing a New Pancreas<br>*Sir Roy Calne* | 187 |
| 23 | A Lifestyle Plan for Long Lasting Weight Loss<br>*Shari Lieberman Ph.D.* | 193 |
| 24 | Cutting-Edge Technology in the Prevention and Treatment of Cardiovascular Disease: A Picture Tells a Thousand Words: The Case for IMT Heart™ Scan<br>*Jacques D Barth, M.D., Ph.D.* | 199 |
| 25 | Event-Related Potential (P300) Prolonged Latency Is Differentially Negatively Correlated with Sex Hormones and Insulin Growth Factors as a Function of Gender: A Preliminary Study of Hormones in Neurocognition<br>*Eric R. Braverman MD, Thomas JH.Chen PhD, Arpana Rayannavar, Neeta Makhija, John Schoolfield MSc, Matthew S. Stanford PhD, and Kenneth Blum PhD* | 205 |
| 26 | Developing an Anti-Aging Clinical Operation: The European Model<br>*Heather Bird, MBA* | 223 |
| 27 | Melatonin: More Than Just a Brake for Jet-Lag<br>*Dr. Jan-Dirk Fauteck* | 231 |
| 28 | Clinical Study in Patients with Sleep Disorders Treated with a New Chronobiotic Melatonin Formulation Compared to Normal-Release and Delayed-Release Formulations: Effects on Sleep Parameters<br>*Dr. M. Gervasoni and Dr. B.M. Stankov* | 235 |
| 29 | Nutritional Factors Including Antioxidants in Dementia and Anti-Aging<br>*Luis Vitetta, B.Sc. (Hons), Ph.D.* | 243 |

Chapter 1

# Anti-Aging Medicine at Eleven Years (2004): Reflections and Projections as a New Era Begins

*Dr. Robert Goldman, Chairman and Dr. Ronald Klatz, President*
*American Academy of Anti-Aging Medicine (A4M)*

## INTRODUCTION

The American Academy of Anti-Aging Medicine (A4M) is a non-profit educational medical organization dedicated to the scientific premise that diseases and disabilities of human aging are largely preventable, treatable, and perhaps even reversible. Anti-aging medicine is the fastest-growing medical specialty throughout the world and is founded on the application of advanced scientific and medical technologies for the early detection, prevention, treatment, and reversal of age-related dysfunction, disorders, and diseases. It is a healthcare model promoting innovative science and research to prolong the healthy lifespan in humans. As such, anti-aging medicine is based on principles of sound and responsible medical care that are consistent with those applied in other preventive health specialties. The phrase "anti-aging" is, as such, a euphemism for the application of advanced biomedical technologies focused on the early detection, prevention, and treatment of aging-related disease. Anti-aging medicine is scientifically based and well documented in leading medical journals.

The American Academy of Anti-Aging Medicine (A4M) is a non-profit educational medical organization dedicated to the scientific premise that diseases and disabilities of human aging are largely preventable, treatable, and perhaps even reversible. The A4M is an international body of physicians, scientists, academicians, and government- and university-affiliated officials. A4M's membership numbers 12,500 in over 70 nations worldwide.

A4M is the:
- First to create the anti-aging medical movement.
- Founder of the world's fastest-growing medical specialty.
- Foremost leader in a $50 billion marketplace.
- Frontier technologies for early detection & disease prevention.

## "THE END OF THE BEGINNING"

The American Academy for the Advancement of Science (AAAS) proclaims in *Science* magazine's February 28, 2003 issue that current aging research has reached its concluding point. Explaining that "[Scientists who study aging] have focused on physiological mechanisms underlying the processes of aging, rather than on the large array of debilitating and costly disorders that so commonly emerge during the latter half of the lifespans of human beings," AAAS points to "the 'one disorder at a time' approach" as "having limited power to ... extend the human lifespan." Rather, Dr. Martin et al submit while curing individual diseases can achieve a gain in life expectancy on the order of 30-40 years , slowing down aging offers "the biggest bang for the buck" by adding 60-70 years. As a result, those who celebrate their 50th birthday attain the opportunity to live to 120 years.[1]

The American Academy of Anti-Aging Medicine (A4M, Chicago IL USA; www.worldhealth.net and www.a4minfo.net) salutes this declaration because it hails a new era for preventive medicine specifically aimed at improving health as we age that is consistent with the anti-aging medical model. Since its inception eleven years ago, the A4M has advanced an innovative healthcare model involving the detection, prevention, and treatment of aging-related disease and the promotion of research into methods to retard and optimize the human aging process. A4M's model for anti-aging medicine embraces a multi-disciplinary approach for wellness-based healthcare, as our membership includes specialists in areas such as endocrinology, neurology, oncology, gynecology, pain management, and cosmetic surgery; as well as general and family practice physicians. A4M continues to unite physicians and scientists across specialties in a spirit of cooperative research and application to promote a scientifically-validated whole-body approach to aging intervention.

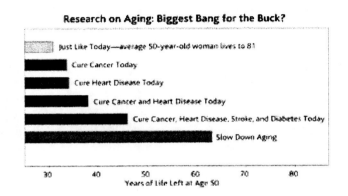

Indeed, *Science* magazine's special Aging issue (February 28, 2003) contains important testimonial to the important near-term applicable advancements being made in human aging intervention. Dr. Valter Longo and colleagues at University of Southern California reported that animal research on longevity is very near its transference to human application. Dr. Longo's article in *Science* remarks that viable techniques to extend the human lifespan by 20 years of more could be "standard procedure 30 or 40 years down the road," but by prompting "as many people as possible to get into this novel way of looking at disease prevention, anti-aging drugs could be available in the next ten years."[2]

## PRESTIGIOUS RECOGNITION

A4M continues to be the world's leading professional organization dedicated to advancing research and clinical pursuits that enhance the quality, and extend the quantity, of the human lifespan. The 12,500 physician, scientist, and health practitioner members from over 70 countries who belong to the A4M are forging an innovative model of healthcare that alleviates the mounting social, economic, and medical woes otherwise anticipated to arrive with the rapidly growing volume of an aging population. This movement is no longer denied, rather it is becoming a widely embraced resource being explored by many public health and public policy experts who seek to minimize the impact of old-age disability and dependence to burden individuals and societies at-large.

The February 2003 issue of *San Francisco Medicine*, published by the San Francisco Medical Society, was devoted entirely to the subject of anti-aging medicine. Featured was an article authored by A4M's president Dr. Ronald Klatz, in which he reviewed the broad-ranging benefits of anti-aging medicine. Dr. Klatz's article concluded that we are now "ushering in a new reality ... in which 75 years old may well be considered middle age."[3] San Francisco Medical Society's all anti-aging issue continues the affirmation of this medical specialty that was conferred by the San Francisco-based American Society of Aging one year ago in that organization's all anti-aging issue of *Generations*, that society's bimonthly journal.

"Winning the War Against Aging" by Dr. Joao Pedro Magalhaes at the University of Nemur (Belgium) and appearing in the March-April 2003 issue of *The Futurist* extends the ongoing recognition of anti-aging medicine by The World Future Society, a nonprofit, nonpartisan educational and scientific organization of 30,000 individuals who are interested in how social and technological developments are shaping the future. A microbiologist studying the biology of aging, Dr. Magalhaes reports that "many advances in antiaging science have been made at the cellular level," and suggests that "aging may soon become nothing more than a scary bedtime story."[4] Commenting in Dr. Magalhaes article, Dr. Steven Austad, biology professor at the University of Idaho remarked that "the prospects of dramatically increasing human longevity are excellent." [4] Dr. Austad is one of anti-aging's most ardent independent supporters, previously expressing that by January 1, 2150 it will be documented that a human has reached the age of 150 or more. His confidence in this prediction is so steadfast that he's wagered $500 million dollars to that effect.[5]

## INTERNATIONAL PARTICIPATION

At the Second World Assembly on Aging that was convened by the United Nations last year, much concern was focused on the growing number and proportion of older persons affecting every nation around the world. The Assembly reported that while one 1 of every 10 persons is 60 years or older, that ratio accelerates to 1 out of every 5 by 2050 and 1 out of every 3 by 2150. Global life expectancy now stands at 66 years, a gain of 20 years being made in just the last half of the 20$^{th}$ century.[6] As a consequence, a universal dilemma of how to provide and care for the world's aging residents has emerged.

In reaction, many nations have adopted a new reality of aging. From Europe to Asia, national health ministries, universities, and public policy officials are now recognizing that aging is a treatable condition that need not relegate a swelling demographic of adults ages 60+ to disability and dependence.

A4M's training and education initiatives have been responsible for expanding the availability of leading-edge preventive healthcare around the world. In its eleven-year history, A4M has trained over 25,000 physicians and scientists in the new science of anti-aging medicine. A4M's 12,000 members now provide advanced preventative and prospective clinical healthcare to over 200,000 men and women around the world. Each day, the ranks of A4M's membership and their patient population grows steadily. In addition, millions of people have embarked on their own anti-aging regimens that do not require regular physician supervision, a testament to the safety of anti-aging therapies.

A4M has witnessed nations that embrace anti-aging medicine as a clinical specialty undergo rapid and positive transformations in their approach to aging as a political, economic, and social issue. To continue this trend, over the course of the next twelve months, A4M will organize, sponsor, or coordinate anti-aging training programs in new venues in China, Brazil, Germany, Spain, Australia, and the Middle East. A4M also looks forward to continued involvement in France and Singapore as established anti-aging educational forums.

## PRESIDENTIAL VALIDATION

In March 2003, the United States President's Council on Bioethics issued a working paper on the status of aging intervention.[7] The A4M commends the Council's outline of the science of life extension because the principles contained in the working paper are consistent with A4M's multi-modal model for anti-aging and include the following:

(1) "Allow more individuals to live to old age by combating the causes of death among the young- and middle-aged":

Improvements in basic public health, sanitation, and immunization resulted in the marked gains in life expectancy of the 20$^{th}$ century, rising from 48 years (1900) to 78 years

(1999) in the US. The President's Council observes that "This approach has been so successful that almost no further gains in life expectancy can be expected from efforts to improve the health of the young." To continue making gains in life expectancy "would require a much greater feat: extending the lives of older people."

(2) "Extend the life of the elderly by combating particular causes of death or reversing some of the damage done by senescence"

The President's Council reports that this approach "has already contributed to the improved health of the elderly and to moderate extensions of life." Most compelling is the Council's observation that "if diabetes, all cardiovascular diseases, and all forms of cancer were eliminated today, life expectancy at birth in the US would immediately rise to about 90 years, from the present 78."

(3) "Direct age retardation to extend the average and maximum lifespans":

The President's Council acknowledges two key anti-aging interventions in which A4M has played a pivotal role in advancing worldwide, namely:

(a) Prevention of oxidative damage: "For many years, there has been ample evidence that oxygen free radicals ... cause gradual deterioration of the body's cell's and tissues. Our bodies produce or obtain through diet, antioxidants ... such as vitamin E, vitamin C, coenzyme Q10, and alpha lipoid acid, that destroy many, but not all, of these free radicals." The President's Council observes that "naturally occurring and synthetic antioxidants in humans [may] retard the degeneration of cells, reduce and slow the accumulation of errors in DNA replication, and thereby extend the human lifespan, perhaps significantly."

(b) Methods of treating ailments of the aged, including hormone therapy: "In the past 15 years, researchers have investigated the possibility of slowing or reversing the effects of aging by the replenishment of certain hormones to more youthful levels, with particular focus on Human Growth Hormone, DHEA, Testosterone, Estrogen, Pregnenolone, Progesterone, and Melatonin." Most notably in this discussion, the President's Council cites Dr. Rudman's 1990 HGH study, commenting specifically that the elderly men who received HGH "experienced increased muscle mass, a loss of fat, improved skin elasticity, and decreased cholesterol levels." As such, the Council states that "hormone treatments may play an important role in unlocking the secrets of the aging process, and in future aging [intervention] techniques."

Additionally and in alignment with A4M's forecast for the role of biotechnology in future aging intervention, the President's Council acknowledges the significance of advancements in stem cell research, tissue and organ replacement, and nanotechnology to extend life as well as halt degeneration of physical and mental performance. Included in this realm the President's Council also recognizes the potential for genetic manipulation to apply single-gene alterations that dramatically extend life in animal models, to humans.

Concluding the scientific review portion of the President's Council on Bioethics' working paper on the status of aging intervention, the group writes: "Scientists may indeed be able to retard the human aging process and significantly extend the maximum and average human lifespan in the foreseeable future."

# SAFETY AND EFFICACY OF ANTI-AGING MEDICINE

Core anti-aging therapies are medically proven and based on sound medical principles derived from published medical research in established peer-reviewed scientific journals. Considered by many to be the next evolution of preventative medicine, anti-aging therapies that are now widely accepted and prescribed by even the most conservative physicians include:

- Calcium for the prevention and treatment of osteoporosis
- Vitamin E for the prevention of heart disease and Alzheimer's Disease
- Daily multivitamin/multimineral supplementation to promote immune function in the elderly
- Early detection screenings for cancers
- Noninvasive scans for organ health, including the heart and brain

Indeed, it would be considered by many to be low-level, substandard medical care were physicians not to recommend many anti-aging therapies as part of their approach to preventative medicine.

Today, each American spends more on health care than anyone else in the world. And yet, we aren't much healthier as a society. Instead, it is up to every one of us as individuals to invest in our health as our number one personal priority. Those "in the know," have known this and are applying the principles to themselves to live longer and more healthful lives:

- A number of reputable scientists have been personally consuming antioxidants for years: at the US National Institutes of Health, Dr. Trey Sunderland, age 50, takes Vitamin E and anti-inflammatory drugs such as ibuprofen, while he conducts work as the Chief of Geriatric Psychiatry at the Institute of Mental Health into Alzheimer's prevention. At Case Western Reserve University (Cleveland, OH USA), Dr. Craig Atwood takes Vitamin E and drinks blueberry shakes while conducting research commissioned by the Alzheimer's Association to find antioxidant compounds to decrease plaques in brain tissue.[8] Such conduct begs the question: If such nutrients were of no preventive or therapeutic value, why would these experts on aging-related diseases continue to consume them?

- Dr. James Jessup at the University of Florida found that older men and women who exercised regularly and took vitamin E supplements became healthier and significantly decreased their levels of free-radical induced oxidative stress, a known contributor to aging and disease. Remarks Dr. Jessup: "The results of this study suggest that people who are over 40 can benefit from regular moderate exercise and vitamin E to protect … their aging bodies."[9]

- From the University of Illinois to Ball State University (Indiana), human performance scientists are in universal agreement that the one thing you can to do slow the aging process, and feel good afterwards, is to keep yourself physically active.[10] A landmark study published in 1995 tracked 9,777 men ages 20-82 and found that physically unfit men who became fit had death rates 44% lower than those who remained unfit. Exercise experts are now revising their definition of "aging" to reflect that aging for most people equates to inactivity. Today, thanks to high-tech sports medicine and rehab advancements, men and women in their 90s and 100s are regaining strength and mobility from muscle training. The take-home lesson: it's never too late to start exercising, but getting a jump start while you're still agile is best.

## CONCLUDING REMARKS

The public is evolving into what the Robert Wood Johnson Foundation calls the "top-tier healthcare consumer," capable of making its own educated decisions regarding all purchases including those relating to medical care. The report states that top-tier healthcare consumers, due to their financial stature, level of education, and employment, "will have the greatest ability to effect change."[11] The A4M, as a non-profit educational medical organization dedicated to the scientific premise that diseases and disabilities of human aging are largely preventable, treatable, and perhaps even reversible, serves as an advocate for this new science and as a conduit to physicians, scientists, and the educated public who wish to benefit from the almost daily breakthroughs in biotechnology which promise both a greater quality as well as quantity of life. A4M has devoted itself to education thousands of doctors and other professionals in the health-related field throughout the world in the area of anti-aging. A4M presents annual educational programs, written materials, and ongoing updates via accredited joint sponsored Category 1 Physician Recognition Award-Approved Continuing Medical Education scientific conferences and symposiums around the world, its educational Internet websites, and print publishing mediums, in order to keep medical professionals and scientists aware of the progress being made throughout the world on anti-aging medicine.

## REFERENCES

1 Martin GM, LaMarco K, Strauss E, Kelner KL. "Research on aging: the end of the beginning," *Science*, Feb. 28, 2003.
2 Mitchell S. "Scientists developing drugs to extend life," NewsFactor Sci-Tech, Feb. 28, 2003.
3 Klatz RM. "Human Growth Hormone," San Francisco Medicine, 76(2), February 2003, 14-16.
4 deMagalhaes JP. "Winning the war against aging," The Futurist, March-April 2003, 48-50.
5 "How long have you got," *Scientific American--The Quest to Beat Aging*, Summer 2000
6 "UN-Ageing: Second World Assembly on Aging," IRNA, http://www/irna.com/newshtm/eng/19214553.htm, accessed April 9, 2002.
7 The President's Council on Biotechnics, Age Retardation: Scientific possibilities and moral challenges, http://bioethicsprint.bioethics.gov/background/age_retardation.html, accessed March 12, 2003.
8 Jaffe S., "Scientists test theories on aging and their resolve," The Plain Dealer, Dec., 16, 2002.
9 "Researcher finds vitamins, exercise may slow harmful effects of aging," Breakthrough Digest, July 30, 2003.
10 "The simple answer for defying age: exercise," Newsday.com, August 20,2003.
11 Morgan CM, Levy DL. *Marketing to the Mindset of Boomers and Their Elders*, The Brewer House, 2002.

## ABOUT THE AUTHORS

Dr. Robert Goldman and Dr. Ronald Klatz are the physician co-founders of the anti-aging medical movement and the American Academy of Anti-Aging Medicine (A4M; Chicago, IL USA), a non-profit medical organization dedicated to the advancement of technology to detect, prevent, and treat aging related disease and to promote research into methods to retard and optimize the human aging process. A4M is also dedicated to educating physicians, scientists, and members of the public on anti-aging issues.

Correspondence: Postal c/o American Academy of Anti-Aging Medicine; 1510 West Montana Street; Chicago, IL 60614 USA.

Chapter 2

# Putting It All Together: A Look at the Best Combination of Planning, Testing, Supplements, and Follow-Up For the Anti-Aging Clinician

*Eric Braverman, M.D.*
*Medical Director, PATH Medical; President, Total Health Nutrients*

**ABSTRACT**

When considering setting up an anti-aging practice, there are four core principles that need to be taken into account: the brain, the pauses, being able to combine conventional and alternative medicine and provide patients with an effective non-drug alternative, and finally making the decision whether or not to prove diagnostic services. In this chapter, we will also briefly discuss the Brain Electrical Activity Map (BEAM) medical diagnostic technology.

**Keywords:** brain; organ pauses; pharmacology; nutritional medicine; brain electrical activity mapping

**INTRODUCTION**

The core principle to remember when considering setting up an anti-aging practice is that the brain is the most important organ. The thyroid can be replaced by a little pill. With parathyroid, one injection and you have replaced the parathyroid. If a man loses his testicles, their function can at least partially be replaced with a little AndroGel cream. If a woman loses her ovaries, one pill of progesterone, estrogen, and testosterone will restore the ovaries' hormonal functions. The heart can be replaced with a donor organ. The function of the adrenal gland can be replaced with two hormones. But if we scoop out the human brain, what is left of the person? Nothing, except a corpse. So dealing with the health of the brain should be central for every doctor.

The second principle is that there are many pauses of the body, that include everything from the menopause of the ovary; adrenopause of the adrenal gland; thymopause of the immune system; somatopause, the loss of growth hormone; pinealpause, the loss of melatonin; vasculopause, the change in blood vessels. The whole human body is going through what is now called geripause.

Pauses have two forms: the ovarian menopause represents complete death of the ovary, whereas the thyroid pause is partial death. Approximately 25% of the thyroid dies as we age. Men with normal testicles have a blood testosterone level of approximately 1,000 when they're 20. This drops to around 300 by the time they reach 70 or 80. If a man were castrated, he would have a blood level of 150 or even 200 because the adrenal gland would still make some testosterone. So the testicles do not decline in function completely in most men. Roughly 70% to 80% of testicular function diminishes with age. So all these different organs are dying at different rates. Some move into a total pause, and some into a partial pause.

The third principle, which is a cornerstone, is providing a non-drug alternative, and combining conventional medicine and drug alternatives. If you take a look at the study of medicine, every time we know a drug works we know of a nutritional equivalent as well. If we know that calcium channel blocker lowers blood pressure we can imitate a calcium channel blocker with magnesium. If we know diuretics lower blood pressure, we know that primrose oil is a mild diuretic. So we can use herbal diuretics. If we know that all the antidepressants work through dopamine: all the ones that work do, such as Wellbutrin and Effexor, we can imitate them with the amino acid tyrosine. We know that digoxin is an herb. We know that other types of agents used for heart failure are ionotropes. They make the heart pump better; but so does growth hormone, and so does testosterone. We know that steroids are used to treat lupus, and arthralgia. But we also know that natural steroids may improve those conditions. As physicians, we should be looking at how drugs work at the pharmacological level and using our knowledge to select a natural agent.

The fourth principle is a very important one, and a challenging one, because there are two models that people can use to set up an anti-aging practice. The first is a model of cash, where the clinic does not do any tests and does not accept any insurance. That model is problematic basically because it is important to scan people to make a decision on what is the most important thing to treat. One patient may have terrible bone density but their brain might be in great shape; whereas another patient may have good bone density and a somewhat unhealthy brain. The only way that you can take care of a patient properly is to find out exactly what the problem is with blood testing, ultrasound scans, PET scans, CAT scans, DEXA scanning (Dual Energy X-ray Absorptiometry), etc.

## DELIVERING HEALTHCARE HEAD-FIRST

The brain is the most important organ in the body. The brain is a central computer, it is the server, and thus it is everything. All the other endocrine systems are very, very simple in comparison. They are all replaceable by simple hormonal replacements. Nobody can replace the brain yet.

Obesity is a metabolic disorder of the brain. Studies on obesity suggest that the metabolism of the brain goes down. Studies on heart disorders suggest that people with brain chemical problems: for example depression, anxiety, and other psychiatric problems, will die faster than other heart patients. So you have patients who die of heart disease with no coronary artery disease, and other patients that will come to see you with 99% blockages and they are still alive. How could that be? The answer is that the brain controls the body. There is a basic principle that attitude, mood, and brain states are the most important issue in aging and quality of life. There is no point in getting people to live to 120, only to see them sit around not knowing who they are and what day it is.

The brain is the core focus of all the different conditions, even cancer. Scientists have now discovered oncogenes in the brain, and that attitude can be enormously powerful in fighting off cancer. Expressions of anger help the cancer patient, while the internalization of anger, as depression, is one of the precursors to cancer. People who suffer from chronic anxiety get more cancer, and they also make the wrong food selections. Everybody knows that they should not be craving fatty foods, but they still eat the fat. Everyone knows that they should not be craving sugar, but they still eat the sugar. The entire selection of diet depends on the brain.

Serotonin-based drugs are looking very promising for the treatment of bowel disorders, and the new drugs being used to treat cardiac arrhythmias are essentially GABA (gamma-aminobutyric acid) agents. Dilantin used to be employed to treat cardiac arrhythmias. Calming the brain calms the heart, and vice versa. Some of the new drugs that are being used in asthma and irritable bowel syndrome are serotonin agents. These are working on the same principle: calming the person down. If the brain is irritated, it can cause irritable lung, irritable bladder, frequent urination and other symptoms. The brain is a component of every aging person and every disease.

## THE PAUSES

Another core principle of conventional medicine to consider is that aging itself is really rapid disease acceleration. It is helpful to think of all the pauses of the body as a ladder. All these pauses can be lined up, and they go from life to death. If a patient's brain goes into electropause and short-circuits and he gets Alzheimer's, it is of no importance that you treated him with growth hormone and testosterone, and he had biceps of 18 inches. What good is it if you have great bones, great muscle mass, but forget who you are, or have major psychiatric problems? Brain electrical problems are antecedent to psychiatric disturbances. The same thing goes with patients who are on hormones who cannot achieve a sleep cycle, which is controlled by the pineal gland. The number one predictor of who is going to live or die has nothing to do with taking testosterone, growth hormone, or estrogen. The number one predictor is body weight, and that has to do with brain metabolism. The second predictor is smoking. The treatments of choice for smokers trying to quit are dopaminergic agents; from electrical devices, to Zyban/Wellbutrin, to Effexor, to tyrosine. What are the number one treatments for obesity? Dopamine and adrenaline. According to some studies, the third predictor of who is going to live or die, regardless of body weight or smoking habits, is sleep. What agents are used to aid sleep? Serotonin agents. From this it can be seen why a mastery of the brain is critical.

The pauses really tell you what needs to be measured if you want a complete clinic. Nearly thirty years ago, doctors were beginning to treat thyropause with Armour thyroid. These doctors were considered quacks because they used two forms of thyroid; T-3 and T-4. Psychiatrists had been using T-3 because it improved mood, and T-4 was being used for metabolism. But using both together was simply not done. However, in the year 2000 the *New England Journal of Medicine* carried an article saying that the best form of thyroid supplementation is the natural thyroid that contains T-4 and T-3. This is just one example of how physicians subscribing to the tenets of anti-aging medicine have been medically prophetic on where hormonal supplementation would lead.

The parathyropause is not thought of very often, although at first instance you would think that it would be quite important. The main reason why nobody has really tried to tackle the parathyropause is that it is very difficult to change bone density. When do people start getting short? The average Caucasian has lost a-quarter to a half-inch in height by the time he reaches 40 years old. The majority of people have lost some height by their 40th birthday, and by 50 virtually everyone is a little shorter. By 60, most people have lost somewhere between 1 and 3 inches. When it comes to bone density, there are people with minus-5 standard deviations, minus-4 standard deviations, and minus-3 standard deviations. The ideal deviation for bone density is plus-1.

The pineal gland producing melatonin starts to go into pause at age 5. Thyroid and melatonin are measured in blood: plasma melatonin, TSH (thyroid stimulating hormone), T-4, and T-3. Basically, every patient should have his or her TSH and T-4 levels checked. Now we get to parathyroid. Parathyroid can be measured in blood, and you can follow bone density. If you do not own a bone density machine it can still be followed to some degree. Refer the patient to a clinic for a bone density scan every one to two years, and follow it with urine telopeptides.

The thymus gland also goes into pause. The thymopause is the pause of the immune system. The thymus gland goes into pause at puberty, and the thymopause is the hardest one to fix. Everyone is experimenting with thymic proteins. At New York University, researchers conducted studies on transfer factor. It is suffice to say that exactly how to deal with the failing immune system of aging is debatable. What is certain though, is that the first thing to do when you want to deal with the failing immune system is measure immune function.

An immune function test determines the T-helper/suppressor ratio. A T-helper/suppressor ratio of 0.1 means that the patient has very few helper cells, and probably has AIDS. A ratio of 0.4 is suggestive of ARC, 0.6 of cancer, and a ratio of 0.9 indicates a viral infection. The normal ration is 1.8. A ratio of 2 suggests an autoimmune condition, and a ratio of 3 indicates MS, lupus, or another advancing autoimmune condition. Basically, the immune system function test is your first basic evidence of immune dysfunction. So before you prescribe a patient a pile of pills, check the status of his immune system. A lot of people get chronic colds because they have sinus problems. There is nothing wrong with their immune system. These people may be taking several pills in an attempt to boost their immune system, yet their immune system is perfectly normal. They have damaged sinuses and allergies. It is an autoimmune problem not an immune deficiency problem. So measure the immune system, and carry out allergy tests.

The next pause to consider is DHEA-pause, or adrenopause. As DHEA levels go down, aldosterone can increase, and the end result is hypertension. Adrenopause is generally treated with 50 mg DHEA for women, and 100 mg DHEA for men (these doses are for people in their sixties). The adrenal gland can be deficient in DHEA in 30 to 40-year olds. Dosages in the medical literature range from 600 mg for advanced lupus, to 5-10 mg for 30 and 40-year-olds. Almost everyone gets pimples when they take too much DHEA, so it has got a nice feedback loop. It is easy to determine whether or not a dose needs adjusting by measuring a patient's blood levels. Remember, with DHEA you have to measure levels of both DHEA and DHEA-sulfate. Furthermore, if a patient has a liver disorder he will not be able to metabolize DHEA.

The next pause is really called nephropause, which is a decline in erythropoietin. Erythropoietin is measurable in blood. Erythropoietin is injectable. It is especially important to people with chronic kidney failure and chronic anemia as it increases the blood count. It may also have a role in the treatment of a patient with a declining blood count. More research needs to be done, but it has promise.

One of the most often talked about pauses in anti-aging medicine is somatopause, the decline in growth hormone levels (GH). When considering somatopause, it is best to measure a patient's IGF-1 levels. GH can be given as people age. GH levels typically drop from 1,000 to 500 between the age of 10 and 20. Acromegaly patients do not get any additional cancer, and children who are treated with GH do not get any additional cancer. Remind every patient that asks about GH that it is a Schedule V drug. It is an insulin derivative. Diabetics are not at an increased risk of cancer from taking insulin. GH makes bone and muscle grow, and when it is being supplemented properly 70 and 80-year-old patients should have levels of 100 or 200. A good dose of GH in the range of 15 mg to 45 mg a month will give IGF-1 increases of 100 to 200 points. Other supplements may raise IGF-1 levels by 10% at best, which is almost trivial.

Everyone who has treated hypothyroid should know that a patient with a TSH of 90 was not treated correctly if after treatment with thyroid his/her TSH levels dropped to 80. TSH needs to be brought down to a level of two or three. Three is probably too high, so two or less is optimal. It turns out that if you are treating someone with GH you need to get his IGF-1 levels into the 300 range at least. The 200 range is just about tolerable, but it is possible to get IGF-1 into the 500 range. The average 80 to 90-year-old's IGF-1 level is in the 70's or 80's. So that provides a nice benchmark.

Therefore, for somatopause, measure IGF-1. GH antibodies can also be measured. Another option is a DEXA scan. A DEXA scan enables you to simultaneously scan bone density and body fat in just 6 minutes. Throw the calipers in the garbage. It is worthwhile investing in evidence-based equipment. By accurately monitoring muscle mass you can see if your treatment for somatopause has been effective.

The medical literature calls somatopause a number of different things. In 2003, *Nutrition Reviews* and *JAMA* called it sarcopause, as in sarcopenia. Somatopause is preferable at it covers what GH preserves in the body: bone and muscle.

Moving on, let us discuss the andropause and how it is treated. Once again, the anti-aging movement has been prophetic. Methyltestosterone used to have black box warnings on it. Everyone knew it caused liver cancer. So now the only testosterone treatment that anyone uses, even conventional doctors, is bioidentical testosterone. Doctors used to have men shaving their scrotum to put testosterone on or using a patch. But now you can get a cream from a compounding pharmacy, or an AndroGel. The important thing is that it is bioidentical. If something is bioidentical, your body is used to having it. This is debated, but it appears that if a transsexual takes estrogen his prostate will shrink. So when treating andropause, men may need a little drop of estrogen to block testosterone from becoming dihydrotestosterone. Time will tell if this theory is correct.

In the case of women, that is most women and not all, because some have polycystic ovaries and some have virilization due to a problem with their adrenal glands, they have to take progesterone, estradiol, and testosterone. The concept is that women are made, like men, with male parts and female parts, but they are dominantly female. Women need to take a little testosterone to keep their sex drive, so that their brain does not get emotionally labile from the estrogen and anxiety does not increase. They have to take the progesterone so they sleep at night. To offset the effects on the brain, the blood sugar, the mind, the sleep pattern, and the bones you have to make sure a woman takes all three hormones.

Next on the ladder is osteopause. It is vital to take care of bone density. If we don't it puts people at risk of fracture and potentially fatal complications. This is just another reminder that if you fail to treat the entire geripause, your clinic might be profitable for you, but not profitable for your patient.

Dermatopause occurs when the skin begins to lose collagen, and therefore its elasticity. Skin really is skin-deep. A good reminder of this is the fact that facelifts tend to look terrible in 70- and 80-year-old people. Facelifts look bad in seniors because of the muscle loss, and changes in facial bone structure. Skin is easy to repair: it is easy to clip some away. The problem is in what lies underneath. So having really great skin depends on many other factors.

Cardiovasculopause is the rusting and hardening of blood vessels. No anti-aging practice can function without an ultrasound. The ultimate in imaging technology is Doppler imaging. Many patients who come into a practice will have normal carotid arteries. However, approximately 10% of patients that have normal carotids have abnormal transcranial Doppler with changes in blood flow to their brain. These changes can be seen on a MRI of the brain as ischemia and brain atrophy. Now know that the brain literally dries up with age. Galen said that people lose the moist humor as they get older. Today we say that people lose acetylcholine and water as they get older. But the bottom line is that the blood flow is changing everywhere. A person may have a terrible ankle-brachial index, but healthy coronary arteries. However, we can predict that they are still going to have a heart attack because they have got a high coronary calcium score. Another person may think he has got great vasculature, but he actually has circulation problems in his feet. He gets fungal infections, which leads to ulcers, and he dies of an infection.

So you can conduct Doppler ultrasound scans on your patients. Despite the current recognition that you can scan people with CAT scans head-to-toe, if you want to set up an anti-aging clinic you can, more economically, ultrasound people head-to-toe. Either make the decision to charge them and bill insurance for a piecemeal ultrasound, or you can just make a one-package deal, for example an ultrasound of the thyroid, or an ultrasound of the feet. There are two types of ultrasound: the Doppler for the heart, the carotids, the brain, the abdomen, the kidneys, the scrotum, the uterus, ovaries and the prostate, and then there are the machines for ankle-brachial and all the small blood vessels.

The pauses tell us what diagnostics are critical for the anti-aging practice. It is important to remember that they occur at different rates and you have to assess that. The ovary dies on virtually all women by 60, but testicular or andropause in men is a gradual pause. Some people have advanced vasculopause. Some people have an early vasculopause. Your job as an anti-aging clinician is to work out exactly what is going on in the patient's body.

## NUTRIENTS AND DIETARY SUPPLEMENTATION

The whole movement of anti-aging began with the recognition that old people do not absorb nutrients. When a baby is born, s/he comes complete with an IV, the umbilical cord and the placenta. I submit that the future of anti-aging is going to include nutritional feedings and supplements given intravenously. The blood of most 60- and 70-year-olds will be deficient in at least one nutrient, so there is no better way to test a person's nutritional status than testing their blood.

People take a hodge-podge of nutrients. There are simply too many supplements to choose from. You can take amino acids, which balance and re-balance your protein. And you are using amino acids to do what? To either treat a condition or supplement a neurotransmitter or a brain function. You can take all the vitamins you want. You can use a vitamin like niacin at 2 g as a therapeutic drug for treating cholesterol, or you could take a B-complex vitamin like folate at 400 mcg as a supplement. So every nutrient choice is either a therapeutic drug use, or a supplement use. All of the amino acids could be useful therapeutically. Vitamins can be useful therapeutically or as supplements. Fatty acids can be useful therapeutically. There are also all the minerals to consider.

The sheer choice of supplements available often means that people interested in their health end up taking a wide variety of pills. Patients will walk into a practice and say that they have been taking calcium for 40 years. Yet these patients are still osteoporotic. Why? To understand this it is necessary to look at the principle of the pauses. Human beings are a complete integrated system. Like a ladder, the brain is at the top, the higher power, down to the genes. If you do not fix one part, your person dies anyway. So without hormones, the calcium the patient had been taking for the last 40 years was not absorbed. Generally, the least important factor of osteoporosis is calcium intake. Cigarette smoking, menopause, GH loss, estrogen loss, and testosterone loss play a far bigger role in osteoporosis than calcium intake.

You are only as young as your oldest part. Below is a list of the different pauses that occur in the human body during the aging process.:

| **PAUSE** | **DECLINE IN** |
|---|---|
| Electropause | Brain memory, metabolism and rest |
| Psychopause | Personality stability and mood, increased anxiety |
| Pineal Pause | Melatonin, increase in sleep disturbances |
| Pituitary Pause | Brain - body hormone balance |
| Sensorypause | Hearing, sight, touch, smell, sensitivity |
| Thyropause | Thyroid and body metabolism |
| Parathyropause | Parathormone and bone density |
| Thymopause | Glandular function and immune system |
| Cardiopause | Pumping power, valves and blood flow |
| Pulmonopause | Lung elasticity and function with increase in blood pressure |
| Gastropause | Nutrient absorption with increase in stomach acidity, gallstones, diverticulosis |
| Adrenopause | DHEA, fight-or-flight response |
| Nephropause | Erythropoietin, filtering of toxins |
| Somatopause | Growth hormone, muscle strength and fibers |
| Pancreopause | Glucose tolerance and insulin sensitivity |
| Andropause | Testosterone, sex drive |
| Menopause | Estrogen, progesterone, testosterone and more |
| Vasculopause | Blood flow to hands, feet and sexual organs |
| Osteopause | Bone density |
| Uropause | Bladder control, infection resistance |
| Dermopause | Collagen, vitamin D, skin health |
| Genopause | DNA repair, cell integrity |

## NON-DRUG ALTERNATIVES

The next step is treating the patient. Here, the important principle is finding a nutrient non-drug alternative to conventional medications. For example, replace statins with red yeast. Statin-like substances can be found in certain herbal supplements. Quinine, N-acetyl cysteine, Gabapentin, tyrosine, phenylalanine, and tryptophan, are all neurotransmitter precursors. Also, don't forget that every medical office uses digoxin, which is an herb. The way anti-aging medicine should start is that the doctor should offer and inform the patient about drugs that can be used to treat their condition. However, a wise anti-aging doctor should also tell the patient that there are a number of nutrients, herbs, and bioidentical hormones that can imitate the effects of these drugs. Thus meaning that the patient will not have to take the drugs, or s/he will have to take less of them. Alternatively, the nutrients will increase the effectiveness of the drugs. So every medication is either going to get more effective, be reduced, or eliminated, and East meets West at a new path with natural and conventional approaches merging.

Why is this so important? It is not possible to be a doctor and not draw from healing of the conventional. If a person says to you that they will not take any conventional manmade approaches, it suggests that they have resentment towards humanity in general and cannot accept humanity's help. On the other hand, if you get a doctor who thinks that there is nothing natural that will ever help them, they have too much of an attitude that human beings are here on this earth to dominate nature and to take over nature. So, ultimately, our selections of a multimodal approach of spiritual, nutritional, our own internal resources, and manmade chemicals reflect our own internal wellness and balance in life.

One natural agent that should be considered in depth is gabapentin, or Neurontin. The average dose of clonidine is 0.1 mg; Xanax 0.5 mg; Klonopin goes up to 16 mg; Tegretol ranges from 200 mg to 800 mg. Most drugs are in the range of less than 200 mg, so why is the average dose of gabapentin 3,600 mg? Gabapentin is a combination of gamma-aminobutyric acid (GABA) and inositol, which passes freely through the blood brain barrier and raises levels of GABA in the brain. Thus, gabapentin is not really a drug in the conventional sense. You either can fix the brain by adding more neurotransmitter precursors such as tyrosine, phenylalanine, tryptophan, arginine (a precursor of nitric oxide), or gabapentin (a precursor and stimulator of GABA). Or you can use something that blocks the receptors. For example, antidepressants are drugs that block receptors. They preserve the neurotransmitter. Tricyclic antidepressants block one receptor, and Selective Serotonin Reuptake Inhibitors (SSRIs) block the uptake of the neurotransmitter.

## DIAGNOSTIC SERVICES

You have to conduct the correct diagnostic tests, and you have to deal with the fact that no one diagnostic system covers everything. To cover absolutely everything you need: a brain map for the brain; an ultrasound for the body; a DEXA scan for bone and muscle; a backup Ultrafast CT for positive stress thalliums; a PET scan for cancer patients; an MRI for MS patients; and blood analysis. The important thing is knowing when and how to use them.

### *Testing the Brain*

Brain function is important in every single condition. As we age, the creative and alert brain starts to decline. Beta and alpha waves diminish, and theta and delta waves increase. As a result, the mind starts to present symptoms of stress, anxiety, and depression.

A variety of instruments and tests are needed to assess the health of the brain:
- A brain map, which can determine a person's likelihood of going senile;
- A Millon profile, which can determine whether or not a patient has a severe psychiatric disorder or if the patient is too anxious, or too blue, or too hysterical to benefit from you
- A Myers-Briggs test, which can tell you whether the patient the type that can handle 49 supplements six times a day and a GH injection daily; or if s/he would be better suited to taking three vitamins, a brain energy supplement, antioxidant, and a multivitamin, and having a GH injection and a testosterone injection once a month. Be mindful that some people are not going to be organized enough to take large numbers of supplements, but some are. Thus, a quick assessment of your patient will help you to determine what sort of regimen they can cope with.
- A Wechsler Memory Scale-III (WMS-III): this test can be done in approximately half-an-hour, and anyone can be trained as a technician to do it. What you may find is that most people who complain of a memory problem actually have an anxiety problem. They are getting irritated, they are getting worried, and they are getting stressed out. That does not mean that they are not going to develop a memory

problem in the future, but the brain has to slow down. Memory is basically a wave and a particle. If the neurons slow down, they keep dropping the biochemical balls of memory. Half of the patients that come for a consultation at my medical practice are suffering from attention loss. Older people miss things and they drop things. Young people become impulsive, and children can be distractible.

Brain waves are the key to life. They are what distinguish the living from the dead. When we measure brain waves we are measuring consciousness, brain speed, brain chemical depression, and brain chemical rhythm. As a doctor, what you are really measuring is whether your treatment worked or not. If a change in brain electricity is the sum result of all of your treatments, the proof that you are successful is the patient saying that their memory is much better. The final end point marker of successful treatment of a patient is a juiced-up, stable, energized, sharp brain. This is why you need to measure the brain with a BEAM (brain electrical activity map).

## *The Brain Electrical Activity Map (BEAM)*

Conventional doctors used to say that EEG was the cornerstone of electrical evaluation of the brain. However, the truth is that EEG is the least valuable thing you could possibly do in terms of gathering information. No sensible doctor would rely solely on the EKG to detect heart disease. They would measure HDL, LDL, and total cholesterol levels, homocysteine levels, C-reactive protein levels, fibrinogen levels, and they would use Holter Monitoring, echocardiography etc. Fortunately, everyone now realizes that if you want to find out a lot about the brain an electrical stress test is required.

The Brain Electrical Activity Map (BEAM) provides us with a way of measuring brain function. The BEAM is the cornerstone because the P-300 voltage tells us about a patient's brain energy, power, and metabolism. If a patient is obese, fatigued, or depressed, it will tell you about the severity of his condition. So, new tools like the BEAM can be used to decide which patient is going to respond to an amino acid, and which patient is going to require treatment with both medications and amino acids.

Thus, the BEAM enables us to discover the root of a brain disorder. This root may be caused by low energy: dopaminergic, low memory processes; acetylcholinergic, arrhythmias; GABAergic; or bad mind-body relaxation, mood, or sleep (serotonergic). The EEG shows almost nothing in cocaine abusers. That is why we use the BEAM. 100% of cocaine-users present with abnormalities the BEAM. In comparison, MRI cannot detect abnormalities caused by cocaine abuse. The issue here is brain chemistry, and electricity. The electrical status of the brain is actually more central than the mix of biochemicals, and the BEAM picks this up.

Basically, every part of the human body has a maximum age of 120. Thus, when it comes to Alzheimer's, the question here should not be "does the patient have Alzheimer's?"; rather, it should be "how far away is this patient from getting Alzheimer's?" Everyone's brain slows down with age. So what a 60-year-old patient needs to know whether he is 40 years away from developing Alzheimer's or 10 years. We will eventually all develop Alzheimer's if we slow down, but new studies suggest that it might be reversible in the early stages. This brings us to another paradigm principle of every anti-aging practice: the early detection of disease. If osteoporosis is detected in the early stages, a patient will not become 3 inches shorter. If muscle cachexia of aging is caught early, a patient will not lose his biceps. If breast cancer or a breast cyst is caught early enough it hopefully will not progress to breast cancer. So, if Alzheimer's is detected in the first stages and it is treated as best as we can, with all our medical resources, the hope is that the patient will not develop full-blown Alzheimer's.

## CONCLUSION

In the future, we may have a computer that can say the brain is 20, the bones are 40, the heart is 90, the adrenals are 60, and the genitals are 50. Thus making it possible to fix the 90-year-old part of the patient first, and then work your way through the body and making them younger. That really is all medicine is about. It is finding the oldest, most worn out part, or pause, and fixing it.

However, at present we do not have such a computer, thus we have to rely on blood tests, imaging technology, psychological assessment, and other relevant evaluations. By using the most high-tech devices available, anti-aging clinicians can detect disease in its earliest stages and therefore intervene before serious problems arise.

## ABOUT THE AUTHOR

Dr. Eric Braverman is the Director of The Place for Achieving Total Health (PATH Medical), with locations in New York, NY, Penndel, PA (Metro-Philadelphia), and a national network of affiliated medical professionals. Dr. Braverman received his BA Summa Cum Laude from Brandeis University and his M.D. with honors from New York University Medical School, after which he performed postgraduate work in internal medicine with a Yale Medical School affiliate in Greenwich, Connecticut. Dr. Braverman is a recipient of the American Medical Association's Physician Recognition Award.

Dr. Braverman has published and presented more than 90 research papers to the medical community. His lectures include topics on Melatonin, Tryptophan, and Amino Acids (given at Los Alamos National Laboratories), and The Core Neurotransmitters and Hormones and How They Affect the Aging Process (given at Brookhaven National Laboratories). One of his most recent lectures was on P-300 Evoked Response as a Predictor of Alzheimer's Disease at Oxford University in England.

Dr. Braverman is the author of five medical books, including the *PATH Wellness Manual,* which is a user's guide to alternative treatment. He has appeared on CNN (Larry King Live), PBS, AHN, MSNBC, FOX News Channel and local TV stations. Dr Braverman has been quoted in the *New York Post, New York Times*, and the *Wall Street Journal*. Dr Braverman's 26 years of medical education, training, and clinical practice have focused on the brain's overall health.

Chapter 3

# Is Growth Hormone Replacement for Normal Aging Safe?: Analysis of Current Medical Literature

*Ronald Rothenberg, M.D.*
*Clinical Professor & Course Director, Preventive & Family Medicine,*
*University of California San Diego (UCSD) School of Medicine;*
*Founder, California HealthSpan Institute*

## ABSTRACT

The purpose of this paper is to discuss whether or not growth hormone replacement therapy (GHRT) for the treatment of somatopause of normal aging is safe and effective. In order to determine this it is important to learn about growth hormone (GH), the benefits of GHRT, and its side effects. We will also discuss whether or not pathological GH deficiency is the same as GH deficiency caused by "normal aging." The links between GHRT and cancer and insulin resistance are also debated.

**Keywords:** growth hormone; growth hormone replacement therapy; growth hormone deficiency; inflammation

## INTRODUCTION

The purpose of this paper is to discuss whether or not growth hormone replacement therapy (GHRT) for the treatment of somatopause of normal aging is safe and effective. This paper is not going to deal with the basics of GHRT, i.e. doses and optimal delivery techniques. Instead it will address the following important questions:
- What are the benefits of GHRT?
- Is "Normal Aging" GH deficiency the same as "Pathological" GH deficiency?
- Does GHRT increase the risk of cancer?
- Does GHRT cause insulin resistance?
- Are the possible side effects of GHRT manageable nuisances or serious problems?

## GROWTH HORMONE, SOMATOPAUSE, AND AGING

Growth hormone (GH) exerts a wide variety of physiological effects on the body. Endogenous peptide ligands such as ghrelin, growth hormone releasing hormone (GHRH), and growth hormone releasing peptide (GHRP) all stimulate the interior pituitary to release GH. GH migrates to the liver to produce insulin-like growth factor 1 (IGF-1). Sixty percent (60%) of the effects that GH has on the body are exerted via IGF-1. For example, GH's anabolic effect upon muscle, bone, and cartilage, and its lipolytic effect on fat, are all mediated by IGF-1. GH and IGF-1 can both pass through the blood-brain barrier.

Somatopause signifies the gradual decline in growth hormone production by the pituitary gland. Somatopause can begin anywhere between the ages of 35 and 50, however when it does occur a person's GH levels will drop significantly. In an article published in *Hormone Research* in 2000, Savine et *al* concluded that life without growth hormone is poor both in quantity and quality. The emphasis here should be placed on quality as maintaining a good quality of life is the goal. Savine found that GH peaks at puberty and starts decreasing at 21. At the age of 60, most adults have the same 24-hour secretion rate indistinguishable from those hypopituitary patients with organic lesions in the pituitary gland. Thus, a normal 60-year-old is the same as a sick 25-year-old in terms of GH levels. Savine also concluded that if an IGF-1 level of 300 is mean normal for a 20 to 30-year-old, almost everybody over the age of 40 has an IGF-1 deficit.

However, what does GH have to do with aging? The important factor here is inflammation. Chronic inflammation is the cause of many age-related diseases. Thus doing whatever we can to decrease chronic inflammation is important in the quest to stay healthy. A number of things can be done to help combat chronic inflammation. For example: keeping glucose and insulin levels under control, taking regular exercise, and eliminating the visceral abdominal fat. Abdominal fat is a living, throbbing endocrine organ that produces inflammatory cytokines, like IL-6. So carrying extra fat is not just a cosmetic issue. By eliminating visceral abdominal fat the person is also getting rid of a very dangerous inflammatory-producing organ. It is also possible to lower inflammation by controlling the Omega-3 to Omega-6 ratio and eliminating infections: most health professionals are now aware of the connection between heart disease and periodontal disease and chlamydia. Another way of combating inflammation is stress reduction, as stress produces inflammatory cytokines. Control of free radicals, homocysteine levels, advanced glycation end products, and youthful hormones, such as testosterone, estrogens, growth hormone, IGF-1 all decrease these inflammatory cytokines. Inflammation induces GH insensitivity, however GHRT decreases inflammation. Thus, reducing inflammation also improves the body's sensitivity to GH.

We know that a person's C-Reactive Protein (CRP) levels are the strongest predictor of whether or not they are going to have a myocardial infarction or not. CRP is far superior to LDL-cholesterol. Thus, it makes sense to keep CRP levels as low as possible. Where does CRP come from? Interleukin-6, (IL-6) tells the liver to produce CRP. So to keep CRP under control, IL-6 levels also need to be kept at a minimum. Homocysteine raises inflammation, therefore it needs to be kept low. Too much insulin induces inflammation as does tumor necrosis factor-a (TNF-a), as does interleukin-10 (IL-10): these are all things that need to be kept under control. Inflammation is linked to many chronic illnesses, from heart disease, to syndrome X, to dementia, to depression, cancer, osteoporosis, and autoimmune disease: all have high inflammatory mediators. Maybe the question should be: "Why are we so inflammatory?"

Insulin resistance provides us with a good analogy for understanding why the body is prone to inflammation. Insulin resistance was a good thing for our Paleolithic ancestors. If you could store fat and make it through famine, you would live long enough to pass on your DNA. No one lived long enough to develop Type II diabetes and its numerous complications, so that was not a problem. It is the same thing with inflammation. If a person's body is geared towards making inflammatory cytokines, they will get by when a saber tooth tiger bites them. White cells will rush to the infection and their blood will clot. Being prone to inflammation is a bonus when faced with acute trauma and acute infectious disease. As these two things were the main challenge to our ancestors, it is in the genome. We have evolved to be prone to inflammation. Now, since trauma and infection are not such a great threat to most people, and now that we are living significantly longer lives, this inflammatory state is killing us. Just as the insulin resistance is killing us.

Moving back to the original question of GH and aging. We age because our hormones decline, not the other way around. GH is vital in order to live a healthy adult life. Why? GHRT improves quality of life. What other benefits does GHRT have? GHRT is beneficial to the brain, the cardiovascular system, the immune system, aerobic capacity, body composition, and bone.

It is interesting to compare the viewpoints of anti-aging specialists and conventional endocrinologists have on GH. Both groups agree that pathological GH deficiency is a disease that should be treated. Both groups agree that GH secretion declines with age, and both groups agree that GH decline is responsible for part of the clinical syndrome of aging. This is where anti-aging and endocrinology's agreement on GH ends. Anti-aging specialists believe that aging and GH decline is a deficiency disease, which can and should be treated. But the vast majority, if not all, of endocrinologists believe that aging and GH decline are normal and should not be treated.

Cappola *et al* carried out a study to investigate what factors were associated with a better quality of life in women aged 70 and over. The results showed that women who had the best quality of life in terms of functional capability (that is walking limitation, mobility, activities of daily living, cognition and so on) had high IGF-1 levels and low IL-6. Thus they had high GH levels and minimal inflammation. The concept is that decreased GH levels and decreased IGF-1 levels lead to frailty. Somatopause is the entry into frailty.

So, does GHRT provide us with the long searched for fountain of youth? No, it does not. But we are on a programmed course of destruction and GHRT could help slow it down a little and improve our quality of life. If the benefits outweigh the risks, then something is worth doing. GHRT is a work in progress. It may not be perfect, but it is the best we have at present.

## BENEFITS OF GROWTH HORMONE
### Growth Hormone and the Brain

GH deficiency is associated with neurocognitive decline, and GHRT improves memory, alertness, and concentration. It is quite amazing that GH can pass through the blood brain barrier, as it is a very large molecule made up from 191 amino acids. The brain needs GH and it needs IGF-1. Many people think that GH is good, whereas IGF-1 is bad, and that we want to increase GH without increasing IGF-1. This is not the case. More than half of the action of GH is exerted through IGF-1, and the general consensus is that both are necessary. So growth hormone improves cognitive capabilities, memory, motivation, and work capacity. There are GH-receptors situated all over the brain. Aleman *et al* correlated IGF-1 with cognitive function in men, with higher IGF-1 levels being linked to better cognitive function. GH deficiency was correlated with poor emotional and psychosocial functioning.

### Growth Hormone and Bone

GH increases the strength and formation of cortical bone. Logobardi linked GH deficiency with reduced bone density, and GHRT with reversal of osteoporosis. Patients who sustain hip fractures tend to have lower IGF-1 levels. GH is synergistic with exercise, thus to get the maximum effect from GHRT it has to be combined with regular exercise. Van der Lely *et al* treated patients over 75 with hip fractures with GH at the time of fracture for six weeks. The end point was return to pre-fracture living arrangements. Results of the double-blind placebo-controlled trial showed that 94% of patients treated with GH returned to pre-fracture living within just six weeks, compared with 75% of control patients.

GH increases bone mineral density. Gillberg *et al* treated men with idiopathic osteoporosis with GH. Participants were randomly assigned to treatment with GH, either as continuous treatment with daily injections of 0.4 mg GH or as intermittent treatment with 0.8 mg GH for 14 days every 3 months. All patients were treated with GH for 24 months, with a follow-up period of 12 months. No positive effects of treatment were noted at the 12-month follow-up. But after 12 months there was a continued increase in bone mineral density and no significant adverse effects were reported. After two years of GH treatment significant improvement in bone mineral density were observed in both groups.

### Growth Hormone and the Cardiovascular System

GH deficiency is associated with increased cardiovascular mortality, while GHRT is associated with improved cardiovascular function. Research suggests that GHRT may help to reverse atherosclerosis, improve cardiomyopathy, and reduce carotid intima media thickness.

Pro-inflammatory cytokines contribute to chronic and acute heart failure. Adamopoulos *et al* treated patients with idiopathic dilated cardiomyopathy (IDC) with GH. Results showed that GH treatment led to a significant decrease in both TNF-a and IL-6 levels, and significant improvements in exercise capacity.

GH also corrects endothelial dysfunction. Too much emphasis is placed upon the cholesterol model of atherosclerosis. Inflammation and endothelial dysfunction are very important factors. Cholesterol may be present at the scene of the crime, but it did not trigger the whole process going. GH improves endothelial dysfunction, which plays a significant role in both heart failure and arteriosclerosis.

What about homocysteine? We know that homocysteine is a strong predictor of cardiovascular disease. Sesmilo *et al* randomly assigned 40 men with GH deficiency to treatment with GH or a placebo for a period of 18 months. Homocysteine levels fell significantly in those treated with GH.

What about CRP, which is the strongest predictor of cardiovascular events that we have? CRP is very high in GH deficiency. With GHRT, CRP decreases and visceral and subcutaneous fat decreases. As we know, visceral fat produces IL-6, which in turn produces CRP.

Thus, the cardiovascular improvements seen with GHRT, appears to be down to its effect upon the inflammatory pathway. IGF-1 is a cardiac hormone. It improves cardiac contractility, stroke volume, and ejection fraction. It improves insulin levels: intracardiac insulin levels, and increases insulin sensitivity. So the heart needs IGF-1. Certainly, after myocardial infarction, IGF-1 is critical in the remodeling of the heart and recovery.

### *Growth Hormone and the Immune System*

When considering GH and the immune system we have to look at the bigger picture, that is, we have to consider the neuro-endocrine-immune system as all part of one system. IGF-1 is vital for lymphocyte maturation. It will restore age-related thymic involution in rodents. IGF-1 is needed to develop T-cells and B-cells, and the age-related decline in these important cells can be reversed with GHRT.

### *Growth Hormone, Body Composition, and Obesity*

It is a well-documented fact that GHRT can decrease visceral abdominal fat, a cytokine-producing organ, by as much as 50%. According to Christiansen, GH deficiency is linked to:
- Abnormal body composition
- An increase in adipose mass and decrease in muscle mass
- Insulin resistance
- Decreased muscle strength

Long-term GHRT can normalize these abnormalities.

GH secretion is impaired in obesity. Johannsson *et al* studied middle-aged men with low GH and abdominal obesity. After nine months of treatment with GH, abdominal visceral fat decreased by 18%, insulin sensitivity improved, total cholesterol, LDL, and triglyceride levels dropped, and diastolic blood pressure decreased. The men did not make any lifestyle changes during the study. An 18% decrease in visceral abdominal fat without making any life-style alterations is quite impressive.

Blackman *et al* studied the effect of treating healthy men and women with sex steroids and GH. The women received HRT, which was Estraderm (transcutaneous estradiol), plus Provera: this was not a wise choice, as Provera increases insulin resistance. The men were given 100 mg of testosterone once every two weeks. One group of men and women were treated only with the sex steroids, while another were also treated with GH at a fixed dose per weight, which is not a good way treat people with GH in terms of producing side-effects. Anyway, a fixed dose was used and the patients were given GH three times a week. Results showed that visceral abdominal fat decreased by 14% in men treated with GH alone, and 16% in those given GH and testosterone. Interestingly, women who were treated with GH alone did not lose abdominal fat, but when GH was combined with the HRT they did. A second study by the same group was published a year later in 2002. The participants were treated with the same regimen as in the 2001 study. Lean body mass increased in women treated with HRT and GH by an average of 2.1 kg, and in men treated with testosterone and GH by an average of 4.3 kg. Fat mass decreased in both groups of men and women. $VO_2$ max increased in both men and women, and muscle strength increased by 6.8% in men treated with both GH and testosterone. These changes occurred within six months, and once again, the participants made no life-style changes: imagine what results you may achievei by implementing positive life-style changes. However, not all the results were beneficial: 38% of women suffered from edema; 32% of men treated with both GH and testosterone suffered from carpal tunnel syndrome; and 41% of men treated with GH suffered from arthralgias. Diabetes or glucose intolerance was noted in 18 men treated with GH, compared with just 7 men who were not treated with GH. Unfortunately, the press picked up on the adverse effects reported by the research team, and the resulting headlines read: "Growth Hormone Replacement Therapy Causes Diabetes." People who use GH in clinical practice know that this is simply not true. In terms of insulin resistance, GH can make it worse if the patient's life-style is not managed correctly. If lifestyle is managed correctly insulin resistance could improve dramatically. The very high rate of side-effects seen with this study might be related to the dosage schedule: the fixed dose per weight, and the three times a week; and not titrating the dose. This side-effect profile is not seen in clinical practice. In clinical practice, approximately 10% of patients may suffer from such side-effects, however these are manageable simply by decreasing the dose.

*Other Benefits of Growth Hormone*

Every study of GH and exercise capacity shows that GH increases $VO_2$ max. Gibney *et al* found a link between GH deficiency and chronic fatigue and depression. Meanwhile, GHRT was found to improve a person's sense of well-being and was associated with an improved quality of life. Gilchrist *et al* concluded that GH deficient adults have a poor quality of life, but that this poor quality of life could be altered with GHRT. Gilchrist found that GHRT significantly improved energy levels, vitality, anxiety, depression, well-being, and self-control.

## GROWTH HORMONE AND INCREASED MORTALITY IN PATIENTS IN ICU

One study that is often brought up when people talk about GH is a study by Takkala *et al* that was published in the *New England Journal of Medicine* in 1999. In this study, critically ill patients: half of whom were on ventilators, a lot of whom were suffering with acute respiratory distress syndrome, were treated with large doses of GH, 16 to 24 units per day. The average anti-aging dose can vary from 4 to 12 units a week or 1 unit a day. The outcome was not good. Significantly higher numbers of patients treated with GH died. So we can conclude that an overdose of GH is not good. A rebuttal to this study by Bengtsson *et al* in the *Journal of Clinical Endocrinology* looked at a meta-analysis of over 2,000 patient years, none of which was associated with increase in mortality.

## GROWTH HORMONE AND CANCER

Does GHRT increase the risk of cancer? Vance *et al* concluded that there is "No evidence that GHRT affects the risk of cancer or cardiovascular disease." Meanwhile Molitch concluded: "Although there has been some concern about an increased risk of cancer [with GHRT], reviews of existing, well-maintained databases of treated patients have shown this theoretical risk to be nonexistent." Shalet *et al* concluded that there is "No evidence of an increased risk of malignancy, recurrent or *de novo*." On the package insert on GH it says don't use in active malignancy. However, the Growth Hormone Research Society published a paper in the *Journal of Clinical Endocrinology* saying that there is no data to support this labeling, and that current knowledge does not warrant additional warning about cancer risk. They say that this line should be removed from the package insert because no evidence that GH increases cancer recurrence or *de novo* cancer or leukemia.

When the issue of GH and cancer is being discussed, the Chan study is always referenced. Blood was drawn for IGF-1 and IGF binding protein-3 (IGFBP-3), and other studies, on a group of men. The blood was stored, and then 15 years later the investigators followed-up the participants to see which men developed prostate cancer. Men who had the IGF levels in the highest quartile had the most prostate cancer. There are some interesting aspects to this study. Firstly, the blood was stored for 15 years. Secondly, the IGF levels in the highest quartile were between 300 and 500. The average age of the men at the start of the study was 59. Now, it is unlikely people in clinical practice will ever have seen someone of that age with IGF levels of 400 or 500. This is why these study findings seem very unusual.

IGFBP-3 is one of the binding proteins that carries IGF. This seemingly simple system is actually very complex. All the binding proteins are hormones in their own right; they do not just provide storage for the hormones. So the highest quartile had a 2.4 times increased relative risk of prostate cancer. When a patient is treated with GHRT, IGF-1 levels increase and levels of IGFBP-3 also increase. Thus, GH stimulates the production of both IGF and IGFBP-3. In the study by Chang *et al* the men with more IGFBP-3 had a decreased risk of prostate cancer.

IGFBP-3 has been called the guardian of the genome. IGF-1 does have a mitogenic effect: it does cause cellular replication and renewal. However, the mitogenic effect of IGF-1 is balanced by the apoptotic effect of IGFBP-3. IGFBP-3 triggers apoptosis in cancer cells. Thus IGFBP-3 plays an important role in cancer control. However, too much apoptosis would cause cellular aging. So it is important that the body gets the balance just right.

A study of 765 men by Scheafer *et al* found no association with IGF-1 and prostate cancer. However, another study by Baffa *et al* linked low IGF-1 levels with prostate cancer. It is clear that we have conflicting evidence. However, if the Chan study is the one and only reason to link GH with increased risk of cancer rates are increased, that reason is not valid.

## GROWTH HORMONE REPLACEMENT AND SIDE-EFFECTS

The most common side-effects of GHRT are edema, arthralgia, and insulin resistance. Vance *et al* concluded that edema and arthralgia are related to the dose schedule. Patients that are affected by edema or arthralgia are often being treated on a low-frequency, high-dose schedule. They are also associated with mg/kg doses instead of a gradually increasing dose. Both are reversible by simply decreasing the dose.

Another side-effect of GHRT is paresthesia. If a patient complains of paresthesia, or edema, or arthralgia, the best thing to do is stop their treatment for a few days, decrease the dose, and maybe treat them symptomatically with some NSAIDs or mild diuretics. Potassium replacement can also help to ameliorate these symptoms. In rare cases, a patient cannot tolerate GH. If their arthralgia or other adverse effect keeps recurring, GHRT is not for them and should be discontinued

GHRT can cause insulin resistance. But this can be avoided if the patient is managed correctly. It is vital that the patient eats correctly. We have the Atkins' diet, the Zone diet, and the Paleolithic diet. All three of these diets are pointing towards the same thing: that we need protein, good-quality fats, and that we have to choose our carbohydrates carefully, that is, obtain them from vegetables. So before a patient embarks on an anti-aging program, it is vital that they eat properly. Testosterone replacement therapy decreases insulin resistance. And so a patient with borderline insulin resistance who wants to be treated with GHRT may benefit from being treated with testosterone first. Diabetics need to be advised that their insulin requirements could go up or down.

Nam *et al* evaluated the effects of low-dose GH therapy combined with diet restriction on changes in body composition and insulin resistance in newly diagnosed obese type 2 diabetic patients. The findings led them to conclude: "Low-dose GH treatment combined with dietary restriction resulted not only in a decrease of visceral fat but also in an increase of muscle mass with a consequent improvement of the insulin resistance observed in obese type 2 diabetic patients." Remember, obesity is another inflammatory disease. Abdominal fat makes IL-6, and IL-6 causes insulin to go up and store more fat: thus creating one big cycle.

## CONCLUSION

In conclusion, given the state of scientific medical knowledge today, GH is safe. GHRT is associated with less morbidity and mortality, less cardiovascular disease, less inflammation, improvements in body composition, improvements in exercise capacity, and a better quality of life. In the word's of Peter Sonksen: "GH is essential for normal adult life, and without it life expectancy is shortened, energy and vitality are reduced, and the quality of this life is impaired. The medical case for GH replacement is now proven beyond any reasonable medical and scientific doubt. "

## REFERENCES

Adamopoulos S, Parissis JT, Georgiadis M, Karatzas D, Paraskevaidis J, Kroupis C, Karavolias G, Koniavitou K, Kremastinos DT. Growth hormone administration reduces circulating proinflammatory cytokines and soluble Fas/soluble Fas ligand system in patients with chronic heart failure secondary to idiopathic dilated cardiomyopathy. *Am Heart J*. 2002;144:359-364.

Aleman A, Verhaar HJ, De Haan EH, De Vries WR, Samson MM, Drent ML, Van der Veen EA, Koppeschaar HP. Insulin-like growth factor-I and cognitive function in healthy older men. *J Clin Endocrinol Metab*. 1999;84:471-475.

Baffa R, Reiss K, El-Gabry EA, Sedor J, Moy ML, Shupp-Byrne D, Strup SE, Hauck WW, Baserga R, Gomella LG. Low serum insulin-like growth factor 1 (IGF-1): a significant association with prostate cancer. *Tech Urol*. 2000;6:236-239.

Blackman MR. Age-related alterations in sleep quality and neuroendocrine function: interrelationships and implications. *JAMA* 2000;284:879-881.

Borson-Chazot F, Serusclat A, Kalfallah Y, Ducottet X, Sassolas G, Bernard S, Labrousse F, Pastene J, Sassolas A, Roux Y, Berthezene F. Decrease in carotid intima-media thickness after one year growth hormone (GH) treatment in adults with GH deficiency. *J Clin Endocrinol Metab*. 1999;84:1329-1333.

Burgess W, Liu Q, Zhou J, Tang Q, Ozawa A, VanHoy R, Arkins S, Dantzer R, Kelley KW. The immune-endocrine loop during aging: role of growth hormone and insulin-like growth factor-I. *Neuroimmunomodulation*. 1999;6:56-68.

Cappola AR, Bandeen-Roche K, Wand GS, Volpato S, Fried LP. Association of IGF-I levels with muscle strength and mobility in older women. *J Clin Endocrinol Metab*. 2001;86:4139-4146.

Cappola AR, Xue QL, Ferrucci L, Guralnik JM, Volpato S, Fried LP. Insulin-like growth factor I and interleukin-6 contribute synergistically to disability and mortality in older women. *J Clin Endocrinol Metab*. 2003;88:2019-2025.

Chan JM, Stampfer MJ, Giovannucci E, Gann PH, Ma J, Wilkinson P, Hennekens CH, Pollak M. Plasma insulin-like growth factor-I and prostate cancer risk: a prospective study. *Science* 1998;279:563-566.

Christiansen J. Effects of GH upon body composition. *Growth Hormone in Adults*, 1196. Cambridge University Press.

Clark R. The somatogenic hormones and insulin-like growth factor-1: stimulators of lymphopoiesis and immune function. *Endocr Rev*. 1997;18:157-179.

Gibney J, Wallace JD, Spinks T, Schnorr L, Ranicar A, Cuneo RC, Lockhart S, Burnand KG, Salomon F, Sonksen PH, Russell-Jones D. The effects of 10 years of recombinant human growth hormone (GH) in adult GH-deficient patients. *J Clin Endocrinol Metab*. 1999;84:2596-2602.

Gillberg P, Mallmin H, Petren-Mallmin M, Ljunghall S, Nilsson AG. Two years of treatment with recombinant human growth hormone increases bone mineral density in men with idiopathic osteoporosis. *J Clin Endocrinol Metab*. 2002;87:4900-4906.

Gilchrist FJ, Murray RD, Shalet SM. The effect of long-term untreated growth hormone deficiency (GHD) and 9 years of GH replacement on the quality of life (QoL) of GH-deficient adults. *Clin Endocrinol (Oxf)*. 2002;57:363-370.

Hedstrom M. Hip fracture patients, a group of frail elderly people with low bone mineral density, muscle mass and IGF-I levels. *Acta Physiol Scand.* 1999;167:347-350.

Johannsson G, Marin P, Lonn L, Ottosson M, Stenlof K, Bjorntorp P, Sjostrom L, Bengtsson BA. Growth hormone treatment of abdominally obese men reduces abdominal fat mass, improves glucose and lipoprotein metabolism, and reduces diastolic blood pressure. *J Clin Endocrinol Metab.* 1997;82:727-734.

Molitch ME. Diagnosis of GH deficiency in adults--how good do the criteria need to be? *J Clin Endocrinol Metab.* 2002;87:473-476.

Munzer T, Harman SM, Hees P, Shapiro E, Christmas C, Bellantoni MF, Stevens TE, O'Connor KG, Pabst KM, St Clair C, Sorkin JD, Blackman MR. Effects of GH and/or sex steroid administration on abdominal subcutaneous and visceral fat in healthy aged women and men. *J Clin Endocrinol Metab.* 2001;86:3604-3610.

Nam SY, Kim KR, Cha BS, Song YD, Lim SK, Lee HC, Huh KB. Low-dose growth hormone treatment combined with diet restriction decreases insulin resistance by reducing visceral fat and increasing muscle mass in obese type 2 diabetic patients. *Int J Obes Relat Metab Disord.* 2001;25:1101-1107.

Nyberg F. Growth hormone in the brain: characteristics of specific brain targets for the hormone and their functional significance. *Front Neuroendocrinol.* 2000;21:330-348.

Pfeifer M, Verhovec R, Zizek B, Prezelj J, Poredos P, Clayton RN. Growth hormone (GH) treatment reverses early atherosclerotic changes in GH-deficient adults. *J Clin Endocrinol Metab.* 1999;84:453-457.

Ren J, Samson WK, Sowers JR. Insulin-like growth factor I as a cardiac hormone: physiological and pathophysiological implications in heart disease. *J Mol Cell Cardiol.* 1999;31:2049-2061.

Rothenberg R. Quality of Life Improves with GH Therapy. *Anti-Aging Medical News* 2002;Summer-Fall:34.

Rudman D, Feller AG, Nagraj HS, Gergans GA, Lalitha PY, Goldberg AF, Schlenker RA, Cohn L, Rudman IW, Mattson DE. Effects of human growth hormone in men over 60 years old. *N Engl J Med.* 1990;323:1-6.

Schaeffer A. *Science* 1998;281:1285.

Sesmilo G, Biller BM, Llevadot J, Hayden D, Hanson G, Rifai N, Klibanski A. Effects of growth hormone (GH) administration on homocyst(e)ine levels in men with GH deficiency: a randomized controlled trial. *J Clin Endocrinol Metab.* 2001;86:1518-1524.

Shalet SM, Brennan BM, Reddingius RE. Growth hormone therapy and malignancy. *Horm Res.* 1997;48 Suppl 4:29-32.

Slonim AE, Bulone L, Damore MB, Goldberg T, Wingertzahn MA, McKinley MJ. A preliminary study of growth hormone therapy for Crohn's disease. *N Engl J Med.* 2000;342:1633-1637.

Sonksen PH. Growth hormone replacement in adults with GH deficiency-- the first 10 years. *Growth Horm IGF Res.* 1998;8:275-276.

Swerdlow AJ, Higgins CD, Adlard P, Preece MA. Risk of cancer in patients treated with human pituitary growth hormone in the UK, 1959-85: a cohort study. *Lancet.* 2002;360:273-277.

Swerdlow AJ, Reddingius RE, Higgins CD, Spoudeas HA, Phipps K, Qiao Z, Ryder WD, Brada M, Hayward RD, Brook CG, Hindmarsh PC, Shalet SM. Growth hormone treatment of children with brain tumors and risk of tumor recurrence. *J Clin Endocrinol Metab.* 2000;85:4444-4449.

Tacke J, Bolder U, Herrmann A, Berger G, Jauch KW. Long-term risk of gastrointestinal tumor recurrence after postoperative treatment with recombinant human growth hormone. *J Parenter Enteral Nutr.* 2000;24:140-144.

Takala J, Ruokonen E, Webster NR, Nielsen MS, Zandstra DF, Vundelinckx G, Hinds CJ. Increased mortality associated with growth hormone treatment in critically ill adults. *N Engl J Med.* 1999;341:785-792.

Van der Lely AJ, Lamberts SW, Jauch KW, Swierstra BA, Hertlein H, Danielle De Vries D, Birkett MA, Bates PC, Blum WF, Attanasio AF. Use of human GH in elderly patients with accidental hip fracture. *Eur J Endocrinol.* 2000;143:585-592.

Vance ML, Mauras N. Growth hormone therapy in adults and children. *N Engl J Med*. 1999;341:1206-1216.

Verhelst J, Abs R. Long-term growth hormone replacement therapy in hypopituitary adults. *Drugs* 2002;62:2399-2412.

Weltman A, Weltman JY, Veldhuis JD, Hartman ML. Body composition, physical exercise, growth hormone and obesity. *Eat Weight Disord*. 2001;6:28-37.

## ABOUT THE AUTHOR

As a pioneer in the field of Anti-Aging Medicine, Ron Rothenberg, M.D., was one of the first physicians to be recognized for his expertise to become fully board certified in the specialty by the American Board of Anti-Aging Medicine (ABAAM). Dr. Rothenberg founded the California HealthSpan Institute in Encinitas, California in 1997 with a commitment to transforming our understanding of and finding treatment for aging as a disease. Dr. Rothenberg is dedicated to the belief that the process of aging can be slowed, stopped, or even reversed through existing medical and scientific interventions. Challenging traditional medicine's approach to treating the symptoms of aging, California HealthSpan's mission is to create a paradigm shift in the way we view medicine: treat the cause.

Dr. Rothenberg received his M.D. from Columbia University, College of Physicians and Surgeons in 1970. He performed his residency at Los Angeles County-USC Medical Center and is also board certified in Emergency Medicine. He received academic appointment to the UCSD School of Medicine Clinical Faculty in 1977 and was promoted to full Clinical Professor of Preventive and Family Medicine in 1989. In addition to his work in the field of Anti-Aging Medicine, Dr. Rothenberg is as Attending Physician and Director of Medical Education at Scripps Memorial Hospital in Encinitas, California.

Dr. Rothenberg travels extensively to lecture on a variety of topics, which include Anti-Aging Medicine and Wilderness Medicine. He has published in the fields of Anti-Aging Medicine and Emergency Medicine, and is the author of *Forever Ageless*. He has recently been featured in the University of California MD TV series in the shows on Anti-Aging Medicine.

Chapter 4

# "Fire in the Heart": New Developments in Diagnosis, Prevention & Treatment of Cardiovascular Disease

*Stephen Sinatra, M.D., F.A.C.C., F.A.C.N., C.N.S., C.B.T.,*
*& Graham Simpson, M.D.*

## ABSTRACT

The aim of this paper is to discuss the integration of conventional cardiology and alternative cardiology. The world of cardiology is moving fast and in multiple directions. In this paper we will discuss the importance of inflammation and how nutraceuticals can be used in the fight against cardiovascular disease.

Keywords: inflammation; insulin; detoxification; nutraceuticals; omega fatty acids; CoEnzyme Q10

## INTRODUCTION

Most of us have some idea of what inflammation is. If a wound gets hot, turns red, hurts, and swells, we recognize that inflammation is at work. In this instance, inflammation is a beneficial process, serving to immobilize and rest the area of injury as the rest of the immune system mobilizes to heal.

Regardless of the source of assault on our bodies, inflammation is the "first alert" mechanism that calls into action the cells responsible for surveillance and protection, heralding them to go to work and limit the damage. These cells attack and destroy the invaders, and clean up the damaged cells, repairing and clearing as they go until a healthy state is restored. As such, inflammation is your body's first line of defense against injury or infection.

Researchers now recognize another kind of inflammation: silent inflammation, or SI, which is very different from the type of inflammation described above. This type of internal inflammation has an insidious nature and is the culprit behind the many chronic diseases that are primarily caused by poor lifestyle habits and environmental pollutants. The chronic and continuous low-level demand that silent inflammation places on the body's defense systems results in an immune system breakdown. In SI there is no regulated progression of a healthy inflammatory response, no planned sequence from the first alarm to the formation of the last new cell. Many of these reactions become intermingled and hamper one another.

The body tissues themselves may lose their ability to recognize cells that are "self" from those that are not, and the body may mistakenly identify its own cells as foreign invaders. This internal programming error, if you will, continues to trigger and re-trigger immune responses, setting the stage for what we call autoimmune diseases, such as lupus, multiple sclerosis and scleroderma. The result is chaos, and what is even more disturbing is that this process may be happening year after year without us even being aware of it.

We now know that SI also plays a central role in the chronic illness that remains our number 1 killer: coronary artery disease. In fact, elevated markers of silent inflammation: such as homocysteine, C-reactive protein (CRP), lipoprotein a (Lp(a)), and interleukin-6 (IL-6), have been found to be more predictive of heart disease than traditional risk factors such as elevated cholesterol levels. In fact, 50% of patients hospitalized for heart disease have normal cholesterol levels.

A landmark study showed that people with high levels of CRP, one of the cardinal markers of inflammation, were over four times more likely to have heart attacks than those with low levels of CRP. Researchers then began to link CRP, along with other markers of inflammation, to a wide range of chronic diseases including Alzheimer's disease, arthritis, Parkinson's disease, and even cancer. It is now accepted that chronic SI is a warning that something is drastically out of balance with one's overall health.

Although chronic SI can cause a variety of disorders, many of us (and unfortunately this includes many physicians) are not aware of the warning signs of this kind of inflammation, or of the best ways to treat it. This knowledge is critical because should a person have one inflammatory condition, the odds that they will develop another skyrocket drastically. Researchers have discovered, for example, that a woman with rheumatoid arthritis has a 100% increased risk of experiencing a myocardial infarction. Very recent research has now demonstrated that higher CRP levels are also associated with age-related macular degeneration. Thus, the same individual may suffer from more than one condition caused by SI. For all these reasons, slowing down this chronic inflammation syndrome is also a major factor for age management, therefore it is crucial that everyone is aware of SI, and that they understand its causes, and now how to take measures to stop it.

## CAUSES OF INFLAMMATION

The many factors that trigger SI are found in both our internal and external environments and include over-consumption of hydrogenated oils, excessive insulin levels, obesity, cigarette smoking, radiation exposure, environmental toxins (mercury, heavy metals), free-radical damage, bacterial and viral infections like nanobacteria and cytomegalovirus (CMV), spirochetes such as the borrelia that causes Lyme disease, periodontal disease, emotional stress, and even some pharmacological drugs.

*Insulin*

The most powerful drug you can consume is the food you eat each day. Depending on the ratio of macronutrients (carbohydrates, fats, proteins) you take in at each meal, your daily diet will either keep you in an optimum "zone" for good health, or it won't.

The "zone" is a physiological state in which the hormones (especially insulin) influenced by the diet are within ranges consistent with optimal health. A "zone meal" is comprised of macronutrients that are kept within ideal balance. The perfect zone meal is proportioned as follows:

  Carbohydrates 40-45%
  Fat 30%
  Protein 25-30%

Combining macronutrients according to the ratio listed above, will keep you "in the zone." The goal is to keep fasting insulin levels lower than 12 µIU/ml, although an ideal level is 5 µIU/ml. We now know that a diet that follows this ratio helps keep weight, insulin, and eicosanoids (hormone-like substances) at ideal levels, which in turn assuages SI in the body. It is important to remember the health consequences of failing to keep insulin levels at bay (<17 µIU/ml): insulin resistance, obesity, Type II diabetes, and heart disease are just a few of the many health complications that may arise from this condition.

### *Controlling Insulin*

Insulin control is achieved through balancing the ratio of protein and carbohydrates at each meal to maintain stable blood-sugar levels for four to six hours. We agree with our colleague Dr. Barry Sears who states, "Hormonally, you are only as good as your last meal, and you will be only as good as your next meal." This means that, for optimal health, you have a dietary choice to make every four to six hours. Accordingly, the following is advised:

- Try to eat a Zone meal within one hour of waking.
- Every time you eat, aim to balance protein, carbohydrates, and fat.
- Try to eat five times a day: three meals and two light snacks.
- Eat more vegetables and fruit, less bread, pasta, rice, and potatoes.
- Always supplement your diet with fish oil and other nutraceuticals.
- Eat a serving of slow-cooked oatmeal topped with seasonal fruit twice a week for fiber, phytonutrients and gamma linolenic acid (GLA).
- Use monounsaturated oils (olive oil) whenever possible on salads and vegetables.
- Use low glycemic carbohydrates whenever possible.

Besides excess insulin, increased blood sugar, free radicals, and elevated cortisol levels accelerate heart disease and aging. All these contributing factors can be modified by the Zone diet, which works to establish hormonal equilibrium in the body.

The essential fatty acids omega-6 and omega-3 are also key dietary components. When these two types of essential fatty acids are metabolized, they produce eicosanoid hormones, which can have dramatically different physiological reactions. Eicosanoids have been labeled as either "good" or "bad", depending upon their effect on the body. "Good" eicosanoids, which are produced from omega-3 fatty acids, are anti-inflammatory by nature, while "bad" eicosanoids, for example arachidonic acid, cause inflammation within the body. The synthesis of each type of eicosanoid depends upon the types of dietary fat we consume as well as endogenous production and metabolism.

Essential fatty acid metabolism is ultimately controlled by one particular enzyme found in the body, delta-5-desaturase, which produces arachidonic acid (AA), a long-chain omega-6 fatty acid that is the precursor of the proinflammatory eicosanoids.

Two dietary constituents profoundly affect the activity of delta-5-desaturase: levels of long-chain omega-3-fatty acids, such as eicosapentaenoic acid (EPA), and levels of insulin. The AA/EPA balance, as measured in the blood, represents the balance of "bad" and "good" eicosanoids throughout the body. Arachidonic acid causes platelet aggregation by triggering the release of thromboxane A2. This kind of endothelial cell unfriendly process is the perfect scenario to set the stage for chronic SI, while promoting blood clotting at the same time. High levels of EPA will counteract the negative effects of AA production and keep inflammation at bay. The ideal AA/EPA ratio is 1.5.

Too much insulin in the body exacerbates AA production and therefore catalyzes inflammation. If you eat an imbalance of (too many) carbohydrates, refined sugars, and proteins at each meal, you will provoke a greater insulin response. Chronic excess insulin will accelerate inflammation, heart disease, obesity, and Type II diabetes; as such hyperinsulinemic patients also have elevated CRP levels.

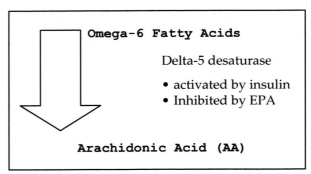

*Figure 1. The Production of Arachidonic Acid by Delta-5 Desaturase*

## Heavy Metals

There are numerous published papers describing adverse clinical effects with aluminum, cadmium, copper, iron, lead and mercury. According to data from the US Toxics Release Inventory, in the year 2000 industry in the United States released 4.3 million pounds of mercury and mercury compounds into the environment, and generated 4.9 million pounds of mercury compounds in toxic waste. This toxic metal burden increases low-grade inflammation at the cellular level, which interferes with mitochondrial function and energy production, and therefore has a very negative effect on the endocrine (glandular), immune, and metabolic systems.

The cardiovascular system is extraordinarily sensitive to mercury. In one small study of 13 biopsied patients with idiopathic dilated cardiomyopathy, investigators found mean mercury concentrations in excess of 22,000 times that of normal levels. Higher mercury levels were thus implicated as causes of this form of cardiomyopathy. Researchers speculated that toxic mercury levels adversely affected mitochondrial activity and the subsequent decrease in myocardial metabolism was a profound metabolic factor in the etiology of idiopathic dilated cardiomyopathy. And how do we become mercury toxic in the first place? Quite simply: breathing contaminated air and eating contaminated fish.

Most mercury vapors arise in the atmosphere from the industrialization of coal. Mercury is then inhaled into the lungs, and transmitted to tissues. And the precipitation of mercury vapors in the water supply is another important factor. Rainfall precipitates mercury into ponds, lakes and streams. Bacteria and algae (your main entree if you're a fish) sequester mercury. First, small (bait) fish ingest algae-laden methylmercury, and then the bigger fish eat these smaller fish. Thus, the larger the fish, the more time it has had to accumulate more mercury from its diet of smaller fish. When we enjoy a dinner with a mercury-overloaded fish, that heavy metal has made it into our food chain.

Salonen and colleagues studied the association between fish intake and myocardial infarction, using hair analysis and urinary excretion to measure mercury levels in 1,833 men. Their results showed that men in the highest tertile for hair mercury content had twice the incidence of acute myocardial infarction and almost 3 times the incidence of cardiovascular death as those with lower hair mercury content. Both hair and urinary mercury increase immune complex oxidized LDL, and high levels of oxidized LDL prime the pump for further inflammation.

Although somewhat controversial, dental amalgams are another source of unwanted mercury toxins in the body. The removal of old, tired, and cracked amalgams by a biological dentist should be strongly considered by anyone with signs and symptoms of mercury overload, such as headache, tremor, cardiac disease of unknown etiology, confusion, weakness, weight loss, insomnia, joint pain, and fatigue to mention a few.

The easiest way to diagnose heavy metal toxicity is to ingest a dose of oral DMSA (dimercaptosuccinic acid) and collect the urine for twenty-four hours. In our respective practices, we commonly perform this test on patients with unexplained fatigue, fibromyalgia, neurological, and emotional problems, in addition to cardiac disease.

## Free Radicals

Free radicals are highly reactive, imbalanced molecules produced during oxidation that steal electrons from cells to neutralize their charge. Free radicals interfere with enzymatic reactions, and cause significant metabolic stress, and thereby damaging cells and DNA. Oxidation may occur within the body through simple metabolic processes like eating, drinking, and breathing, which generate free radicals as byproducts of energy (ATP) production. Alcohol, drugs, poor diets, radiation, and other catalysts all accelerate the production of free radicals in the body. The danger of free radicals is that they fan the fires of inflammation and attack cell membranes, ultimately disrupting cellular communication. When free-radical damage disturbs the integrity of cell membranes, they leak, and excessive waste builds up inside the cells.

One of the primary ways we can protect ourselves from free-radical damage is to take oral antioxidants. Because cell membranes are composed mostly of fat, fat-soluble antioxidants like alpha lipoic acid, CoEnzyme Q10, and vitamin E can best penetrate into the cell. Antioxidants slow the aging process by promoting cellular repair, inhibiting inflammation, and preventing production of the inflammatory substances that accelerate aging.

Cardiologists frequently cite the process of lipid peroxidation as a focal point for the origin of atherosclerosis. Many antioxidants, particularly CoEnzyme Q10 and quercetin (found in onions), actively block the oxidation of LDL that contributes to SI.

## Nanobacteria

Although oxidized LDL cholesterol helps to set the stage for atherosclerosis, there are other causes of cardiovascular disease. Oxidized LDL may be part of the story, but it's not the entire explanation. The controversial Nanobacteria Story may well be an important initiating event behind atherosclerosis.

Nanobacteria, formally known as *nanobacterium sanguineum*, are so minute that they eluded researchers for decades. They are $1/100^{th}$ of the size of normal bacteria, and until recently, nobody believed that anything so small could even be alive. It turns out, however, that nanobacteria are not only very vital and thriving, but may cause damage to our health in more ways than we could imagine.

One of our missions has been to explain how and why heart disease occurs in people who do not exhibit the traditional risk factors. If we can identify the cause, then we can help prevent thousands of unexplained deaths each year. There have been numerous hypotheses, but so many never pan out. Take *Chlamydia pneumoniae*, the pathogen that causes acute respiratory disease, for example.

In news reports, from just a few years ago, authorities proclaimed that infection with this bacterium probably accounted for much of the unexplained plaque in people. They hoped that doctors could treat the *C. pneumoniae* and thereby eradicate the plaque. Well, further research uncovered that *C. pneumoniae* was only found in a small percentage of all plaque and was certainly not pervasive enough to be a major cause for it.

### **_An Apt Analogy_**

To help illustrate what the discovery of nanobacteria could ultimately mean for our health, it is important to consider the relationship between *Helicobacter pylori* and ulcers. It was only after years of having patients undergo gastric surgery that doctors learned the real culprit in many ulcers was a bacterium known as *helicobacter pylori*. Surgeons were putting their patients with ulcers through major surgery, cutting their vagus nerve, and revamping part of their small intestine when, in most cases, the only treatment needed was antibiotics.

In the same way in another alarmingly common procedure, cardiac surgeons have been cutting and pasting blood vessels to "bypass" plaque-filled arteries. We may learn, instead, that a course of the right antibiotic is all that is needed for severely calcified arteries.

Scientists from the Hungarian Academy of Sciences have reported finding nanobacteria in more than 60% of carotid artery-clogging plaques studied. The Hungarians also validated previous research reports of how truly miniscule these bacteria are, and how easily they can enter the body via blood exchange and blood products. Their protective calcified apatite coat makes nanobacteria highly resistant to heat, radiation, and all antibiotics with the exception of tetracycline. Nanobacteria have been implicated in nephrolithiasis, polycystic kidney disease, and renal stone formation.

More research will determine whether nanobacteria are the real culprit behind coronary arteriosclerosis. For now it's prudent to keep in mind that microbes could play a substantial factor in the genesis of silent inflammation that could culminate in cardiovascular disease. We'll now discuss some of the research that looks at other viruses and spirochetes as well as the relationship of periodontal disease and the heart.

### *Spirochetes*

In 1982, Willy Burgdorfer discovered the cause of Lyme disease when he isolated spirochetes of the genus *Borrelia* from the mid-gut of Ixodes ticks. Some researchers believe that as many as 60 million people in the US are infected with *Borrelia*, but that Lyme disease occurs in them only when their immune systems become overloaded.

Lyme disease has been reported in forty-seven states and on four continents, and ticks are not the only sources. Blood transfusions, fleas, mosquitoes, sexual intercourse, and unpasteurized cow's and goat's milk have also transmitted the disease. People with Lyme disease are often simultaneously co-infected with other viruses and bacteria.

The spirochetes responsible for Lyme disease do best in an anaerobic (low-oxygen) environment and cannot tolerate large quantities of oxygen. They can change their shape and chemical structure, and are more evolved than bacteria in many ways. Furthermore, these spirochetes can turn off several surface proteins, which have the effect of keeping the immune system from being able to detect them. This stealth-type camouflage prevents antibodies from attaching to them, and prevents the enzymes in the blood from finding and destroying them. In this way, the spirochete can penetrate virtually any tissue in our body including blood vessels, heart, brain and oral cavity.

### *Periodontal Disease*

Multiple microbes including spirochetes, bacteria, and viruses can be cultured in and around the teeth and periodontal sections of the oral cavity. There is a significant relationship between gum disease and chronic inflammation. Low-grade inflammation, particularly in the periodontal areas of the mouth can cause immune system decline. Chronic persistent low-grade inflammation can raise CRP levels. In one study of 50 patients referred for angiography and assessed for periodontal disease, there was a significant relationship between the extent of coronary atherosclerosis and periodontal disease.

Cardiologists are especially cognizant of the relationship between oral hygiene, edentulous teeth, gum disease, halitosis and a strong probability of subsequent cardiovascular disease. Practicing good oral hygiene, taking antioxidants, magnesium, essential fatty acids and CoEnzyme Q10 can help support gum health, thereby reducing chronic inflammation.

*Toxic Blood Syndrome*

Many heart attacks and strokes occur when arteries are only one-third narrowed, so it is not the blood vessels that are of interest to us, but the blood flow when it is compromised by plaque rupture. Inflammation is the primary culprit responsible for vascular disease. In fact, 95% of chronically sick patients are hypercoagulable. Many of these patients have "toxic blood syndrome," which is characterized by elevated levels of oxidized LDL, CRP, fibrinogen, homocysteine, Lp(a), and ferritin. Elevated CRP was the most significant of 12 markers in 28,263 healthy postmenopausal women as a predictor of future cardiac events. It was the strongest risk factor associated with an acute coronary event such as plaque rupture and myocardial infarction. In acute myocardial infarction there has also been an increased mortality in patients with higher CRP levels when compared to age-matched cohorts with lower levels.

## *Homocysteine*

Hyperhomocysteinemia is not only a risk factor for cardiovascular disease; it has also been implicated in osteoporosis, low birth weight, neural tube defects, certain cancers, and Alzheimer's disease. Homocysteine is directly toxic to blood vessels in the brain and heart. Elevated levels wreak oxidative stress, and cause endothelial dysfunction, neuronal DNA damage, and even mitochondrial membrane weakening. High homocysteine levels in the brain cause cerebral microangiopathy and apoptosis of neural cells.

Hyperhomocysteinemia has been shown to double the incidence of Alzheimer's disease. In one study of 1092 people who were "dementia free" over an eight-year follow-up, 111 developed dementia and 83 developed full-blown Alzheimer's disease. Those with homocysteine levels of 14 µmol/L and above doubled their risk, and for every 5µmol/L increase their risk of developing Alzheimer's disease rose by 40%. The correlation between homocysteine levels and Alzheimer's was independent of age, gender and APOE genotype.

One of the most important factors in lowering homocysteine is the use of various B vitamin components including folic acid, calcium folinate, vitamin B6, vitamin B12, pyridoxal phosphate, and betaine hydrochloride (trimethylglycine). Garlic, beets, broccoli, and SAMe are also potent methyl donors in reversing toxic homocysteine back to harmless methionine.

It is important to be aware that approximately 40% of the population has genetic polymorphisms of 5,10-methyltetrahydrofolate reductase (MTHFR). What this means is that a large percentage of people, particularly those of European and French Canadian decent, cannot adequately metabolize synthetic folic acid. For these patients, refractory homocysteine levels will persist despite the use of B vitamin components and natural methylators.

People with hyperhomocysteinemia, that are resistant to usual B vitamin and methylator treatment, need Metafolin (HS Fighters: 877.877.1970), a very highly bioavailable form of methyltetrahydrofolate that also readily crosses the blood brain barrier.

What are acceptable levels of homocysteine? A homocysteine level of less than 7 µmol/L is ideal. Levels over 10 are unacceptable, especially in those with presenile dementia or arteriosclerotic cardiovascular disease. High homocysteine levels are treacherous, especially in the company of elevated Lp(a) because together they can induce the binding of Lp(a) to fibrin, a clot promoting mechanism . On an anecdotal note, Dr Sinatra has seen elevated homocysteine in the company of high Lp(a) in many of his patients who have heart disease, and treats it aggressively in them as well as those at risk for developing it.

## *Lipoprotein (a)*

Lipoprotein (a) is a cholesterol particle with a disulfide bridge that is highly inflammatory and thrombotic. In a ten-year follow-up of myocardial infarction in 5,200 participants, those with the highest Lp(a) levels had a 70% increased incidence of myocardial infarction. For the clinical cardiologist Lp(a) is probably the most difficult risk factor to neutralize. Because statin therapy is known to increase Lp(a), it is important that physicians track Lp(a) levels whenever treating hypercholesterolemia with statin therapy.

We have found that targeted nutraceuticals, especially liver supporting nutrients, CoEnzyme Q10, policosanol, and Omega-3 essential fatty acids, i.e., fish oils, in combination with niacin, and/or Niaspan will often neutralize the toxic effects of Lp(a).

### *Fibrinogen*

Fish oils, garlic, bromelain, and natural Cox 2 inhibitors such as ginger and green teas will also help to alleviate high fibrinogen levels, a phenomenon observed in smokers and postmenopausal women with more frequency. Levels greater than 360 mg/dl are undesirable and have been associated with coronary calcification. This coagulation protein has been successfully neutralized with the nutrients mentioned above as well as enzymes that will be discussed later in this chapter.

### *Ferritin*

Serum ferritin (high levels of stored iron) is also associated with increased risk for myocardial infarction. The high levels of iron that can oxidize LDL cholesterol may reflect iron overload or hereditary hemochromatosis. In the setting of high iron overload it is important to cut iron consumption to a minimum and use high-dose vitamin C with caution, as mega doses of greater than 500mg daily may enhance iron absorption from the diet.

In summary, it is important to assess all these "toxic blood" components, particularly when treating an individual with a family history of early-onset, or what we call premature, cardiovascular disease. Certainly, homocysteine and Lp(a) associations can have a genetic predisposition. The assessment of arteriosclerosis needs to go beyond cholesterol and triglyceride monitoring, and the toxic blood components cited are a good place to start in light of the fact that these inflammatory and thrombotic components are the most undesirable factors in the generation and promotion of plaque.

Younger plaque is soft and covered by a thinner fibrous cap, loaded with cholesterol. It is also quite volatile. It is this young plaque that so often goes unnoticed on angiograms. To some extent many of us have atherosclerosis; thus the real question should be, "Do you have an unstable plaque?" Inside fatty plaques, macrophages can become engorged, becoming incompetent to do the job they are designed to do. Instead, they evolve into angry foam cells, releasing pro-inflammatory toxic substances that may result in further instability to the plaque.

It used to be thought that cholesterol was the major marker for atherosclerosis. This is no longer the case. Pro-inflammatory messengers, referred to as cytokines and leukotrienes, are now recognized as behind-the-scene culprits. When inflammation is present, specific cytokine messengers are heralded into service to instruct the liver to increase intermediary inflammatory substances that are released into the blood and serve as measures of underlying chronic inflammation. CRP is one of those intermediary substances. By interrupting and arresting inflammation we can help to prevent atherosclerosis, hypertension, heart disease, stroke, and even sudden death. Let us look at what we can do to lower inflammatory mediators and minimize SI in the body.

## WAYS TO REDUCE INFLAMMATION

### *Detoxification*

The chemical cocktail of stress, pesticides, industrial wastes, poor diet, heavy metals, chronic infections, and drugs greatly contribute to the SI in our bodies as we age. As the toxic load increases, so does the incidence of chronic disease (Figure 2).

We believe that regular detoxification should become part of a healthy lifestyle. Although you should always avoid obvious toxins whenever possible, it is extremely difficult to avoid many toxins that are present everywhere in the environment today.

That is why each of us should incorporate certain daily detoxification strategies to help flush out the toxins that are circulating in the blood or are lodged in soft tissues and vital organs.

These strategies should include diets such as the Omega Zone diet, bathing, infrared saunas, massages, and liver and colon cleansing on a regular basis. Also, a detoxifying nutraceutical formula can provide additional protection from the various toxins. Such detox formulas should include liver supporting nutrients like milk thistle, artichoke, and L-Carnitine. Alpha lipoic acid and other sulfur-containing nutraceuticals will help chelate heavy metals. Indole-3-carbinol will also assist in the conjugation of the metabolites of petrochemicals like xeno-estrogens out of the body.

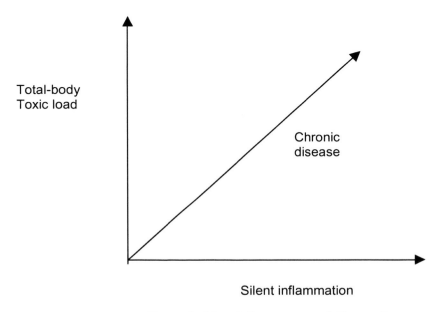

*Figure 2. Silent Inflammation and Chronic Disease*

## *Diet/Weight Loss*

More than 65% of the US population is now overweight. Researchers speculate that obesity will replace tobacco as the major risk factor for disease and death in America today. Recent research suggests that adipocytes have become the "home" for inflammatory cytokines. This is probably one of the major reasons obese people tend to get more cancer, Type II diabetes, and heart disease, as well as other inflammatory disorders. The obesity and diabetes epidemics are linked to the "metabolic syndrome," with its deadly quartet of:
 a. High insulin levels
 b. Weight gain (apple shape)
 c. Elevated triglycerides (TG) and decreased HDL
 d. Elevated blood pressure

Metabolic syndrome also places patients at a much-increased cardiovascular risk. In fact, the most important finding in treating hypertension in the last decade has been an understanding of metabolic syndrome and its relationship with insulin resistance, a condition that can only be reversed through diet and exercise. Hippocrates knew best, many years ago, when he proclaimed: "Let food be your medicine."

For a diet to become a lifestyle, it must be convenient and not too complex. Most people become overwhelmed deciding what they should and should not eat, based on the latest medical news. Designing a Zone meal is simple and involves dividing a plate into three sections. First, fill one-third of it with a protein (a typical portion is approximately the size of the palm of your hand), and fill up the other two-thirds of the plate with low-glycemic vegetables (broccoli, cauliflower, dark leafy greens, and others that won't raise your blood sugar rapidly), and fruit. Finally, add a dash of heart-healthy fat like olive oil to your salad or greens, avocados, or almonds. This is the way we have been genetically designed to eat. Dr. Sinatra prefers a Pan Asian Modified Mediterranean (PAMM) way of eating using the Zone principles because cultural societies following traditional Asian and Mediterranean diets have the lowest rates of cancer and heart disease in the world.

## *Nutraceuticals*

Nutraceuticals are components of foods or dietary supplements that support healing. They include antioxidants, enzymes, vitamins and minerals, Co-Q10 and L-carnitine, garlic, green tea, and fish oil to mention a few. At the microscopic level, many of these nutrients and antioxidants penetrate into the cell and help eradicate free-radical damage, while decreasing inflammation at the same time.

Flavonoids and carotenoids are nutraceuticals that can have a positive impact on the body. For example, dietary antioxidant flavonoids, especially quercetin, were studied in the Zutphen Elderly Study. In this European study reported in the *Lancet*, researchers looked at mortality in elderly men. Results showed that a higher death rate was associated with a lower flavonoid intake. The dietary flavonoids consumed by the male subjects came primarily from onions, green tea, and green apples. Their results confirmed that all-cause mortality was reduced in those men consuming greater than 30 mg of flavonoids per day.

The cardiovascular benefits of similar oligomeric proanthocyanidins (OPCs), which add the bright colors to many fruits and vegetables, and also belong in the flavonoid class of nutrients, have also been noteworthy. OPCs inhibit xanthine oxidase, a promoter of the superoxide radical, platelet aggregation, and the oxidation of LDL. They improve blood vessel elasticity and integrity, and additionally have an "ACE effect" on lowering blood pressure. In animal research, OPCs have also demonstrated a cholesterol lowering effect.

Most people have heard of the "French Paradox," a term that describes the discrepancy between the traditional pate-rich, high-fat French diet and their comparatively low incidence of heart disease. It has been suggested that red wine consumption offsets the evils of a high-fat diet. But why, you ask? Researchers believe that OPCs named quercetin and resveratrol, as well as other flavonoids, present in grape skins are responsible for this victory over heart disease.

## *Magnesium*

Magnesium is a mineral with favorable cardiovascular benefits: it acts like a calcium channel blocker to prevent spasm in blood vessel walls. Magnesium has a profound positive influence on vascular tone and reactivity, as well as platelet aggregations. In fact, a magnesium deficiency has been observed in those with insulin resistance and the diabetic syndrome. Taking 400-800 mg of bioavailable sources is recommended to anyone looking to lower blood pressure, block coronary artery spasm and Raynaud's, and even relieve symptoms of mitral valve prolapse.

In one study, magnesium supplementation decreased many symptoms associated with mitral valve prolapse including weakness, chest pain, shortness of breath, palpitations, and anxiety. Because many patients with mitral valve prolapse have an associated diastolic dysfunction of the heart's left ventricle (LV), CoEnzyme Q10 therapy, which improves LV cardiodynamics, is also instrumental to help improve quality of life for these patients.

### *CoEnzyme Q10*

CoEnzyme Q10 is an essential biological cofactor produced endogenously in the body that is also found in the food chain. As a critical component in the electron transport chain in mitochondria, CoEnzyme Q10 has a crucial role in cellular energy production (by recycling adenosine triphosphate (ATP) as well as being a cofactor in its production) as an electron and proton carrier. Because CoEnzyme Q10 is vital to mitochondrial energy production, it has become the cardinal nutrient in metabolic cardiology.

Since it takes more energy to fill the heart than to empty the heart, CoEnzyme Q10's ability to support heart cell bioenergetics translates into improved diastolic dysfunction. Because of this action, CoEnzyme Q10 is instrumental in addressing diastolic dysfunction, and subsequent systolic dysfunction, that could lead to heart failure. Those with hypertensive cardiovascular disease, mitral valve prolapse, infiltrative cardiomyopathy, and especially those with statin-induced diastolic dysfunction, have improved with the simple co-administration of CoEnzyme Q10.

Other potential therapeutic uses of CoEnzyme Q10 include treating stable and unstable angina, ventricular arrhythmia, mitral valve prolapse, hypertension, congestive heart failure and toxin-induced cardiotoxicity (such as that seen in Adriamycin therapy). CoEnzyme Q10 is also appropriate in the setting of myocardial ischemia, and should be used as a myocardial-preserving agent during chemical thrombolysis for reperfusion, urgent angioplasty, and coronary bypass surgery. In fact, pretreatment with CoEnzyme Q10 for weeks before elective coronary artery bypass grafting surgery has been shown to assist patients in weaning off of heart-lung bypass with improved cardiodynamics.

Since its discovery in 1972, there have been multiple controlled trials on the use of CoEnzyme Q10 with more than 40 showing some benefit, and 4 showing none. In one double-blind study of 641 patients receiving CoEnzyme Q10 (2 mg/kg or placebo for one year), a 20% reduction in hospitalizations in the CoEnzyme Q10 group was realized compared to those taking placebo. The CoEnzyme Q10 group had a better quality of life as well as lowered bills for medical care.

Another topic of special emphasis is statins: the number of these drugs prescribed every year is astounding, and may have a link to the increase number of cases of idiopathic cardiomyopathies that abound. Statin drugs can cause profound deficiencies in CoEnzyme Q10 because the HMG-reductase inhibitors "kill" cholesterol so successfully by interfering with the same biochemical pathway that produces endogenous CoEnzyme Q10 in the body. So, CoEnzyme Q10 should be supplemented by anyone receiving 3-hydroxy-3 methylglutaryl coenzyme A-reductase inhibitors (statins). CoEnzyme Q10 treatment has been noted to counteract the side effects of myalgias associated with statin therapy, and is appropriate to treat this side effect.

CoEnzyme Q10 production drops off with aging, and while its side effects (nausea, abdominal discomfort, and excess energy or anxiety) are rare, it is contraindicated for healthy pregnant or lactating women because the unborn and newborn produce sufficient quantities of the compound on their own. For further information on CoEnzyme Q10, the reader is referred to *BioFactors*, Volume 18, 2003. This journal is a peer-refereed review of original papers arising from the 3$^{rd}$ Conference of the International CoEnzyme Q10 Association held in London UK, November 2002. Several investigations discussed the complex biochemical and metabolic functions of CoEnzyme Q10.

### *Metabolic Cardiology*

We believe that a new subspecialty in cardiology, i.e., "metabolic cardiology", will be driven by the biochemical interventions that will be utilized to optimize metabolism in cardiac myocytes. By supporting cellular function, such as ATP production, Coenzyme Q10 and other similar agents defend precious heart cells from the ravages of aging, toxins, and the myriad of other conditions that ultimately wear down mitochondrial function and eventually cause cardiovascular pathology. Metabolic cardiology is going to be one of the next great emerging fields, arising from a new emphasis on the relationship between ATP and energy in the heart. Coenzyme Q10, L-Carnitine, and D-ribose, will be the most significant players.

The synergism of CoQ10 and L-Carnitine, for example, has been known for approximately 15 years. Italian researchers have demonstrated an extraordinary synergistic effect of these nutrients in several conditions, such as ischemia, reperfusion injury of the heart, fatty infiltration of the liver induced by alcohol, and hyperbaric oxygen toxicity in experimental animals. These nutraceuticals offer remarkable biochemical and metabolic complementary roles.

L-Carnitine has the unusual ability to enhance fatty acid oxidation in cells while removing excess harmful substances, such as acyl groups and free radicals, from inner mitochondrial membranes. Since 60% of cardiac energy comes from the beta-oxidation of fats, employing L-Carnitine is instrumental in treating angina, myocardial infarction, congestive heart failure, and peripheral claudication.

In the setting of acute and/or chronic ischemia, Coenzyme Q10 and L-Carnitine offer significant clinical advantages with absolutely no risk to the patient. These nutrients, while supporting cardiovascular function, also preserve the inner mitochondrial membrane and may even support vulnerable cells, particularly senescent myocardium from apoptosis. Recently, another new emerging compound has been gaining increasing support among our fellow "metabolic cardiologists."

D-ribose is a biochemical, five-sided sugar that has been extensively investigated in both animal and clinical models. Investigators believe that under certain cardiac conditions, especially during ischemic episodes like angina and myocardial infarction when the heart is deprived of oxygen, there is a profound depression of energy compounds such at ATP. A drop in ATP means a subsequent decrease in myocardial function causing the heart to struggle as a pump. This is probably one of the reasons that we see so-called "stunned myocardium" following acute coronary artery syndrome and myocardial infarction. Researchers are now learning that D-ribose plummets during ischemia, and that it takes considerable time to recover and regenerate ATP compounds. D-ribose helps to replenish the severely depleted adenosine nucleotide pool in the ischemic monocytes, a process that is critical to ATP synthesis.

It has been previously noted that coenzyme Q10 and L-carnitine increase exercise time and delay the onset of electrocardiographic evidence of ischemia during exercise stress testing of angina subjects. The pentose sugar D-ribose (15 grams daily) has been similarly noted to protect cardiac cells from ischemic episodes and increase exercise time before symptom onset due to angina. The combined antioxidant, membrane-stabilizing and metabolic activities of CoQ10, L-Carnitine, and D-ribose will play a significant role in the setting of silent and overt myocardial ischemia.

As new research unfolds, these nutraceuticals provide an exciting platform in cardiovascular disease to improve quality of life for patients suffering from progressive angina, unstable angina, acute coronary syndrome, diastolic dysfunction, and congestive heart failure. Metabolic cardiologists will upgrade the level of patient care as they gain further insight into this new great emerging field in cardiovascular medicine.

*Enzymes*

Within a single cell there are roughly 100,000 genes, the majority of which house enzymes, the workhorses of the living cell. All enzymes are proteins, and are also composed of long chains of amino acids. Also recognized as the corporeal life force, enzymes are involved in nearly every metabolic process in the body. As we age, or develop a disease, our body has fewer and fewer enzyme stores at its disposal. For example, a sixty-year-old has 50% fewer enzymes than a thirty-year-old.

Enzymes function as catalysts and make things work faster. They have the ability to initiate, accelerate, and terminate biochemical reactions in the body. Enzymes increase the activity of the cells that are important to a healthy immune system, and they are integral in maintaining homeostasis. Provided there are sufficient enzymes, cases of acute inflammation may be healed within a few days. With chronic SI, however, the continued shortage of enzymes leads to an eventual breakdown of the reactions needed to remove diseased tissue from the body and return it to normal health. Enzymes are important biological response modifiers and play a vital role in controlling inflammation and promoting heart health.

Although wobenzyme has been used exclusively by Olympic athletes over the years to reduce inflammations in tendons, muscles and joints, newer inflammatory mediators such as nattokinase have been gaining popularity for reducing inflammatory mediators such as CRP. In the future enzymes such as nattokinase and wobenzyme as well as fish oil will be utilized in reducing the total "inflammatory load" in the body.

## Omega-3 Fatty Acids

Leading medical institutions worldwide have confirmed that daily supplementation with pharmaceutical-grade fish oil, rich in omega-3 essential fatty acids, is your most powerful weapon for assuaging inflammation.

Although the evidence in the cardiovascular literature resounding that omega-3 essential fatty acids are appropriate in the treatment and prevention of cardiovascular disease, the most recent noteworthy trial appeared in the *Lancet*. In this study of approximately of 11,000 Italian participants who suffered a myocardial infarction, the group given fish oil had a 45% lower incidence of sudden cardiac death and a 20% reduction in all-cause death over a three- year period. Those receiving fish oil also appreciated a reduction in blood pressure, suppression in platelet activity, drop in triglyceride levels, and a marked attenuation in cardiac arrhythmia. Perhaps the most noteworthy way fish oil seems to attain its beneficial effect is its favorable impact on heart rate variability (HRV). Omega-3 essential fatty acids also reduce plaque rupture by literally "getting inside plaque" to stabilize it and rendering it less vulnerable to rupture. Eating "healthy fish" or taking fish oil supplements is an absolute must, especially for the populations at risk for cardiovascular disease. In fact, just two fish meals per month will reduce an individual's risk of sudden cardiac death by 50%.

Unfortunately, because most fish have become contaminated with toxins, such as dioxins, mercury, and PCBs, consuming fatty cold-water fish as your primary source of omega-3s is now being questioned. To combat this situation, choose a pharmaceutical-grade fish oil that has been concentrated and purified to the highest standards possible. Pharmaceutical-grade fish oils are, as a result, toxin-free and can be ingested without any fear of toxins or contaminants found in the fish we eat, or as may be contained in more commonly available omega-3 supplements.

## Control of Chronic Infections without Antibiotics

Current research from the National Institutes of Health (NIH) and elsewhere shows that while chronic infections are really never eradicated, they can be controlled as long as a person remains on an antimicrobial program. The disadvantages of living on antibiotics, however, do not make this an attractive or plausible way to live.

Research has shown that some people who have taken tetracycline for acne for years have less atherosclerosis. This previously anecdotal observation now makes sense when we recognize that many people have chronic infections, such as CMV and nanobacteria, which contribute to the SI and elevated CRP levels we see. It is our opinion that if we boost the body's natural immunity with select nutraceuticals and practice good oral hygiene, we can thwart many of these chronic infections. These formulas can be taken for an entire lifetime without any substantial risk.

We have already seen how most infections are masked by soluble fibrin monomers such as the ones in the protein coats of the agent that causes Lyme disease, and how useful enzymes like Wobenzyme are in the treatment of these chronic infections.

After studies done in Florida at Hemex Laboratories, researchers are now convinced that the presence of any form of infection is associated with inflammation and severely localized hypercoagulability (toxic blood). Therefore, to help get adequate blood flow to the infected tissues to completely extirpate these stubborn infections, we believe it is essential to take targeted nutraceuticals.

Garlic is also important because many microbials cannot grow well in its presence. Malic acid helps bind iron so that many harmful organisms requiring iron for their reproductive cycle are kept from replicating. We have found TOA-Free Cat's Claw, or Samento, to be very helpful for Lyme disease. Samento (*uncaria tomentosa*), is extremely potent and able to significantly strengthen the immune system. Samento also has powerful anti-inflammatory, antioxidant, and anti-tumor properties. Research shows that Samento eliminates dependence on steroids and inhalers, reduces HIV and hepatitis-C levels, drops CRP levels, and lowers some tumor markers, such as prostate specific antigen (PSA).

Other nutraceuticals, such as elements of colostrum, grapefruit seed extract, rice bran, rhodiola rosea (found in Northern Alpine regions), and many different mushrooms like shiitake and reishi, also have powerful effects in fighting chronic infections and inflammation.

## *Pharmacology*

While many physicians are unaware of the important role of eicosanoids, the pharmaceutical industry is very cognizant of these powerful hormones because many of the more popular drugs used today alter eicosanoid levels. Most of these drugs inhibit the enzymes that synthesize eicosanoids and have little therapeutic effect in altering the balance of "good" and "bad" eicosanoids.

As an example, the cyclooxygenase enzymes (Cox-1 and Cox-2) are responsible for the synthesis of prostaglandins and thromboxanes, but they can be blocked by aspirin, Cox-2 inhibitors, and non-steroidal anti-inflammatory drugs (NSAIDs). Furthermore, the only drugs that can inhibit all types of eicosanoid synthesis are corticosteroids; while blocking the synthesis of "bad" eicosanoids may reduce inflammation, the anti-inflammatory and other beneficial properties of "good" eicosanoids are obstructed in the process. Unfortunately, the undesirable side effects make long-term corticosteroid usage inadvisable.

Recent research indicates that the cardiovascular benefits of statin drugs (first used to decrease cholesterol levels) may be due primarily to their anti-inflammatory actions that reduce CRP levels. As pointed out earlier, CRP is associated with generalized inflammation and is considered a significant biomarker for the development of heart disease. New research suggests that statin therapy also increases insulin levels and insulin resistance, which may amplify the future risk of heart disease, diabetes, and obesity.

Our position on statins was summarized in an editorial in the March 2003 issue of *The Southern Medical Journal*. Although there is little doubt that statin therapy can significantly reduce the incidence of coronary morbidity and mortality, especially for those who are at the greatest risk of developing coronary artery disease, over-utilization of statins in the population that does not have overt coronary artery disease or silent inflammation should be avoided.

However, recent interventions using electron beam computerized tomography (EBCT) to demonstrate an association between high coronary calcium burden (score greater than 1,000) and cardiac events suggest that statin therapy may prove to be a good intervention. In other words, in patients with myocardial infarction, coronary artery bypass surgery, stent emplacement, stable or unstable angina, and high coronary calcification, statin therapy should be utilized regardless of their cholesterol levels. In diabetics with high cholesterol and high inflammation indices determined by elevated CRP, homocysteine, LP(a), and other inflammatory cytokines, statin therapy is also beneficial. The use of statins in high-risk coronary patients, especially those with inflammatory markers, is good medicine.

However, overuse of these potent pharmacological agents with known and unknown side effects in otherwise healthy people is not considered smart medicine. We also do not know the long-term effect of statin therapy, especially since longitudinal studies for those taking statins for more than 10 years are lacking. Carcinogenicity and cardiomyopathy (diastolic dysfunction) associations with statin therapy may cause us to rethink our posturing on statin therapies in the future. For now, we implore physicians to select statin therapy to address the individual risks and health needs of each patient, and avoid prescribing them simply to treat high cholesterol numbers alone.

### *Exercise and Stress Management*

There is no doubt that exercise should be an indispensable part of any person's total health promotion program, not only because of its many benefits, but also because of the sense of well being that exercise provides.

The biological basis of all these benefits is that they are mostly a consequence of the hormonal and weight loss changes that various types of exercise induce. The real key is that the higher the intensity of exercise, the more the hormonal responses are affected. Moderate to higher-intensity aerobic exercise reduces insulin (and therefore inflammation), and increases glucagon levels: exactly as a Zone-favorable diet does. However, high intensity exercises such as marathon running, wrestling, boxing, and other professional and Olympic sports, to mention a few, can cause enormous oxidative stress and subsequent antioxidant insufficiency. The most common antioxidants that are depleted with regular intense exercise include CoEnzyme Q10, magnesium, and vitamin E. In a premenopausal female athlete severe iron deficiencies may also been noted. High intensity exercise, like emotional stress, can enhance the oxidation of LDL.

Emotional stress can cause inflammation just as easily as oxidized LDL. The medical community now recognizes that a supercharged sympathetic nervous system (SNS) can set you up for cardiac events and sudden death. Heart rate variability, an assessment of sympathetic and parasympathetic nervous system balance or imbalance, can now be performed in an office setting. Anger, hostility, and the inability to express feelings are also serious cardiovascular risk factors. In addition to exercise, various mind-body approaches can be very effective in altering SNS response and inflammation.

## CONCLUSION

To underscore the importance of the concept of "fire in the heart," a front page article in the February 23, 2004 issue of *Time* magazine highlights the link between inflammation, cancer, heart attacks, Alzheimer's disease, and other diseases. Everywhere we turn we are facing evidence that inflammation plays a larger role in chronic disease than we physicians ever thought. We need to ask ourselves the rhetorical question "is your heart on fire?" To some degree, silent inflammation is insidiously eroding our vital organs.

One of our colleagues, neurologist Dr. David Perlmutter, would agree. His newest book, The *Better Brain Book* with Carol Colman, discusses the inflammatory and toxic environment of the aging brain. Plaque stabilization, whether in the brain, heart or other organs will eventually come under the domain of dietary Cox 2 inhibitors including green tea, ginger, curcumin, oregano, onions, garlic and fish oil. In addition, vital nutraceuticals such as folic acid, fish oil, enzymes, CoEnzyme Q10, magnesium, quercetin, L-Carnitine, D-ribose, and others will continue to be utilized by like-minded physicians as safe alternative options.

More integrative therapies will include statin therapy, ACE inhibitors, low-dose aspirin, antibiotics and leukotriene inhibitors as more conventional approaches to halting the ravages of inflammation. The integration of proven complementary therapies with conventional treatments in heart disease will allow physicians to offer many additional options to their patients.

We urge physicians to keep an open mind and harbor a willingness to support conventional methodologies while investigating alternatives that can improve quality of life and reduce human suffering. Choosing from the best conventional and complementary options is the only logical and ethical thing to do to help douse the inflammatory inferno in the heart.

# REFERENCES

Actis-Goretta L, Ottaviani JI, Keen CL, Fragga CG. Inhibition of angiotensin converting enzyme (ACE) activity by flavan-3-ols and procyanidins. *FEBS Lett.* 2003;555:597-600.

Bertelli A, Bertelli AA, Giovanni L, Spaggiari P. Protective synergic effect of coenzyme Q10 and carnitine of hyperbaric oxygen toxicity. *Inter J Tissue Reactions.* 1990;12:193-196.

Bertelli A, Ronca G. Carnitine and coenzyme Q10: biochemical properties and functions synergism and complementary action. *Inter J Tissue Reactions.* 1990;12:183-186.

Bertelli A, Ronca F, Ronca G, Palmieri L, Zucchi R. L-carnitine and coenzyme Q10 protective action against ischemia and reperfusion of working rat heart. *Drugs under Experimental Clin Res.* 1992;18:431-436.

*BioFactors.* 2003;18.

Breiner M. *Whole Body Dentistry.* Quantum Health Press; 1999.

Burke BE, Neuenschwander R, Olson RD. Randomized, double-blind, placebo-controlled trial of coenzyme Q10 in isolated systolic hypertension. *South Med J.* 2001;94:1112-1117.

Cacciatore L, Cerio R, Ciarimboli M, Cocozza M, Coto V, D'Alessandro A, D'Alessandro L, Grattarola G, Imparato L, Lingetti M, et al. The therapeutic effect of L-carnitine in patients with exercise-induced stable angina: a controlled study. *Drugs Exp Clin Res.* 1991;17:225-235.

Chang WC, Hsu FL. Inhibition of platelet aggregation and arachidonate metabolism platelets of procyanidins. *Prostaglandins Leukot Essential Fatty Acids.* 1989;38:181-188.

Danesh J, Collins R, Peto R. Lipoprotein (a) and coronary artery disease. Meta-analysis of prospective studies. *Circulation* 2000;102:1082-1085.

Duan W, Ladenheim B, Cutler RG, Kruman II, Cadet JL, Mattson MP. Dietary folate deficiency and elevated homocysteine levels endanger dopaminergic neurons in models of Parkinson's disease. *Journal of Neurochemistry* 2002;80:101-110.

Dumesnil JG, Turgeon J, Tremblay A, Poirier P, Gilbert M, Gagnon L, St-Pierre S, Garneau C, Lemieux I, Pascot A, et al. Effect of low glycaemic index-low-fat-high protein diet on the atherogenic metabolic risk profile of abdominally obese men. *Br J Nutr.* 2001;86:557-568.

el Boustani S, Causse JE, Descomps B, Monnier L, Mendy F, Crastes de Paulet A. Direct in vivo characterization of delta 5 desaturase activity in humans by deuterium labeling: effects of insulin. *Metab.* 1989;38:315-321.

Ernest E. Chelation therapy for coronary heart disease: An overview of all clinical investigations. *American Heart Journal* 2002;140:139-141.

Freeman DJ, Norrie J, Caslake MJ, Gaw A, Ford I, Lowe GD, O'Reilly DS, Packard CJ, Sattar N; West of Scotland Coronary Prevention Study. C-reactive protein is an independent predictor of risk for the development of diabetes in the West of Scotland Coronary Prevention Study. *Diabetes* 2002;51:1596-1600.

Ghirlanda G, Oradei A, Manto A, Lippa S, Uccioli L, Caputo S, Greco AV, Littarru GP. Evidence of plasma CoQ10-lowering effect by HMG- CoA reductase inhibitors: A double-blind, placebo-controlled study. *J Clin Pharm.* 1993;33:226-229.

Gorman C, Park A. The Fires Within. *Time Magazine* 2004;163:38-46.

Goyette P, Christensen B, Rosenblatt DS, Rozen R. Severe and mild mutations in cis for the methylenetetrahydrofolate reductase (MTHFRO gene), and description of 5 novel mutations in MTHFR. *Am J Hum. Genet.* 1996;59:1268-1275.

Hankey GJ, Eikeboom JW. Homocysteine and vascular disease. *Lancet* 1999;354:407-413.

Hertog MG, Feskens EJ, Hollman PC, Katan MB, Kromhout D. Dietary antioxidant flavonoids and risk of coronary heart disease: The Zutphen Elderly Study. *Lancet* 1993;342:1007-11.

Kajander EO, Ciftcioglu N. "Nanobacteria: an alternative mechanism for pathogenic intra- and extra-cellular calcification and stone formation." *PNAS* 1998; 95:8274-8279.

Kajander EO, et al. Nanobacteria from blood, the smallest culturable autonomously replicating agent on Earth. *Proceedings SPIE.* 1997; 3111:420-428.

Kajander EO, Ciftcioglu N, Aho K, Garcia-Cuerpo E. Characteristics of nanobacteria and their possible role in stone formation. *Urol Res.* 2003;31:47-54.

Kajander EO, Ciftcioglu N, Miller-Hjelle MA, Hjelle JT. Nanobacteria: controversial pathogens in nephrolithiasis and polycystic kidney disease. Curr Opin Nephrol Hypertens. 2001;10:445-452.

Kamikawa T, Kobayashi A, Yamashita T, Hayashi H, Yamazaki N. Effects of coenzyme Q10 on exercise tolerance in chronic stable angina pectoris. *Am J Cardiol.* 1985;56:247-251.

Langsjoen PH, Langsjoen AM. Overview of the use of CoQ10 in cardiovascular disease. *Biofactors* 1999;9:273-284.

Layman DK, Shiue H, Sather C, Erickson DJ, Baum J. Increased dietary protein modifies glucose and insulin homeostasis in adult women during weight loss. *J Nutr.* 2003;133:405-410.

Lemaitre RN, King IB, Mozaffarian D, Kuller LH, Tracy RP, Siscovick DS. n-3 polyunsaturated fatty acids, fatal ischemic heart disease, and nonfatal myocardial infarction in older adults: the cardiovascular health study. *Am J Clin Nutr.* 2003;77:279-280.

Libby P. Atherosclerosis: the new view. *Scientific American* 2002;May:24-55.

Lichodziejewska B, Klos J, Rezler J, Grudzka K, Dluzniewska M, Budaj A, Ceremuzynski L. Clinical symptoms of mitral valve prolapse are related to hypomagnesemia and attenuated by magnesium supplementation. *Am J Cardiol.* 1997;79:768-772.

Loesche WJ. Periodontal disease: link to cardiovascular disease. *Compend Contin Educ Dent.* 2000;21:463-466,468,470.

Ludwig DS. The glycemic index: Physiological mechanism relating to obesity, diabetes, and cardiovascular disease. *JAMA* 2002;287:2414-2423.

Meunier MT, Villie F, Jonadet M, Bastide J, Bastide P. Inhibition of angiotensin I converting enzyme by flavanolic compounds: in vitro and in vivo studies. *Planta Medica.* 1987;53:12-15.

Miller AL. The methionine-homocysteine cycle and its effects on cognitive diseases. *Alter Med Rev.*2003 8:7-19.

Mokdad AH, Marks JS, Stroup DF, Gerberding JL. Actual causes of death in the United States. *JAMA* 2004;291:1238-1245.

Morita H, Taguchi J, Kurihara H, Kitaoka M, Kaneda H, Kurihara Y, Maemura K, Shindo T, Minamino T, Ohno M, et al. Genetic polymorphism of 5, 10- methylenetetrahydrofolate reductase (MTHFR) as a risk factor of coronary artery disease. *Circ.* 1997;95:2032-2036.

Morisco C, Trimarco B, Condorelli M. Effective coenzyme Q10 therapy in patients with congestive heart failure: a long-term multicenter randomized study. *Clin Investig.* 1993;71(8 Suppl):S134-136.

[No authors listed] Dietary supplementation with n-3 polyunsaturated fatty acids and vitamin E after myocardial infarction: results of the GISSI-Prevenzione trial. Gruppo Italiano per lo Studio della Sopravvivenza nell'Infarto miocardico. *Lancet* 1999;354:447-455. Erratum in: *Lancet* 2001;357:642.

Nygard O, Nordrehaug JE, Refsum H, Ueland PM, Farstad M, Vollset SE. Plasma homocysteine levels and mortality in patients with coronary artery disease. *N Engl J Med.* 1997;337:230-236.

Pauly D, Johnson C, St. Cyr JA. The benefits of ribose in cardiovascular disease. *Med Hypotheses.* 2003;60:149-151.

Pauly D, Pepine C. D-Ribose as a supplement for cardiac energy metabolism. *J Cardiovasc Pharmacol Ther.* 2000;5:249-258.

Pelikanova T, Kohout M, Base J, Stefka Z, Kovar J, Kazdova L, Valek J. Effect of acute hyperinsulinemia on fatty acid composition of serum lipids in non-insulin dependent diabetics and healthy men. *Clin Chim Acta.*1991;203:329-337.

Pliml W, von Arnim T, Stablein A, Hofmann H, Zimmer HG, Erdmann E. Effects of ribose on exercise-induced ischemia in stable coronary artery disease. *Lancet.* 1992;340:507-510.

Pradhan AD, Manson JE, Rifai N, Buring JE, Ridker PM. C-reactive protein, interleukin 6, and risk of developing type 2 diabetes mellitus. *JAMA* 2001;286:327-334.

Retter AS. Carnitine and its role in cardiovascular disease. *Heart Disease.* 1999;1:108-113.

Ridker PM, Hennekens CH, Buring JE, Rifai N. C-reactive protein and other markers of inflammation in the prediction of cardiovascular disease in women. *N Engl J Med.*2000;342:836-843.

Ridker PM, Rifai N, Pfeffer MA, Sacks FM, Moye LA, Goldman S, Flaker GC, Braunwald E.

Inflammation, pravastatin, and the risk of coronary events after myocardial infarction in patients with average cholesterol levels. *Circulation* 1998;98:839-844.

Salonen JT, Nyyssonen K, Korpela H, Tuomilehto J, Seppanen R, Salonen R. High stored iron levels are associated with excess risk of myocardial infarction in eastern Finnish men. *Circulation* 1992; 86;803-811.

Salonen JT, Seppanen K, Nyyssonen K, Korpela H, Kauhanen J, Kantola M, Tuomilehto J, Esterbauer H, Tatzber F, Salonen R. Intake of mercury from fish, lipid peroxidation, and the risk of myocardial infarction in coronary, cardiovascular, and any death in eastern Finnish men. *Circulation* 1995;91:645-655.

Sears B. *OmegaRx Zone*. Regan Books. New York; 2002.

Seddon JM, Gensler G, Milton RC, Klein ML, Rifai N. Association between C-reactive protein and age-related macular degeneration. *JAMA*. 2004;291:704-710.

Seshadri S, Beiser A, Selhub J, Jacques PF, Rosenberg IH, D'Agostino RB, Wilson PW, Wolf PA. Plasma homocysteine as a risk factor for dementia and Alzheimer's disease. *New England Journal of Medicine*. 2002;346:476-483.

Seymour RA, Preshaw PM, Steele JG. Oral health and heart disease. *Prim Dent Care*. 2002;9:125-131.

Shechter M, Merz CN, Paul-Labrador M, Meisel SR, Rude RK, Molloy MD, Dwyer JH, Shah PK, Kaul S. Oral magnesium supplementation inhibits platelet-dependent thrombosis in patients with coronary artery disease. *Am J Cardiol*. 1999;84:152-156.

Simpson G, Sinatra S, Suarez-Menendez J. *SPA-Medicine*. Basic Books. New Jersey; 2004.

Sinatra ST. Alternative medicine for the conventional cardiologist. *Heart Disease*. 2000;2:16-30.

Sinatra ST. Care, cancer and coenzyme Q10. *J Am Coll Cardiol*. 1999;33:897-899.

Sinatra ST. CoEnzyme Q10, L-carnitine, apoptosis and the heart. *Int Journ Anti-Aging Med*. 2000; Winter:15-24.

Sinatra ST. Is cholesterol lowering with statins the gold standard for treating patients with cardiovascular risk and disease? *Southern Med Assoc*. 2003;96:220-222.

Sinatra ST. *The CoEnzyme Q10 Phenomenon*. Keats Pub. 1998.

Sinatra ST, Peterson SJ. Use of alternative medicines in treatment of cardiovascular disease. In: Frishman WH, Sonnenblick EH, Sica DA (eds): *Cardiovascular Pharmacotherapeutics, Manual 2nd ed*. McGraw-Hill. New York;2004:485-512.

Singh RB, Niaz MA, Agarwal P, Beegum R, Rastogi SS, Sachan DS. A randomized, double-blind, placebo-controlled trial of L-carnitine in suspected acute myocardial infarction. *Postgrad Med J*. 1996;72:45-50.

Singh RB, Wander GS, Rastogi A, Shukla PK, Mittal A, Sharma JP, Mehrotra SK, Kapoor R, Chopra RK. Randomized, double-blind placebo-controlled trial of coenzyme Q10 in patients with acute myocardial infarction. *Cardiovasc Drugs Ther*. 1998;12:347-353.

Sullivan, JL. The iron paradigm of ischemic heart disease. *Am Heart J*. 1989;117:1177-1188.

Tanaka J, Tominaga R, Yoshitoshi M, Matsui K, Komori M, Sese A, Yasui H, Tokunaga K. CoEnzyme Q10: The prophylactic effect on low cardiac output following cardiac valve replacement. *Ann Thorac Surg*. 1982;33:145-151.

Turunen M, Olsson J, Dallner G. Metabolism and function of coenzyme Q. *Biochima et Biophysica Acta-Biomembranes*. 2004;1660:171-199

Visser M, Bouter LM, McQuillan GM, Wener MH, Harris TB. Elevated C-reactive protein levels in overweight and obese adults. *JAMA* 1999;282:2131-2135.

Walter DH, Fichtlscherer S, Sellwig M, Auch-Schwelk W, Schachinger V, Zeiher AM. Preprocedural C-reactive protein levels and cardiovascular events after coronary stent implantation. *American Journal of Cardiology* 2001;37:839-846.

Wegrowski J, Robert AM, Moczar M. The effect of procyanidolic oligomers on the composition of normal and hypercholesterolemic rabbit aortas. *Biochem Pharmacol.*1984;33:3491-3497.

Wolfe BM, Piche LA. Replacement of carbohydrate by protein in a conventional-fat diet reduces cholesterol and triglyceride concentrations in healthy normolipidemic subjects. *Clin Invest Med.* 1999;22:140-148.

## USEFUL RESOURCES
- Hemex Laboratories, www.hemex.com
- Nutramedix, www.nutramedix.com and www.samento.com.ec
- The Zone Lifestyle, www.zonecafe.com
- Sinatra S. and Simpson G., *Spa Medicine,* Basic Books, 2004

## ABOUT THE AUTHOR

Stephen T. Sinatra is a board-certified cardiologist, certified bioenergetic psychotherapist, and certified as a nutrition and anti-aging specialist. At his practice in Manchester, Connecticut, Dr. Sinatra integrates conventional medicine with complementary nutritional and psychological therapies that help heal the heart. He is a fellow in the American College of Cardiology and the American College of Nutrition.

His latest book entitled *Eight Weeks to Lowering Blood Pressure* was released by Ballantine in February 2003. Dr Sinatra also writes a monthly national newsletter entitled *The Sinatra Health Report,* which is published by Phillips Health, L.L.C. For more information on the topics contained in this chapter, please visit www.drsinatra.com.

# Chapter 5

# Integrated Anti-Aging: from Medical to Surgical Interventions

*Stephen M Pratt, M.D., A.C.C., A.S.P.S.*
*Private Practice, Southern Plastic Surgery, Nashville, TN*

## ABSTRACT

Increasingly, physicians from all specialties will be called upon to integrate programs which have now become commonplace to the members of the American Academy of Anti-Aging Medicine (A4M) into their daily practices. In no specialty will this be more common than those physicians and surgeons who are engaged in the practice of plastic surgery and cosmetic dermatology. Similarly, as clinical age management physicians, we may also be required by our patients to have a familiarity with techniques available in the plastic surgery realm. As in all other aspects of our practice we should view it as our duty to avail this knowledge to the patient when the patient requests information or when we think that a particular technique or procedure may be of benefit.

**Keywords:** plastic surgery; cosmetic dermatology; aesthetic medicine; facial rejuvenation; liposuction

## INTRODUCTION

Plastic surgery encompasses both cosmetic surgery and reconstructive surgery, and it is important to make clear distinctions between the two. According to the *American Medical Association*, "reconstructive surgery is performed on abnormal structures of the body, caused by congenital defects, development abnormalities, trauma, infection, tumors or disease. It is generally performed to improve function, but may also be done to approximate a normal appearance." Whereas cosmetic surgery, for example breast augmentation, "is performed to reshape normal structures of the body in order to improve the patient's appearance and self-esteem." Another important distinction is that reconstructive surgery has no relationship with anti-aging medicine; however cosmetic surgery makes use of the latest anti-aging technology available.

## COSMETIC SURGERY AND CLINICAL AGE MANAGEMENT

As we know, cosmetic surgery is not necessary and therefore is not usually compensated by third-party payers. Although, recent evidence suggests that a growing number of third-party payers are reconsidering their stance on cosmetic surgery. Therefore, patients coming into a plastic surgery practice are different from the average patient. These people are aware that they will have to pay for their procedure, and they are willing to do so because they want to invest in their betterment. Thus, most cosmetic surgery patients are interested in joining a clinical age management program.

Cosmetic surgery patients are very demanding. They have high expectations and they demand a lot of care. The clinical age management patient is typically very similar. The main problem when trying to enroll a cosmetic surgery patient on a clinical age management program is that such patients are looking for immediate results and are not that willing to try treatments where it takes a long time, in some cases years, until improvements are noticeable. The cosmetic surgery patient simply wants to come in and have their problem fixed, there and then preferably. If they don't like their neck, or their nose, it can be fixed within a month or so. They will heal within three to four weeks of surgery and then begin to consider what they should have done next. This is where the plastic surgeon should step in and try to encourage the patient to improve their lifestyle and introduce the concepts of anti-aging medicine to them.

Physicians are very hesitant to recommend patients for plastic surgery. The majority of patients who turn up at a cosmetic surgery practice will have been referred to the practice by a previous patient. It is likely to be the same with clinical age management practices. The traditional M.D. in this country is there to treat disease, not aging. That is our culture. There may be a paradigm shift, to some extent, in that population, but one that may take a sizeable amount of time.

Some patients will have tried everything except surgery to improve their looks, however in order to achieve the results they want cosmetic surgery is probably their only hope. This is the type of patient we refer to as a "jump-start" patient. This type of patient needs to be offered the full clinical age management program, but in order to make them feel much better about themselves needs a number of procedures that will alter their appearance dramatically. The procedures will boost the patient's confidence and perhaps most importantly give them a new lease of life. This type of patient would not be receptive towards more subtle anti-aging treatments, such as hormone replacement therapy, skin care, nutrition, and vitamin supplements, before surgery as they simply wouldn't have seen the results they wanted, and thus would have quickly lost interest. However, by carrying out a few procedures that produce obvious results it is often possible to capture the patient and keep them in the program and, probably, do a much better job in their overall management for the next 10 to 20 years.

Cosmetic surgery is not for everybody, just like hormone replacement therapy may not be for everybody. But it is for some. Even though we may not want it for ourselves, for instance, we have to accept the fact that it may be needed and it may be beneficial to others. The only need for cosmetic surgery is if that individual patient wants it. There is no other indication for cosmetic surgery whatsoever. It is possible to tell a patient from a surgeon's viewpoint what may make them look better, but the patient needs to forget about other people may think and think only about how they feel about themselves. If the patient perceives a problem, then it is their decision to go ahead and have surgery.

Medical practitioners in any field have to accept the fact that there may be some cosmetic procedures that may actually be beneficial to people. It may increase their well-being and their sense of self, and it may make it easier for us to treat them in the other ways that are necessary. Conversely, plastic surgeons must not forget the fact that they are not doing their patients a service if they simply allow the patient to come in, get the quick fix, and leave.

It is important to introduce patients to all of the aspects of what is a very multidisciplinary field, that being anti-aging medicine, also referred to as clinical age management. It is also important to start with the basics: diet, exercise, nutrition, and skin care.

At my medical practice, we have one surgeon and two dermatologists. Our facility is equipped with a laser center with nine resurfacing, hair removal, sclerotherapy, spider vein, and pigmentation lasers, a skin care center, and a full-service spa. The practice is also affiliated with three salons. From the moment a patient walks in the door everybody in the office is stressing these other things that can be done to improve the patient's appearance and self-esteem. It is a mind-set, from everybody from the receptionist to the nursing staff that the patient needs to be introduced to all of the services offered, not just surgery. The big areas are skin care and weight management. Those are the toughest sell, and for that it is usually best to refer the patient to a nutritionist or an anti-aging specialist.

## COSMETIC SURGERY PROCEDURES

Many cosmetic surgical procedures that patients want, for example many of the noninvasive procedures, and procedures involving resurfacing lasers and other types of lasers, can be conducted by a qualified and aptly trained clinical age management physician.

### Fillers

The biggest boon in plastic surgery in the next decade is probably going to be fillers. If you look at the aging process and how plastic surgeons have approached, for instance, the aging face since the 1950s when the first facelift was actually done, the major problem was seen to be loose skin. However, we now know that that is simply not the case. The problem of the aging face is at least a dichotomy of loose skin and loss of volume. Someone needs a facelift, or their skin starts to look worse on their face, because they lose volume in one area of their face and tend to gain volume, that is, fat, in other areas of their face.

For the last 30 years, plastic surgeons have really been missing the point. They have stretched and stretched and stretched skin, not necessarily making people look better but certainly making them look different, as we all know. Recently, there has been a shift in the plastic surgeon's emphasis. They do not only want to improve skin, but they are trying to improve skin in a noninvasive way, and they are also trying to fill in the deficits that time causes us to lose. The tear trough deformity below the eye is a big one which is usually seen as the first sign of aging. A person can look good for their age at 40, but they're not going to look 20 because of certain subtle changes that occur in their skin and in the volume of their face.

At present, there are a least 20 fillers that are soon to come out on the market. The one that most people are familiar with now is collagen, which has the lion's share of fillers. Its advantage, and disadvantage, is that it is only temporary. If you don't like it, or your practitioner doesn't do a good job or gets over-zealous, it does go away. The patient will only have to put up with it for three months. That is also a disadvantage because the patient has to come back and have repeat procedures, and that can get expensive. There are several permanent fillers coming onto the market in the next year, these include: Restolin, Macrolin, and Holoform. Holoform is actually a temporary filler, but it lasts about four times as long as collagen does. Some of the other fillers available, such as those used overseas, are going to be more permanent and this will probably change the dynamics of what is done from a cosmetic surgical standpoint as far as facial rejuvenation. The good thing about injectable fillers is that the procedure can really done by anybody who's trained in it, whether they be a dermatologist, or an emergency room doctor, or whatever type of specialty is practicing clinical age management.

Fillers are easy to do. Collagen is very popular around the lip area, for instance. It can be done in the office, and with some of the newer topical creams available, these procedures are virtually painless in most people. Making a procedure as pain-free as possible is important because if a patient has a bad or painful experience they will tell their friends, and they will be more hesitant to come in and have more procedures. If you are going to do noninvasive cosmetic procedures, be they Botox®, collagen, or laser resurfacing, it is very important to use a good topical anesthetic agent so that the patient will leave in a relative state of comfort, sing your praises, and tell their friends that the procedure was no problem at all.

### Botox®

Botox® is, without doubt, the procedure of choice at present. Botox® is *Botulinum* toxin type A. It paralyzes the muscle by blocking the end-plate receptors to acetylcholine. Paralyzed muscles shrink, thus Botox® works by shrinking muscles. Of all the cosmetic procedures available, Botox® is by far the one that is the most free of complications. Despite the media hype around Botox®, it is not a new treatment. It has been used to treat blepharospasm since the 1960s, but it is also useful for the treatment of frown lines between the eyes, forehead creases, and crows' feet.

In the thousands and thousands of patients treated with Botox® at my medical practice, we have never seen an allergic reaction. We have also never seen a patient develop muscle weakness, although that is the most common complication. In trained, competent hands, Botox® is quick and easy, and it makes people feel better about themselves.

### *Skin Resurfacing Procedures*

All resurfacing procedures that are ablative, that is which cause damage to the epidermis, are basically the same, whether it is Baker's peel, phenol peel, trichloroacetic acid (TCA) peel, Jessner's peel, $CO_2$ laser resurfacing, or erbium Yag laser resurfacing. All of these procedures work by creating a full-thickness injury to the tissue, and such injuries take a certain length of time to heal. The length of healing is dependent on how deep the injury is. The redness that occurs after ablative skin resurfacing persists for months and months and months. It is not so much of a problem for women as it is easily covered with make-up, however it can be extremely problematic for men.

The good news is that a number of new nonablative laser and light source techniques are becoming available. The main advantage with nonablative resurfacing is that it does not have the burning effect that some of the older lasers do because the epidermis is protected. As the epidermis is protected there is no healing time and no down time. Thus, the patient gets all the benefits of ablative skin resurfacing but none of the side effects.

One of the most promising new technologies is a machine that sprays a cryogen on the surface of the skin to cool the epidermis, while at the same time radio frequency (RF) heat energy passes through the epidermis to the deep dermal layers. The result is that the epidermis is left uninjured, but the heat energy passes through to the deeper layers of the dermis. This does two things. It causes immediate shrinkage of collagen, which is present in the reticular dermis, and it causes a late effect of collagen synthesis by new fibrocyte and fibroblast dedifferentiation that occurs at about six to nine months. The body views this as a full-thickness injury, as an injury to the skin, and treats it as such, and causes us to, again, make collagen.

After about the age of 30 the body stops making collagen. Basically, we have what we have unless we sustain an injury. Nonablative resurfacing fools the body into thinking that it has sustained a deep tissue injury, and therefore triggers it into secreting collagen. Such new technologies are being hyped as the "non-surgical facelift." If someone started out at age 30 and had nonablative resurfacing once a year, it may well be that when they reach 60 they will have as tight a skin, or nearly as tight a skin, as they did when they're 30. However, it will take at least 30 years until we know whether this prophecy will become true.

### *Liposuction*

The typical liposuction patient is female who works out and had two children in her thirties. She tries to eat properly, but probably doesn't and just can't seem to do anything to shift that fat. So she joins one of the designer gyms in town and goes on the boot camp program, and is very dedicated. However, despite what the trainers say you can't exercise away everything. So when the woman notices that her belly, or her thighs, or whatever, are not disappearing, despite all the hard work she is putting in she gets very discouraged.

Even if you do your best, there are just some areas of fat you can't get rid of period. After having two children, you are never going to get rid of that pooch in your lower tummy if you're 38 years old. You don't have the hormones in you to do it. You don't have the anatomy to do it. And generally, that is the last area to go. When women taken up exercise to lose weight and tone up their breasts are usually the first thing to disappear, every spare ounce of fat will disappear from everywhere else, and the secondary fat on the lower stomach will be the very last thing to go. This is where plastic surgical procedures come in, because it is possible, through a relatively small procedure, to get rid of those areas, while at the same time giving the patient a renewed interest in the other healthy aspects of their life.

Obviously, it is best to first talk to a patient about their diet, and if they are not eating healthily, advise them to follow a lower-fat diet that will help them lose weight. Secondly, if the patient does not exercise regularly, getting them to do so is a step in the right direction. However, most liposuction patients have already tried exercise and eating healthily and neither has helped. For these patients, liposuction is probably the best option.

## CONCLUDING REMARKS

Plastic surgery is very *a la carte* now. Ten years ago you could call a plastic surgeon's office and ask the receptionist what the price of a facelift is, and they would tell you. That is impossible now. Today, there are at least 10 varieties of a facelift: from the very minimum liposuction, all the way up to the works, where the patient is given virtually everything available. The key is to individualize.

In the southern United States, most people are interested in their neck and their mid-face. So it is possible to get by with much less surgery. However, in New York people seem to want the works for some reason. Such trends may be a regional phenomenon, or it may just be a practice-oriented trend. But as doctors, we have to listen to our patients and not try to talk them into everything if what they want is only one thing. Because again, the indication for cosmetic surgery is if that person thinks they need it. It doesn't hurt us if a patient's neck looks like that, and it really is no one else's concern. But if the patient has that perception, then it becomes an issue, and only then. A lot of times we try to incorporate what other people think more than what we think.

It is difficult for plastic surgeons to back up and to try to offer a patient something that they don't offer or something that they do offer but that is not as lucrative, so to speak, as what can be done surgically. But it is our duty to do that. It is important to start out with the least invasive treatments, the treatments that a patient can do at home, the treatment that is going to do them the most good in the long term. Skin care, for instance; following up with an aesthetician three or four times a year; taking the right hormone supplements as needed; a dietary regimen that's going to keep the patient's skin looking good; avoiding the sun; drinking lots of water; and all those things that you just have to keep drumming into people. In the preoperative patient, it is our job to cheer the patient on and give them enough self-esteem to change their life-style and to go ahead and do what they need to do to look better. In the postoperative patient, the role of the practice is really to convince the patient that they actually do look better.

It is interesting to see how many people color their hair after they get a procedure done. They will come back in with new wardrobes. It is as if they have developed a renewed interest in themselves. And that is good. People talk about aging gracefully and vanity and all that sort of thing, and all these clichés that you hear. But this is the third millennium now. These things are available. However, no surgery should ever be de-emphasized or considered minor because it is medicine, it is surgery, and things can go wrong

Basically, what the majority of people want is to have a better quality of life for the time we're going to be here. And when we're 80 or 90 we want to feel like we're 40 or 50. That might sound like a pipe dream now, but in 30 or 40 years it might just be possible that we can do that. However, the only way we are going to achieve such a thing is through a combination of different treatments and therapies. There is never going to be one magic pill for this because aging, as we know, is such a multimodality thing. Even with the aging of the face: people start to look older between age 20 and 50 not because of one thing but they have bony atrophy, they have muscle hypertrophy, they have facial dehiscence. They have fat loss in some areas and fat gain in others. They have thinning of the dermis, thickening of the epidermis, sun damage, and melasma. There is no one thing that is going to solve all of those problems.

You have to use numerous therapies: water, good skin care, certain lasers for pigmentation irregularities, certain lasers for fat abnormalities. That is why we all have to work together.

Most of the people who want cosmetic surgery are not looking for a life change. Plastic surgery is not going to change their lives or make them a different person. It is just going to make them feel a little bit better about themselves or one aspect of themselves. If there is something that really bothers you about yourself, when you get rid of that problem you feel better, and you approach life differently: feeling happy increases the chance of living a longer, healthier life.

## ABOUT THE AUTHOR

Dr. Pratt completed his undergraduate degree at Vanderbilt University where he graduated Magna Cum Laude. He then attended Vanderbilt University School of Medicine where he received his Doctorate in Medicine in 1983. Dr. Pratt completed a Fellowship with the Institute of Reconstructive Plastic Surgery, and New York University Medical Center in Plastic and Reconstructive Surgery. He is a member of the American Society of Plastic and Reconstructive Surgeons and the American College of Surgeons. Dr Pratt is currently in private practice at Southern Plastic Surgery in Nashville, Tennessee.

# Chapter 6

# Extreme Sports and Anti-Aging Medicine

*Bradley C. Grant, M.D., M.P.H.*
*Associate Professor, Western University*

## ABSTRACT

Getting older does not mean that we have to start taking it easy. In fact, we should be doing the exact opposite. Research has shown that active seniors tend to live longer, more functional, more fulfilling lives than their inactive peers. If a person has always wanted to take up an adventurous, or extreme sport their age should not stop them from doing so.

**Keywords:** adventure; athletics; physical activity; exercise benefits

## INTRODUCTION

The disciplines of Anti-Aging Medicine and Extreme Sport rarely meet, however in this paper we will discuss how extreme sports relates to anti-aging. The relationship between these two disciplines is truly a question of motion. Motion is a life-giving force. There will be no discussion about nutritional supplementation or anything of that type. This discussion could also be entitled "The Ageless Athlete," or, "If You Don't Use It, You Lose It." Because the aim of this paper is to show that it is possible to keep enjoying sports, even extreme sports, well into old age.

When we talk of extreme sports we are talking about very high-edge activities, such as canyoneering, snowboarding, and rollerblading. Many companies are packaging a lot of these sports to clients as very high-thrill, but very low-risk activities. In other words, these companies are saying that you don't have to be as fit as an Olympic athlete in order to take part in these types of activities.

If possible it is best to try not to package people. It is important to be very honest about the kind of activities offered, and a lot of them are actually very high-skill, and also high-risk. However, it is possible to reduce this risk with preparation and with a lot of work conditioning programs prior to taking part. Again, age is not a necessary factor. Nor are medical conditions. The aim is to show people what there is out there, what they can do with what they have, and how to enjoy the outdoors.

The philosopher William James penned a wonderful phrase for anyone considering taking up an extreme sport. He said: "It's only via risking our person from hour to another that we live at all?" For people involved in extreme sports, that phrase has become a mantra. People involved in extreme sports love to challenge themselves. They love to push themselves, and their boundaries. It is a state of mind for a lot of people, but it is also a way of life for many people.

When we talk about extreme sports, we are talking about activities such as mountain climbing, ice climbing, white-water rafting, kayaking, and snowboarding, and in the case of extreme sporting, doing so on 600-foot high desert dunes. All of these activities are high thrill and high adrenaline activities.

## SENIORS AND EXERCISE
### Facts and Figures
In the US in the 1900's the average lifespan was 48 years for males and 50 years for females. A century later, in the year 2000 life expectancy rise to stand at 70 for males and 76 for females. Much of this gain can be attributed to advances in public health and dramatic improvements in medicine and technology.

However, the increase in life expectancy has led to the development of an ever-increasing population of citizens that are moving into the elderly realm. We know about the graying of America, the aging of the Baby Boomers generation. Right now, approximately 12% of the US population are aged 65 and over. However, it is estimated that by 2030 this population will have doubled, meaning that a staggering 70-million citizens will be over the age of 65.

Statistics suggest that roughly 30% of people between the ages of 45 to 65 engage in regular exercise. Two-thirds of people in this population have been playing their sports of choice for about 20 years, and half of those people practice three to eight hours a week. Furthermore, a third of that population practices eight hours a week. These people are not weekend athletes. These are people that are dedicated to their particular activity, or adventure.

### Medical Conditions
Approximately 88% of seniors (people aged 65 and over) see a doctor regularly. Two-thirds, or 66%, of seniors take at least one medication; and at least 80% have more than one chronic medical condition. Why is that important to us? It is important because we need to know whether medical conditions are a limiting factor for doing activities, sports, exercise, and extreme sports. The answer is that in this day and age, it is not.

There is certainly a compelling body of evidence to suggest that a lack of activity can, to a large extent, encourage aging. There is a direct relationship between activity and physical disability, and functional capability and ultimately musculoskeletal disability.

### Medication
It is clear that many older adults are affected by chronic medical conditions, and that the majority of these conditions require pharmacological treatment. For this reason it is important to be aware that some commonly used medications can trigger exercise-related complications. Briefly:
- Diuretics contribute to dehydration and electrolyte depletion.
- Beta-blockers cause a reduction in exercise capability and capacity.
- Calcium channel blockers can cause problems with post exercise orthostatic hypertension.
- Insulin and oral hyperglycemics carry with them an increased risk of hyperglycemia.
- Anticoagulants increase the risk of bleeding.
- Leukocorticoids increase the incidence of osteoporosis and the fragility of capillaries, thereby increasing the potential for injuries.

## THE EFFECTS OF AGING ON PHYSIOLOGICAL SYSTEMS
How does aging affect specific physiological systems? The primary systems that we need to consider are the cardiac system, the pulmonary system, the musculoskeletal system, the hematological system, and the neurological system.

Aging reduces the efficiency of the heart. As we get older maximum heart volume, stroke volume, $VO_2$ max, and cardiac output, are all reduced significantly. With the pulmonary system, the effects of aging lead to a reduction in vital capacity and residual volume, and an increase in respiratory frequency. We lose muscle mass and muscle strength. The joints also have a tendency to become stiff as tendons become weaker and ligaments lose their tensile strength. Age affects the hematological system by leading to decreases in plasma volume, red cell mass, and blood volume. Finally, the effects of age on the neurological system, which is all-important in assessing a person's functional capability, lead to a decrease in spinal motor neurons, coordination reaction times, balance, and proprioception.

There is one other area that needs emphasis, and that is psychological well-being. As people get older, they tend to feel that they are less in control of their lives. There is also a higher incidence of depression and dementia among seniors. Cognitive function diminishes, and the senses are impaired. Hearing, vision, balance, postural stability, and proprioception all deteriorate with age.

### *Can Exercise Training Limit Age-Related Physiological Changes?*

Can the physiological changes associated with aging be limited through sustained physical activity and exercise training? Yes they can. Research has shown that with a good exercise program that combines both aerobic and resistance exercise, elderly people can develop strength and improve their cardiovascular fitness and overall quality of life.

It is a difficult task to give relatively sedentary seniors the motivation to participate in regular exercise. When someone gets older everybody says, "You've got to start taking it easy because you're not as young as you used to be." We now know that this is simply not the case. Unfortunately, many seniors don't know this, so it is important to educate peoples about exercise. However, it is important to remember that no two people are the same, thus it is best to individually tailor an exercise program to meet each individuals goals and desires. It is also that the exercise program is varied, and that there is an emphasis on enjoyment and socializing.

### *The Relationship Between Aging and Athletic Performance*

Why do athletes who continue to compete into their older years tend to experience a decline in athletic performance? One reason is that it is difficult to maintain the same volume, frequency, and intensity of exercise as you age. Competitive motivation and instincts also change. There are more musculoskeletal injuries that the aging athlete has to face, and there is also the impact of other medical conditions, as previously stated. Things like degenerative joint disease, osteoarthritis, and osteoporosis.

### *The Impact of Regular Exercise Upon Health and Disease*

Can regular exercise actually play a role in disease prevention in older adults? The answer is that it can be very protective. There are a number of maladies that simple exercise can offer protection against, for example, coronary artery disease, hypertension, dyslipidemia, obesity, and cancer.

In addition to disease prevention, what other health benefits can be accrued from regular exercise? Research suggests that engaging in regular exercise can improve cognition, sleeping habits, and psychological well-being, enhance the self-image, and delay functional disability. All of these together with the opportunities for social interaction that group exercise offers reinforces the healthy lifestyle.

### *Aging and Musculoskeletal Problems*

What age-related factors can contribute to the development of orthopedic injuries in older adults? As we discussed, with aging we lose some neurological function, we lose cognition, our senses become impaired and we lose that postural stability. Ultimately, that postural instability causes increased susceptibility to falls and thus more injuries. Obviously a person can opt for low-impact sports, such as kayaking if they are overtly worried about sustaining an injury, or they could throw caution to the wind and choose high-impact activities such as cliff-diving. Alternatively, they could choose a happy medium and enjoy medium-impact activities such as hiking.

What about the relationship between exercise and osteoarthritis in older adults? Osteoarthritis is a multifactorial disease. Genetics, obesity, biomechanical dysfunction, malalignment, previous trauma, and repetitive trauma all play a role in the development of osteoarthritis. There seems to be a particularly high incidence of osteoarthritis in people who have suffered repetitive trauma to a joint, especially in those who have had prior surgery or some type of abnormal alignment. However, it has also been shown that aerobic and resistance exercise does, in fact, benefit those people. Research shows that they have less symptomatology, and that it improves their ability to move and their general outlook on life.

How does advanced age affect the evaluation and management of musculoskeletal injuries? With chronic injuries, people tend to delay visiting their doctor; this delay, coupled with the fact that older people heal at a slower rate, means that there is also delayed healing of the injury. However, elderly people typically have more time to spend on rehabilitation.

When evaluating a person it is important to consider the impact of nonsteroidal anti-inflammatory drugs (NSAIDs). NSAIDs are frequently prescribed for musculoskeletal injuries. As we know, gastrointestinal toxicity is always a problem regarding the dosage, the length of treatment, concurrent use of glucocorticoids and other such medications. In addition, it is important to consider what other concomitant medical conditions a person may have, for example renal insufficiency or congestive heart failure, and how these conditions may impact negatively on these people. Another factor that should never be overlooked is the side-effects of these particular medications. Even though side-effects such as nephrotoxicity and fluid retention, or blood pressure elevations may be rare they still need to be accounted for. But to their benefit, NSAIDs do allow individuals to go into extreme environments and be able to cope with the stresses involved in such environments.

What measures can be taken to reduce the risk of exercise-related musculoskeletal injury in older adults? One of the most important measures is to avoid abrupt changes in the exercise regimen. Cross-training is also very important. Probably the best thing to do is to get the person to try and do a variety of activities and alternate then from day to day. The importance of paying attention to surface conditions cannot be over-emphasized as people with postural instability and neurological impairments are tremendously affected by differing surface conditions. Although it may seem obvious, it is extremely important to employ proper use of equipment and facilities, and to make sure the individual has adequate strength and good neurophysiological capabilities.

## THE IMPACT OF THE ENVIRONMENT

What about the environment? Is the environment a factor that we have to consider in older adults? Clearly it is. Older individuals are more susceptible to extremes of temperatures. Seniors have a reduced total body volume, impaired thirst mechanism, and their kidneys output higher levels of water, thus meaning that they are susceptible to dehydration. Decreases in sweat gland function and attenuated increases in skin blood flow in response to a higher core temperature, also means that they are susceptible to conditions such as heat stroke and heat exhaustion. Conversely, attenuated vasoconstriction in response to a decreased core temperature increases the older person's susceptibility to problems like frostbite and chilblains. The ability to generate heat by shivering, or shivering thermogenesis, also diminishes as with age. Additionally, as we get older our ability to perceive ambient air temperature is impaired, thus meaning that older people tend to make fewer behavioral adaptations to the environment, for example taking clothes off when the temperature climbs and putting more clothes on when the temperature drops. All of these factors, together with the fact that many of the medications prescribed to seniors, for example beta blockers, antihistamines, and antidepressants, have a significant effect upon sweat gland production, mean that seniors are especially susceptible to their environment.

## EVALUATING THE OLDER EXTREME SPORTS ENTHUSIAST

Should older adults undergo formal medical evaluation before participating in athletic activity? The decision whether or not to evaluate someone before they take part in extreme sports, or any other kind of athletic activity, should depend on a number of things: the person's age, past and current medical conditions, and the intensity of the exercise program. However, it is probably wise to always perform a pre-participation examination. The most important aspect of the pre-participation examination is to try and identify any underlying maladies that could negatively impact their experience. The pre-participation examination also provides the opportunity to counsel the individual and to reestablish and identify what their exercise goals are.

What should be included in the pre-participation examination of an older adult? As has already been mentioned, the examination should cover past and current medical conditions. Cardiovascular fitness and body composition should also be determined. It is also important to find out if the individual is taking any medication and to make an overall assessment of current functional capacity. It is very important to assess functional capacity. Always assess flexibility, strength, and postural stability, are those are very important factors when people are going on trips of this nature.

Should diagnostic testing be considered in pre-participation evaluations of older adults? The decision to do diagnostic testing is dependent upon the individual's history and the results of their physical exam. However, just for the sake of review, it may be prudent to check serum electrolytes, in order to see if the person is using diuretic drugs. Other tests that may be of use include lipid profiles and urinalysis. It is useful to determine body composition, as this provides a way of establishing goals and assessing an individual's response to training. Bone density testing can also be conducted to assess the risk of fracture.

Should older adults undergo formal exercise stress testing before participation in exercise? This is controversial. A lot of people feel that stress testing is not necessarily that helpful in being a good predictor of coronary artery disease in the majority of asymptomatic individuals. However, stress testing is definitely advisable in people with a prior history; a family history of heart disease; people with two or more risk factors; and in people with signs and symptoms related to coronary artery disease. Stress testing is also necessary if the individual wants to take part in very high-adrenaline activities, for example bungee jumping.

## **GETTING IN SHAPE FOR EXTREME SPORTS**
### *Resistance Training*

Is there a role in resistance training for older adults? Sarcopenia is the medical term for a reduction of muscle mass. Between 50 and 70 years of age, there is a functional decline in strength of approximately 15% per decade. After age 70, this increases to 30%. Can it be delayed? Yes, indeed, it can. It is possible to retard the decline in muscle mass by resistance training. In fact, simply by exercising two times a week, many individuals can slow the decline. Another easy way of getting older people to do some resistance training is to get them to carry weights while walking. It is isokinetic, but nevertheless it's certainly good resistance.

### *Nutrition*

Do older adults have special nutritional considerations? One thing to remember is that older people have a lower caloric intake, as they have a smaller lean body mass. As a result, the most important thing is the quality of nutrition. Another thing to consider is the efficiency of the gastrointestinal tract. Older people have reduced gastric emptying and secrete lower levels of gastric enzymes. Another thing to consider is medication. As we know, certain medications can have a significant impact upon the absorption, digestion, and utilization of nutrients. It is also important to consider whether any medical condition an individual has may necessitate the need for dietary restrictions.

## CONCLUDING REMARKS

In conclusion, determination, faith, fitness, courage, and teamwork are some of the most important characteristics of successful aging. Heed the old dictum that an ounce of prevention is worth a pound of cure insofar as you need diet, exercise, you want to detect any medical conditions, and any type of pharmacological intervention. So you want to have a balanced program that includes nutrition, exercise, flexibility, postural stability, strength, cardiovascular training, because the individuals that take part in extreme sports seem to have less hospitalization. We find that there is less medical care involved. They obviously have better fitness: cardiovascular, strength, and body composition. And overall, they tend to have decreased physical disability, increased functional capacity, improved quality of life, and overall higher life expectancy. Why? Because they enjoy what they do. These people lend credence to the expression that "you're as old as you feel." These people are involved in the world. They participate. They channel their needs and their desires. And as a result they're able to cope with stresses. And, as we know, stress is deadly when it comes to life expectancy. So why not engage in adventurous sports? Why not just get out and exercise? As Mark Twain said, "Twenty years from now you will be more disappointed in the things that you did not do rather the things that you have done."

## ABOUT THE AUTHOR

Dr. Grant received his doctorate in 1979 from the College of Osteopathic Medicine and Surgery in Des Moines, Iowa. Dr. Grant is an avid outdoorsman and extreme sports enthusiast. He participates in mountaineering, backcountry skiing, alpine skiing, rafting, kayaking, extreme golf, competitive cycling, competitive soccer, gymnastics, diving, tennis, football, and baseball. He has also competed in triathlons and marathons. As such, Dr. Grant is uniquely qualified to speak on extreme sports.

Dr. Grant is an Associate Professor at Western University College of Osteopathic Medicine in Pamona, California, and CEO and Medical Director of Lake Elsinore Family Medical Clinic.

# Chapter 7
# Testosterone, The Male Hormone Connection: Treating Diabetes and Heart Disease

*Michael Klentze, M.D., Ph.D.*
*Medical Director, Klentze Institute of Anti-Aging, Munich, Germany;*
*Member, A4M Advisory Board - Europe*

## ABSTRACT

The purpose of this paper is to examine the links between testosterone, obesity, type II diabetes, and cardiovascular disease. The anti-aging physician approaches and treats obesity, type II diabetes, and cardiovascular disease in a very different way than that of a conventional physician. Here we will focus on testosterone replacement therapy, and will discuss the reasons for recommending a patient for replacement therapy, its benefits and its side effects.

**Keywords:** testosterone replacement therapy; androgen; cardiovascular disease; obesity; insulin

## INTRODUCTION

Is there a link between testosterone, obesity, diabetes, hypercholesterolemia, and cardiovascular disease? Why do men die? What are the leading causes of death in men? What is the relationship between men and women?

Cardiovascular disease (CVD) is the prime cause of death among the elderly in industrialized countries, and a major determinant of chronic disability. Cardiovascular disease, cancer, stroke, accidents, medication, Lyme disease, and murder are the leading causes of death in men.

If a patient gives you $10,000 to estimate his risk of dying from a myocardial infarction (MI) in the next five years, what would you measure? Most doctors would take the patient's blood pressure; others may order an ECG as well. There is a world of difference between how a cardiologist and an anti-aging doctor would respond to such a question. A cardiologist would conduct an invasive exam with a heart catheter, arteriography etc. Anti-aging doctors would turn to the laboratory instead. So what can we do? Insulin is a strong predictor of MI within the next five years. Another is C-Reactive Protein (CRP), a marker of inflammation. CRP is produced in response to interleukin-6 (IL-6). Other predictors of myocardial infarction include DHEA-sulfate, homocysteine, plasminogen activator inhibitor type 1 (PAI1), IGF-1, and lipoprotein-a (Lp(a)).

The lifetime risk of CVD is much larger in men compared to women, suggesting that testosterone or the lack of estrogens play an important role. On the other hand, testosterone levels decrease with age, coincident with the age-related increase in atherosclerotic disease. Results obtained from cross-sectional studies suggest that men with CVD might have lower testosterone levels. While intervention studies with testosterone in older men with CVD suggest an improvement of ECG. In addition, testosterone exerts significant effects on several risk factors for CVD. Studies on intima-media thickness (IMT) of the carotid artery suggest an improvement by administering testosterone. There is a gap in lifespan and in onset of severity of CVD with a male disadvantage. The higher rate of CVD has been attributed to the decrease of testosterone in aging men. Of significant note is that CVD and unfavourable biochemical CVD risk profiles in men (low HDL-cholesterol, high LDL-cholesterol, high triglycerides, high fibrinogen, and high PAI-1 levels) are associated with low rather than normal levels of testosterone.

The number of people in Germany who die from sudden death by MI or non-stable plaque per year is 100,000. In the US this figure is 1.3 million. A German study of approximately one million people showed that obesity is increasing with age. This is a major public health problem, as we know that body mass index (BMI) is one of the major risk factors for heart disease. The average hip-waist ratio is also on the increase. We know that the mean increase of fat mass in men between the age of 25 and 70 is 15 kg; the mean loss of lean body mass over the same period is approximately 8 kg. The reason for this rise in BMI, hip-waist ratio, and obesity is simple: it is attributable to lifestyle.

## PLASMINOGEN ACTIVATOR INHIBITOR TYPE 1 (PAI-1)

The physiological role of PAI-1 is the inhibition of fibrinolysis. Therefore, the increase of PAI-1 levels caused by PAI-1 polymorphism is linked to increased blood clotting and decreased fibrinolysis. PAI-1 polymorphism correlates with high risk of CHD, stroke, embolic disease, and myocardial infarction. Women who are affected by this polymorphism should be treated with estradiol replacement, as it reduces PAI-1 levels. It is important to control aromatase activity by monitoring estradiol levels and SHBG (sex hormone binding globulin) during testosterone administration. The risk of acute MI increases with plasma levels of thrombogenetic factors (fibrinogen, PAI-1, factor VII). Those plasma levels are inversely correlated with endogenous testosterone in men.

### *Insulin is a potent stimulator of PAI-1*

In the arterial wall smooth muscle cells (SMCs) form the extracellular matrix, and play an important role in determining arterial tone. Proliferation and migration of SMCs are important steps in the formation of neointima and stenoses. Apoptosis of SMCs contribute to plaque instability and rupture. Macrophages play a key role in atherosclerosis as they can internalise large amounts of exogenous lipids by phagocytosis. They also form foam cells, cytokines, and growth factors (EGF platelet derived factor, IL-1, TNF-alpha), and stimulate the migration and proliferation of SMCs.

### *Obesity*

Obesity reached epidemic proportions at the beginning of the new Millennium. The prevalence of obesity increases with age and reaches a maximum between the ages of 50 and 59 years. There is a tendency for the mean BMI to decrease in the oldest age group.

Aging is associated with visceral fat accumulation in both genders, with the highest prevalence being in the oldest age group (> 60 years). Energy intake, as well as fat intake, either drops or remains unchanged with age, and thus age-related weight gain is associated with a decrease in energy expenditure due to an increasingly sedentary lifestyle.

Recent figures suggest that Greece has the highest obesity rates in the world. The same figures placed Germany and the US in joint fourth place. However, when Americans are obese, they tend to be severely obese. The reason for that is the carbohydrate problem in the United States. You can say that it is an "American paradox": after removing cholesterol and fat from the diet something was needed to give people the feeling of fullness. As a result the American diet became packed-full of carbohydrate: bread, noodles, rice, potatoes, and so on. This is the reason why the weight and obesity problem in the US is still on the increase, despite the popularity of low-fat or no-fat diets. Of men in the US, 23% have the metabolic syndrome, in which insulin resistance plays a key role. Epidemiological studies indicate that insulin levels and testosterone are inversely correlated.

A study by Hwang examining the correlation between leptin, sex hormones, and fat distribution in middle-aged and aged men, showed that free testosterone, DHEA-S and SHBG levels were significantly different in middle-aged men and their older peers. However, leptin, testosterone, and estradiol levels were similar. The study also revealed that sex hormone levels change steeply during middle-age, but much more steadily in older-age. Testosterone and leptin levels were found to be strongly linked with BMI and waist-hip ratio.

Lipoprotein-a (Lp(a)) levels are affected by levels of thyroxin, human growth hormone (hGH), estrogens, and progestins. Levels of 30 mg/dL and above are considered an independent risk factor for coronary, cerebral vascular, and peripheral atherosclerotic vessel disease. But what about cholesterol? Cholesterol is not a predictive factor of MI. Unfortunately, cholesterol has been relegated to a convenient marketing tool for a lot of industries to sell product. Recent studies suggest that the cardiovascular risk factors we should be concerned about are Lp(a), insulin, homocysteine, fibrinogen, and PAI-1.

## *Fat Cells*

The fat cell, as we know, does not only store fat, it is a very active metabolic cell. Fat cells secrete a number of substances that have a direct effect upon insulin. They also manufacture estradiol, estriol, and estrone by aromatization of testosterone, thus obese people lose their testosterone to their fat cells. Fat cells also secrete angiotensin, which is known to increase blood pressure. Furthermore, there are three hormones that increase the number of fat cells and increase fat storage in these cells, thus making a bad situation worse. These are cortisol, insulin, and estradiol. Estradiol plays a role in pregnancy, and men and women who get high levels of estradiol get fatter and fatter. Estradiol is a fat hormone.

## *Leptin*

Leptin, which stimulates the hypothalamus, is secreted by adipocytes. Leptin by itself is a product of the OB gene, the obesity gene, and is an adipose cytokine. It is secreted by white fat cells, and its primary role is in adaptation to negative energy balance. In normal circumstances, leptin stimulates the hypothalamic satiety center and creates a feeling of fullness. However, obesity increases leptin levels and can cause leptin resistance. If a person has leptin resistance, the concentration of leptin is sufficient to stimulate the hypothalamic satiety center, however, due to the body's resistance to leptin, only some of the leptin stimulates the hypothalamus. This triggers hunger, and thus the person feels the need to eat more.

Leptin also plays a role in the regulation of insulin levels and insulin sensitivity. When we have higher body fat, we also have higher leptin levels and higher insulin levels. This is the correlation between leptin, BMI, and fat. Metformin is used to decrease insulin levels in people with type II diabetes. However, what is interesting is that metformin does not increase leptin levels. Metformin is the only drug that lowers insulin levels without raising leptin levels.

## *Adiponectin*

Another hormone of interest is adiponectin. Adiponectin is interesting because it has a direct correlation with insulin. Adiponectin is an adipose-derived peptide and it acts as a systemic regulator of glucose and lipid metabolism. There is a strong relationship between adiponectin, BMI, and body composition. We also know that adiponectin is a mediator of insulin sensitivity, and an enhancer of fatty acid oxidization. Thus, suggesting that it encourages fat burning and weight loss. If adiponectin levels are low, insulin is not able to phosphorylate the insulin receptor, which normally happens at the tyrosine residuals of the insulin receptors. This phosphorylation stimulates the starting of the insulin effect. This is why we need adiponectin. Low levels of adiponectin have been linked with an increased risk of cardiovascular disease.

### *Athlersclerosis*

Atherosclerosis is a chronic inflammatory disease. In the early stages of all age-related diseases we find the same pathogenesis: inflammation. Inflammation provides us with a link between Alzheimer's disease, heart disease, and cancer. It takes a long time to build up plaques. A fundamental part of the pathology of atherosclerosis or coronary sclerosis is damage to the endothelial wall of the artery. This causes macrophage-stimulating cytokines to migrate to the damaged endothelium and trigger inflammation. Then we start to see the development of plaques. Atherosclerotic plaques begin to develop when oxidized cholesterol molecules accumulate inside the wall of an artery. However, the problem is not caused by cholesterol itself. The problem is the inflammation and the oxidation.

One of the central mediators for inflammation is cyclooxygenase-2 (COX-2). COX-2 expression is exacerbated by omega-6 fatty acids but inhibited by omega-3 fatty acids. Cytokines, such as interleukin-6 (IL-6), and proliferation factors (SMP) that are produced by macrophages all increase the supersensitive CRP. High CRP levels (2.0 or higher) are a predictor for atherosclerosis. Both COX-2 expression and cytokines are inhibited by testosterone.

Coronary atherosclerosis in most men is a chronic disease. Most men have plaques that are very stable. But plaques that are unstable can erupt tomorrow. This is why you cannot predict sudden death, for example, by bike ergometry. So we have to diagnose very early. What is very interesting is that the whole scientific community is now beginning to turn to preventive medicine after years of focusing on curative medicine.

Atherosclerosis is a multifactorial disease. According to the International Task Force for the Prevention of Cardiovascular Diseases, its pathogenesis is favored by non-modifiable risk factors, such as age, sex, and positive family history, as well as:

- Obesity
- Smoking
- Diabetes mellitus
- Hip-Waist Ratio
- BMI increase
- Arterial hypertension
- High blood levels of LDL-C cholesterol
- Low levels of HDL-cholesterol
- High Lipoprotein-a levels
- High insulin levels

### *Insulin and Type II Diabetes*

Insulin levels are on the rise in obese people. Insulin levels can be elevated even when glucose levels are normal. It is possible for a person to have a glucose level of 90 or 100, which is normal for people of around 50-years of age, and an insulin level of 16 or 20.

Insulin levels, serum glucose and lean body mass are very closely correlated. When insulin is increasing, what happens then? This is called insulin resistance. Insulin affects HDL, and fibrinolysis. It also increases the proliferation of smooth muscle cells, which can lead to the development of atherosclerotic plaques and hypertension.

## Type II Diabetes

In the year 2000, the US spent roughly US$2 billion on the treatment of diabetes. There are 20-million people in the US with diagnosed diabetes, and 90% of these people have Type II, not Type I, diabetes. However, there are also a significant number of people with undiagnosed Type II diabetes. Diabetes affects more African-Americans and Hispanics than Caucasians. This is probably due to the fact that African-Americans and Hispanics are more susceptible to obesity.

Type II diabetes mellitus is diagnosed when a person has a fasting glucose of 126 mg/mL or more; and an oral glucose tolerance test result of under 190 mg/mL after one hour, and under 140 mg/mL after two hours. The optimum insulin level is 8 mg/mL or below. People with insulin resistance may present with a fasting glucose of 100mg/mL or more. However, they may also have normal glucose levels. The majority of people affected by insulin resistance are over 30-years old, but the condition is on the increase among younger people, especially in Western countries. They are often overweight by 20% or more of their bodyweight. Typically these people present with high glucose levels, but this is not always the case.

More and more, overweight children are presenting with insulin resistance and this is a real public health problem. These youngsters have increased LDL levels, decreased HDL levels, increased triglyceride levels, raised blood pressure, increased fibrinogen levels, increased CRP levels, increased PAI-1 levels, and increased levels of inflammatory markers. They also have endothelial dysfunction. Basically, they are suffering from metabolic syndrome, which includes obesity, hypertension, hyperglycemia, hyperinsulinemia, and dyslipidemia.

## The Role of Anti-Aging Medicine

Anti-aging medicine should start in a child's first year, or possibly even during pregnancy. Studies have shown that children with a low birth weight have a higher risk of insulin resistance. In adults, obesity leads to insulin resistance. However, in adults the beta cells are usually healthy, thus a person with insulin resistance may have normal glucose levels but high insulin levels. But in children the beta cells are not healthy enough to compensate for this insulin resistance so they have high glucose levels and they develop Type II diabetes.

So what can we do? The first thing is to change the lifestyle. Before we start with hormone treatment or any other medical intervention, the patient should be encouraged to start eating healthily and exercising regularly: exercise is far more effective at treating insulin resistance than any medicine. Patients should be advised to switch to a low glycemic diet, which provides carbohydrates that do not rapidly increase glucose levels. This means no potatoes, no rice, no pasta, and no bread. So what can be eaten on a low glycemic diet? Natural rice, full corn, etc. Men should be encouraged to combine aerobic exercise with strength training. Because if you build up muscle, glucose will be burned better when insulin levels drop. Other things to consider are testosterone and metformin.

Human growth hormone (hGH) could be of great benefit but it is very expensive and it is always better to start first with lifestyle changes and testosterone. These steps will increase IGF-1 levels in most cases. HGH is stimulated by a hormone called ghrelin.

## Ghrelin

Ghrelin is mainly produced in the stomach, and is the only hormone secreted into the blood that stimulates appetite in order to increase the energy balance of the body. Moreover, ghrelin displays several functions, the exact role of these functions is currently uncertain but they are thought to regulate ghrelin receptors in the periphery. The testicles as well as the ovaries belong to the functional area of ghrelin, and the Leydig cells of the testicles produce ghrelin by themselves. Thus suggesting that ghrelin is the link between reproductive function and metabolism in the human species. A study by Pagotto *et al* examining the correlation between ghrelin and testosterone in hypogonadal men revealed that plasma levels of ghrelin are significantly reduced in hypogonadal men compared to eugonadal men. The results also showed that administering testosterone to these men causes ghrelin levels to rise to normal levels. Because hypogonadal men have decreased ghrelin levels they should be very slender because of the reduced appetite. However, decreased ghrelin levels actually do the opposite. Obese men also have low ghrelin levels. None of the studies conducted in this area have been able to link low ghrelin levels in obese men to insulin resistance. However, it is very interesting that ghrelin resistance in hypogonadal men and obese men can be responsible for the low levels of the hormone.

Testosterone may activate the androgen receptor, present on the X chromosome, to increase the gene expression of ghrelin. When considering prescribing a patient with testosterone, it is important to consider andropause. Andropause is the decrease in bioavailable or "free" testosterone that occurs with age: this normally occurs at 2% per year starting at around the age of 25. Therefore a 50-year-old man will have lost about 50% of his testosterone, which is a lot. Measuring free testosterone is quite complicated as it changes from lab to lab, and there are only a few good assays available. Therefore, it is easier to measure total testosterone and sex hormone-binding globulin (SHBG), and then determine the free androgen index.

## *TESTOSTERONE*

The aging process is characterized by a decline of most physiological functions. Among these, the decline in endocrine functions plays an important role in the symptomatology of the aging process. In contrast to women, who experience a rather abrupt termination of the ovarian cyclic hormonal activity, in men both endocrine (testosterone) and exocrine (spermatogenesis) testicular functions are preserved until very old age. Hence, the male equivalent of the menopause: the andropause, does not really exist. Nevertheless, both endocrine and exocrine function decline with age. Whereas it has long been debated whether plasma testosterone concentration decreases with age in healthy men, the occurrence of an age-associated decrease in bioactive testosterone concentration is no longer disputed.

Normal plasma testosterone levels range between 11 and 40 nMol/L, and reach their maximum at 25 to 30 years. Approximately 50% of testosterone circulating in plasma is bound to sex hormone binding globulin (SHBG), a ß-globulin with high affinity but limited binding capacity for testosterone, and the remaining 50% is bound to albumin, which has a low-affinity for testosterone but a high binding capacity. In young healthy males, the concentration of free testosterone in plasma varies between 0.2 and 0.7 nMol/L. Because of the high binding affinity of SHBG, only the free testosterone and part of the albumin bound testosterone is bioavailable. The significance of SHBG bound testosterone is poorly understood. It has been shown, that some tissues (prostatic cells) carry SHBG receptors, the activation of which leads to the stimulation of cyclic AMP. The formula for determining bioavailable testosterone is as follows. The bioavailable index is the total testosterone divided by SHBG multiplied by 100%.

Male sexual function declines with age. It is now clear that the age-associated decrease in testosterone levels has both a testicular and hypothalamo-pituitary origin, but Leydig cell function decrease does not always occur together with an increase of the pituitary hormone luteinizing hormone (LH). However, LH levels in elderly men frequently remain stable or only increase modestly, because of the alteration of neuroendocrine control of gonadal function. Moreover the circadian rhythmicity of LH and testosterone secretion is blunted in elderly men and the amplitude of LH pulses decrease.

Where are the testosterone receptors? If you ask most doctors they would say testosterone is in the testis, in the penis, perhaps in the brain. Nobody would think that the walls of the coronary vessels have the most testosterone receptors. The coronary vessels can convert testosterone to estradiol, and estradiol is the most potent stimulator of nitric oxide (NO). Therefore the walls of the coronary vessels have the most testosterone receptors, next is the brain, then bone, then muscle, and then fat. So why don't doctors prescribe testosterone men with problems in the knees or hips? There is no reason why they shouldn't. Measure it and use it.

Then there is the penis. Testosterone has the same effect on the penis as it does on the walls of the coronary vessels: it stimulates NO production. Thus, it works in virtually the same way as Viagra. Arginine is one of the most potent stimulators of nitric oxide production. If you give a patient arginine it is converted to citraline and then nitric oxide is produced.

## *Testosterone Deficiency*

Testosterone deficiency in men is manifested typically by symptoms of hypogonadism, including decreases in erectile function and libido. One quarter of men over 65 have subnormal testosterone levels. Testosterone also has an important role in the regulation of normal growth, bone metabolism, and body composition. Specifically, testosterone deficiency is an important risk factor for osteoporosis and fractures in men. In men older than 65 years of age, the incidence of hip fracture is 4 to 5 in 1000, and approximately 30% of all hip fractures occur in men. Men with testosterone deficiency have significant decreases in bone density, particularly in the trabecular bone compartment. Testosterone deficiency has been reported in over half of elderly men with a history of hip fracture. Men with testosterone deficiency also have alterations in body composition, which includes an increase in body fat. Quantitative CT scans that assess fat distribution have shown that testosterone deficiency is associated with an alteration in site-specific adipose deposition with increased deposits in all areas particularly in the subcutaneous and muscle areas. Because truncal fat correlates with glucose intolerance and cardiovascular risk, hypogonadism may have important implications with regard to overall health and mortality. Therefore, testosterone deficiency is associated with an enhanced risk for osteoporosis, altered body composition including increases in truncal fat, and, possibly, decreases in muscle performance.

## *Benefits of Testosterone Replacement Therapy*

Administration of adequate testosterone replacement therapy leads to improvements in libido and erectile function. Following testosterone replacement, men note an increase in energy and mood, which may reflect either direct behavioral effects of androgens, and/or, an elevation of hematocrit due to rising testosterone levels.

Testosterone therapy in hypogonadal men is indicated if bioavailable testosterone is below 30% or total testosterone is below 12 nmol/L, and clinical signs of androgen deficiency are evident. The aim of testosterone therapy is to substitute the androgen within normal adult male ranges and keep levels as physiological as possible. Natural testosterone preparations are used, applied either intramuscularly, transdermally, or subcutaneously. The most important thing to remember when prescribing testosterone is to always maintain physiological levels. When we have supraphysiological levels we get problems, such as decreasing HDL levels. However, this only happens with supraphysiological levels. Supraphysiological levels tend to arise if testosterone is administered by intramuscular injection. Thus, the best way to deliver testosterone is via testosterone gels, which have proven effective in studies and clinical practice. Daily application of testosterone gels leads to physiologic testosterone serum levels without serious side effects.

There are some very, very important reasons for hypogonadism and these should be thoroughly investigated before prescribing testosterone therapy. It is very important to determine that there is no disease in the pituitary, or hypothalamus. Symptoms of low testosterone levels include:
- Depressive mood
- Lack of self confidence
- Lack of cognition and memory

- Decrease of vitality and energy
- Hot flashes
- Tendency to cry
- Nausea
- Fast pulse rate
- Sleep disturbances
- Night sweating (rare)
- Lack of libido

Prior to beginning testosterone replacement therapy, contraindications must be excluded, such as existing prostate cancer, or male breast cancer. Therapy must be evaluated regularly at intervals every 3 months in the beginning, and at least 12-month intervals thereafter. Control investigations include clinical signs of androgen deficiency and patient satisfaction, clinical examinations (skin, bone, breast, prostate), and lab parameters such as testosterone, SHBG, dihydrotestosterone, estradiol, PSA, hemoglobin, and hematocrit.

Testosterone therapy also leads to important beneficial effects on the skeleton and lean tissue mass. Testosterone replacement increases bone density in hypogonadal men, with the most dramatic effects seen in the trabecular bone compartment. These effects may be seen as early as 6 months following initiation of testosterone therapy. In one recent study of the long-term benefits of testosterone therapy, the greatest benefits in trabecular bone were seen in the first several years of therapy.

With regard to body composition, testosterone replacement therapy results in a dramatic reduction in adipose content, with the greatest effects seen in the subcutaneous and skeletal muscle areas. Testosterone enhances lipolysis in adipocytes by increasing the expression of beta-adrenergic receptors, adenylate cyclase, proteinkinase A and hormonsensitive lipase (HSL). Androgen therapy also leads to a significant increase in lean skeletal muscle mass and strength. Therefore, there are beneficial effects of testosterone replacement on body composition and bone mineral density in adult hypogonadal men that may serve as indications for therapy in addition to libido and sexual function.

Because testosterone levels decline with age, and aging is accompanied by body changes including loss of muscle and increases in fat, there is a great interest in the potential benefits of testosterone administration in elderly men. In a recent randomized, placebo-controlled trial Snyder *et al* administered testosterone via a scrotal patch to 108 elderly men for 3 years. Results showed that testosterone administration had beneficial effects on both lean body and fat mass. Testosterone increases levels of fast-twitch (type 2) muscle fibers, levels of which decrease with age. Thus, if you add testosterone to your intervention, levels of type 2 muscle fibers will increase and glucose burning will improve. Therefore, there may be a role for androgens in improving body composition and function in elderly men.

Testosterone is an important modulator of insulin sensitivity in men. The relative Hypogonadism in men with insulin resistance is due to impaired Leydig cell secretion of testosterone. Testosterone increases Insulin sensitivity. The apparent protective effects of plasma free testosterone against an atherogenic profile in the physiological male concentration range of free testosterone is probably related to increases in insulin sensitivity by caused by testosterone. Additionally, testosterone administered even in combination with an aromatase inhibitor suppresses Lp(a) levels, and physiological testosterone levels have favourable effects on cardiovascular risk factors (increasing HDL cholesterol and decreasing LDL cholesterol). However, testosterone may have a direct adverse effect on the vessels by interfering with nitric oxide (NO) expression and lowering Lp(a) and HDL-cholesterol levels. Although, results of the PROCAM Study by Assmann *et al*, in which 40.000 men and women were followed for ten years, suggested that HDL cholesterol alone is not easily correlated with cardiovascular risk.

HDL-cholesterol levels appear to be more clearly associated with insulin resistance and hypercholesterolemia than coronary risk, whereas Lp(a) is an important risk factor for myocardial infarction, venous thromboembolism, and stroke. More than 25% of all men and women have high Lp(a) levels: that is, an Lp(a) level of 30 mg/dl and above. Lp(a) levels are largely determined by genetics, however levels are also clearly moderated by hormonal status. Testosterone has also been shown to increase coronary blood flow in elderly men with heart disease. Men with low testosterone levels who had heart disease achieved better ECG scores after being treated with testosterone.

In summary, the benefits of testosterone replacement include:
- Improved muscle mass and muscle strength
- Decreased fat mass
- Improved spatial capacities, cognition, and memory
- Improved bone mineral density
- Improved "well-being"
- Improved sexual function and libido
- Improved energy and mood
- Decreased total-cholesterol and LDL-cholesterol levels
- Improved insulin sensitivity and glucose levels

## *Side Effects of Testosterone Replacement*
### *Gynecomastia*

Gynecomastia describes the enlargement of the male breast, to the extent that it mimics female appearance. Gynecomastia is a cosmetic problem and increases the risk of male breast cancer. Some men undergo surgery to correct the problem, however such procedures often produce insufficient results.

In contrast to young men, the breast of the elderly is composed of diffuse smooth fat and dominated by connective tissue. Although some swellings are more indurate than others or present a more dense aspect in ultrasound, no reliable discrimination between true gynecomastia, which is caused by proliferation of glandular tissue, and lipomastia, which is caused by a proliferation of adipose tissue, is possible. Gynecomastia and lipomastia are also very difficult to distinguish between histologically, as there is only a gradual difference in the relation of fat to glandular tissue. Gynecomastia is suggested if a skin fold below the mamilla or the alveolar mamilla exceeds 3 cm. Another aid to diagnosis is the fact that less than 30% of men with a BMI below 32 display gynecomastia, however this rises to 90% in men with a BMI in excess of 32. It is important to exclude mammary gland cancer in patients presenting with gynecomastia.

Khan *et al* treated 36 men with gynaecomasty with tamoxifen. Results showed that the drug caused a reduction of the gland in 83% of participants and decreased tenderness in 84%. Tamoxifen is a specific estrogen receptor modulator (SERM), which blocks the mammary epithelium from the effects of estrogens in order to increase the androgenic effects. Tamoxifen acts on estrogen receptor alpha as an antagonist, and estrogen receptor beta as agonist. The distribution of both receptor types is organ specific. In breast tissue tamoxifen acts against the alpha receptors that dominate breast tissue, and in bone the drug stimulates the dominating beta-receptors, therefore affecting bone density.

### *Prostate*

The prostate increases in size by 1.6% per year. There is no difference in testosterone levels between men with and without benign prostate hyperplasia (BPH), and men with prostate cancer do not have abnormal hormone levels of testosterone, dihydrotestosterone, free testosterone, SHBG, estradiol, or cortisol, However, there is evidence that estradiol stimulates prostate growth. Thus, the detection of the estradiol alpha receptor and the CYP 19 (aromatase) polymorphism in men could be useful for estimating the risk of a patient developing BPH if they were prescribed testosterone or DHEA, as these are both precursor of estradiol.

Testosterone exerts its effects on gene expression via the androgen receptor (AR). Modulations of the transcriptional activity influenced by the androgen receptor can be assigned to a polyglutamine stretch of variable length within the AR. This stretch is encoded by a variable number of CAG triplets in exon 1 of the AR gene. Longer triplets residues mitigate binding of AR co-activators and, thus, facilitate decreased androgenicity. In eugonadal men with CAG repeat residues of normal length an influence of the polymorphism on androgen target tissues such as the prostate, spermatogenesis, bone, hair, metabolic parameters, and psychological factors has yet been demonstrated. The AR itself seems to be the problem, as it increases its sensitivity to androgens with age due to its loss of methyl groups bound to the CAG triplet repeats, thus shortening the repeats and causing mutations. Polymorphisms with short AR repeats are known. In the case of shortened CAG repeats, peptide growth factors like IGF-1 and EGF are expressed in high amounts. In such cases treatment with finasteride, which blocks 5 alpha-reductase results in a reduction of prostate size as well as a decrease in prostate specific antigen (PSA) levels. Thus it may be of benefit to test patients to see if they have any of the following polymorphisms: CAG repeat, CYP 17 (17-hydroxylase, which leads to high tissue amounts of androgens) and 5 alpha-reductase (which leads to high dihydrotestosterone levels in the prostate). It is also important to regularly check PSA levels and urological controls (TUS). Extending these findings to pharamcogenetic considerations during testosterone administration has to be considered. This aspect could gain clinical significance especially in older men, as they are more likely to develop unwanted side effects. Thus when treating men with testosterone it is important to take into account the AR polymorphism when deciding the dose.

Epidemiological studies show no constant relationship between testosterone levels and prostate cancer. Recently a study by Lunglmayr *et al* showed that low serum testosterone levels were found in patients with high-grade prostate cancers long before cancer was diagnosed, thus suggesting that low serum levels could be considered as an additional marker for prostate cancer.

Can we administer testosterone to men who have undergone treatment for prostate cancer? Older studies showed that administering testosterone to patients with active prostate cancer leads to disastrous results. However today, with widespread PSA screening and aggressive treatment, if prostate cancer is caught early enough it is often curable, as shown by no-detectable PSA. Recent case reports show that men who have been cured of prostate cancer and who are truly hypogonadal men, can be treated carefully with gel without activation of their cancer. Recently, testosterone replacement in hypogonadal men deemed at high risk of prostate cancer (by virtue of having a high-grade PIN (prostatic intraepithelial neoplasia) on prostate biopsy) was shown not to result in an increased risk of prostate cancer or PSA elevation.

*Increased Hemoglobin and Hematocrit*

Testosterone replacement can lead to increased hemoglobin levels and hematocrit (Hct). If Hct rises by more than 50%, testosterone administration should be interrupted and the dosage should be lowered.

## *Testosterone and Type II Diabetes*

How do modern antidiabetic drugs, like rosiglitazone (Avandia) work? Avandia stimulates the PPR gamma receptor, thus improving insulin sensitivity. Thus it does the same as exercise and testosterone. Pioglitazone and metformin have virtually the same effects. Men in contrast to women display a correlation between low testosterone levels and insulin resistance and type II diabetes, while the same inverse relation is known for SHBG and insulin resistance. Low testosterone levels are correlated with type II diabetes and carbohydrate metabolism disorders, and low levels of free testosterone are correlated with obesity, which is the origin of insulin resistance and type II diabetes. It is important to remember that free testosterone is not a real predictor for type II diabetes. When calculating a patient's risk of developing type II diabetes total testosterone and the FTI (free testosterone index) should be considered. There is no difference between the concentrations of free testosterone, DHEA, estradiol, and SHBG in non-diabetic and diabetic men.

To summarize, testosterone administration in men with type II diabetes has shown the following benefits:
- Lowered insulin levels
- Lowered glucose levels
- Lowered HbgA1c levels and decreased glycated endproducts
- Saved insulin in the late stages of the disease

Testosterone is useful in the treatment of Type II diabetes, because it increases the expression of the glucose transporter gene (GLUT4), and increases the sensitivity of peroxisomal PPAR-alpha and gamma receptors. Approximately 85% of the population have PPAR-alpha receptor mutations, and these people develop insulin resistance very, very quickly. The PPAR-alpha and gamma receptors show decline of genetic expression during aging. These receptors are members of the nuclear receptor transcription factors super-family, and play an important role in the metabolism of fat (alpha) and inflammation (gamma). The alpha receptor has anti-inflammatory effects (via suppression of Nfkappa B, and stress-kinases, and inhibition of IL-6, IL-12, and TGF-alpha). Thus, the age-related decline of PPAR alpha results in increased inflammatory processes as well as a decrease of energy levels in mitochondria. The activation of PPAR gamma stimulates the activation of macrophages, which express surface factor CD 36 (LDL scavenger), and foam cells are formed. Furthermore, PPAR gamma inhibits inflammatory cytokines, and stimulates the cholesterol transport protein APCA 1, which eliminates cholesterol.

Because testosterone increases the sensitivity of the peroxisomal PPAR gamma receptor and has similar effects as rosiglitazone, androgen deficiency and estrogen excess shifts the carbohydrate metabolism to insulin resistance and increases SHBG levels. The loss of testosterone in middle and older-age, which in turn increases the risk of obesity and insulin resistance and increases SHBG levels, also increases the risk of type II diabetes.

What happens to the concentration of free testosterone and estradiol as we age? Estradiol levels normally increase, while testosterone levels decrease. Diabetic men typically have lower testosterone levels than non-diabetic men. Hyperandrogenemia is associated with high BMI, high waist-hip ratio, high blood pressure, higher glucose and insulin levels, and higher levels of LDL-cholesterol and triglycerides. One of the reasons why obese men tend to have low levels of bioavailable testosterone, and higher levels of estradiol or estrogens is because they are aromatising a lot of testosterone in the fatty cells. Another is that estradiol increases SHBG levels. SHBG levels increase with age and free testosterone levels decrease with age.

Estradiol is an important hormone and sometimes it is necessary to give men estradiol. If a man is very small, and if he has nearly no fat mass, his estradiol level is typically below 12, which is not measurable. Such low levels of estradiol can lead to osteoporosis. Studies in men with a lack of aromatase enzyme found that men with no estradiol, but normal testosterone levels suffered from osteoporosis. Estradiol is responsible for the inhibition of bone mass loss.

The breakdown mechanism of estradiol has a significant impact upon testosterone. If we are looking at estradiol levels, and we have a patient with high estradiol levels and normal SHBG levels, the problem is likely to be down to breakdown enzymes. If there is a slow breakdown of estradiol it tends to, accumulate in tissues. Estradiol is broken down into water-soluble compounds that can be excreted in the urine. Normally, you would prescribe testosterone to increase estradiol levels, however this will not work in men with not enough aromatase. So in some cases it may well be necessary to prescribe estradiol.

## CONCLUSION

The potential benefits of androgen therapy for older men, include maintenance or improvement in bone density, improved body composition (that is, ratio of fat to lean muscle mass), improved strength, improved libido and sexual function, improved mood, and improvement or maintenance of cognitive function.

Current data on cardiovascular risk suggest that it is better for men to have a high rather than a low testosterone level. In general, higher serum testosterone levels correlate with lower metabolic cardiovascular risk factors, including higher high-density lipoprotein (HDL) cholesterol levels, lower blood pressure, and lower levels of plasma fibrinogen, fasting insulin, and lipoprotein. Nonetheless, concerns about this issue tend to raise basic questions about why men have more cardiovascular disease than premenopausal women: Are estrogens protective, are androgens causative, or both? Recent well-controlled data are insufficient to provide a definitive answer. Generally, parenteral testosterone therapy in older men results in a decline in serum levels of total cholesterol and low-density lipoprotein (LDL) cholesterol, and no change in HDL cholesterol, although a few new studies show a decline in HDL cholesterol with treatment.

Thus, most of the available evidence suggests that testosterone replacement is potentially beneficial to aging men, particularly in the areas of bone density and body composition. However, the magnitude and longevity of the beneficial effects of testosterone replacement are currently uncertain.

## REFERENCES

Abate N, Haffner SM, Garg A, Peshock RM, Grundy SM. Sex steroid hormones, upper body obesity, and insulin resistance. *J Clin Endocrinol Metab*. 2002;87:4522-4527.

Andres R, Blackman MR, Harman SM, Metter EJ, Muller DC. Aging, androgens, and the metabolic syndrome (MS). Paper presented at: The 4th World Congress on the Aging Male; February 28, 2004; Prague, Czech Republic.

Blouin K, Richard C, Belanger C, Dupont P, Daris M, Laberge P, Luu-The V, Tchernof A. Local androgen inactivation in abdominal visceral adipose tissue. J Clin Endocrinol Metab. 2003;88:5944-5950.

Gooren LJG. Testosterone therapy in aging males and effects on lipid metabolism. Paper presented at: The 4th World Congress on the Aging Male; February 27, 2004; Prague, Czech Republic.

Katznelson L, Finkelstein JS, Schoenfeld DA, Rosenthal DI, Anderson EJ, Klibanski A. Increase in bone density and lean body mass during testosterone administration in men with acquired hypogonadism. *J Clin Endocrinol Metab*. 1996;81:4358-4365.

Kauffman LM. Testosterone therapy and its influence on growth and malignancy of the prostate gland. Paper presented at: The 4th World Congress on the Aging Male; February 28, 2004; Prague, Czech Republic.

Khan HN, Rampaul R, Blamey RW. Management of physiological gynaecomastia with tamoxifen. *Breast* 2004;13:61-65.

Morales A. Oral administration: a preferred route of testosterone intake. Paper presented at: The 4th World Congress on the Aging Male; February 27, 2004; Prague, Czech Republic.

Nieschlag E, Zitzmann M. Pharmacogenetics of testosterone action. Paper presented at: The 4th World Congress on the Aging Male; February 26, 2004; Prague, Czech Republic.

Oh JY, Barrett-Connor E, Wedick NM, Wingard DL; Rancho Bernardo Study. Endogenous sex hormones and the development of type 2 diabetes in older men and women: the Rancho Bernardo study. *Diabetes Care* 2002;25:55-60.

Rolf C, Knie U, Lemmnitz G, Nieschlag E. Interpersonal testosterone transfer after topical application of a newly developed testosterone gel preparation. Clin Endocrinol (Oxf). 2002;56:637-641.

Simon D, Charles MA, Nahoul K, Orssaud G, Kremski J, Hully V, Joubert E, Papoz L, Eschwege E. Association between plasma total testosterone and cardiovascular risk factors in healthy adult men: The Telecom Study. *J Clin Endocrinol Metab*. 1997;82:682-685.

Swerdloff RS, Wang C. Androgen deficiency and aging in men. *West J Med*. 1993;159:579-585. Review.

Snyder PJ, Peachey H, Hannoush P, Berlin JA, Loh L, Lenrow DA, Holmes JH, Dlewati A, Santanna J, Rosen CJ, et al. Effect of testosterone treatment on body composition and muscle strength in men over 65 years of age. *J Clin Endocrinol Metab*. 1999;84:2647-2653.

van den Beld AW, Muller M, Bots ML, van der Schouw YT, Grobbee DE, Lamberts SWJ. Testosterone and cardiovascular disease, epidemiological aspects. Paper presented at: The 4th World Congress on the Aging Male; February 27, 2004; Prague, Czech Republic.

Wang C, Swedloff RS, Iranmanesh A, Dobs A, Snyder PJ, Cunningham G, Matsumoto AM, Weber T, Berman N. Transdermal testosterone gel improves sexual function, mood, muscle strength, and body composition parameters in hypogonadal men. Testosterone Gel Study Group. *J Clin Endocrinol Metab*. 2000;85:2839-2853.

## ABOUT THE AUTHOR

Dr. Klentze received his medical degree from the University of Munich Medical School and is board certified in psychiatry and gynecology. He is Medical Director of the Klentze Institute of Anti-Aging Medicine in Munich, Germany and is an advisory member of the American Board of Anti-Aging Medicine for Europe. In addition, Dr Klentze holds memberships in the Endocrine Society (USA), European Committee of Anti-Aging Medicine, German Society of Gynecology and Obstetrics, and the European Menopause Society. He is the author of several scientific articles on aging-related topics, including: androgens in women, neurosteroids and the aging brain, and vitamins and antioxidants.

# Chapter 8

# Current Status of Estrogen Therapy

*Seung-Yup Ku, M.D., Ph.D.; and Seok Hyun Kim, M.D., Ph.D.*
*Dept of OB/GYN, College of Medicine, Seoul National University*

## ABSTRACT

Replacement of deficient hormones is an important axis of anti-aging medicine since aging is caused and manifested by various hormonal declines. Somatopause has been treated with growth hormone; andropause with testosterone; thyropause with thyroid hormones; and menopause with estrogen or other natural substances (including isoflavone and black cohosh), whereas facial flush, genital atrophy and other menopausal symptoms have been controlled with estrogen therapy (ET). Many studies have reported that ET helps to prevent cardiovascular disease, osteoporosis, and Alzheimer's disease. Recently, however, the increased risk of breast cancer and insignificant preventive effect of ET on cardiovascular disease was revealed by the Women's Health Initiative (WHI) study. Thus, it is appropriate to review the risks and benefits associated with ET when managing postmenopausal women. The efficacy of ET and natural estrogen surrogates in relieving postmenopausal symptoms will also be discussed. We will also consider the possible antioxidant properties of ET.

***Keywords:*** menopause; Postmenopausal Estrogen Progestin Intervention (PEPI) Trial; The Women's Health Initiative (WHI) Study; Heart and Estrogen Replacement Study (HERS); North American Menopause Society (NAMS)

## INTRODUCTION

The subject of estrogen therapy (ET) has become very controversial since the findings of the Women's Health Initiative (WHI) study. This paper will cover some of the basics of ET and relevant societies' guidelines and recommendations for its use.

The average human lifespan has increased dramatically over the last century, and recent projections expect this trend to continue for the foreseeable future. According to a recent report, the index of aging in Korea as of 2001 was 35%. Korean studies have revealed that the average lifespan of Korean women is approximately 78 years; this figure is projected to rise to 87 by 2010. The average woman usually outlives the average man by 7 to 8 years, and this is a significant social issue that has to be addressed.

## MENOPAUSE

Despite significant increases in female life expectancy, the age of menopause has remained relatively constant. Therefore, the menopausal period has been growing since the 1950's. As can be seen in Figure 1, the women of today endure the symptoms and long-term complications of the menopause for 20 years or more of their life.

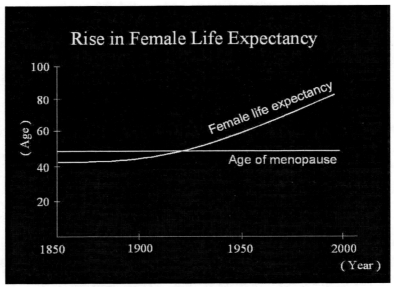

*Figure 1. The rise in female life expectancy over the last 150 years, in comparison with the relative stability of the age of menopause.*

Menopause means the stop of menstruation. It is accompanied by the decline of ovarian function, and typically occurs at around 50 years of age. Perimenopause usually begins in a woman's mid-40s and is indicated by irregular shortened menses. Because the transition from reproductive age to menopause, or climacteric, begins several years before menopause itself, anti-aging physicians and health practitioners should be concerned with the problems these women have much earlier than at the beginning of menopause.

The changes that occur at menopause include a decrease in reserve of follicles. Declining estradiol and inhibin levels lead to a rise in FSH levels, and the follicular phase becomes shorter. This means that follicles do not mature adequately. Together, this combination of events leads to luteal phase insufficiency, anovulation, oligomenorrhea (very light or infrequent menses), and eventually the cessation of menstruation.

The role of the anti-aging physician is to prevent or delay menopausal symptoms by keeping the risk of menopausal complications under the threshold level.

## *Symptoms of Menopause*

As a woman enters into menopause, the cyclic FSH fluctuation disappears, and the increasing FSH levels accelerate follicle maturation. This acceleration shortens the menstrual period: this is the first sign of perimenopausal transition. The level of FSH is approximately 40 mIU/ml at menopause and can rise to as high as 100 mIU/ml within a year of menopause.

The symptoms of menopause include vasomotor symptoms such as hot flashes or night sweats: these symptoms tend to be more severe in women who smoke and those with a higher body mass; some women may also experience psychogenic manifestations such as depression. Other symptoms include genitourinary tract atrophy, skin and skeletal changes, and sexual symptoms.

Hot flashes are the most common menopausal symptom. They are experienced by 50% to 75% of women. The average duration is about 4 minutes, and the interval between episodes can vary from every few minutes to several days. Hot flashes, or night sweats, can cause sleep disturbance and this is thought to be at least partially responsible for psychogenic manifestations of menopause, such as depression, decreased concentration, and mood swings.

The genital atrophy that occurs with menopause results from the thinning of vaginal epithelium. In addition, vaginal rugae disappear, vaginal secretion decreases, and the vagina becomes short and narrow. Vaginal sensation also decreases because of peripheral neuropathy. Women may also suffer with dyspareunia, leukorrhea, and occasionally vaginal spotting. Sexual problems may be caused by decreased lubrication.

Menopause causes atrophy of the urethral mucosa and a drop in urethral closure pressure. Together this can lead to a friable urethra. As such, postmenopausal women may experience urinary incontinence, burning sensation on urination, urgent and/or frequent need to urinate, and residual urine.

Lipid metabolism also changes with menopause. Postmenopausal women have higher LDL and lower HDL cholesterol levels, which increases their risk of cardiovascular disease. As can be seen in Figure 2, cardiovascular disease is the leading cause of death in Korea, and in many other countries including the USA. The increase in LDL cholesterol and drop in HDL cholesterol levels is caused by the decrease in estrogen levels that occurs at menopause. Every woman is exposed to the risk of cardiovascular disease in the postmenopausal period; however, these changes can be reversed by estrogen replacement. Without replacement, these metabolic changes may lead to the pathogenesis of atherosclerosis or coronary heart disease.

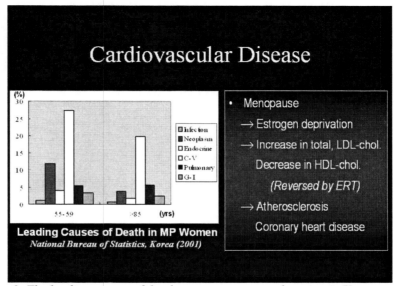

Figure 2. The leading causes of death among menopausal women in Korea, and how changes in lipid metabolism that occur at menopause lead to an increased risk of cardiovascular disease.

Bone metabolism is also affected by menopause. As a woman ages, her estrogen levels decrease and bone loss accelerates. Decreasing estrogen level leads to a decrease in calcium intake and absorption, thus serum ionized calcium levels drop. The resulting low levels of calcium stimulate the secretion of parathyroid hormone, and calcium is then mobilized from bone by excessive osteoclastic activity. The end result of this cascade of events is osteoporosis.

Postmenopausal women lose up to 5% of trabecular and 1% of cortical bone mass per year. The largest bone loss occurs in the first 8-10 years of menopause. Approximately 30% of postmenopausal women fall in the fast bone loser category; they lose more than 3% of bone mass per year. If a woman has an inadequate peak bone mass, her bone mineral content becomes less and less as time goes on, thus leaving her vulnerable to fractures.

## ESTROGEN THERAPY

The use of ovarian extract was first suggested by Charles Edouard Brown-Sequard in 1889. Eight years later, the first report on the effectiveness of ovarian extract for hot flushes was published.

Estrogen was first isolated in 1929, progestin in 1934, and estradiol in 1936. Three years later, conjugated estrogen was isolated. Premarin was first used and approved in Canada in 1941, and in the USA one year later.

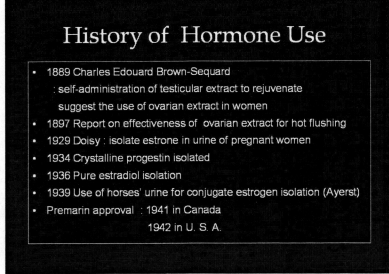

*Figure 3. History of Hormone Replacement Therapy*

Recent figures indicate that 46% of naturally postmenopausal women, and 71% of bilaterally oophorectomized women use ET in the USA. In Korea in 2002, these figures were 23% and 30%, respectively.

## *Estrogens and Progestins*

There are two categories of estrogens, natural and synthetic. Some of the natural estrogens available include, conjugated equine estrogen (e.g. Premarin®), estradiol valerate, piperazine estrone sulfate (e.g. Ogen®), micronized estradiol, and 17ß-estradiol hemihydrate. Synthetic estrogens are not used for ET because of their side effects. The most common route of administration of estrogens is orally. However, there are also a number of methods of transvaginal and transdermal administration.

Progestins are prescribed for the purpose of endometrial protection. Both synthetic (for example, medroxyprogesterone acetate (MPA)) and norethisterone acetate, and natural progestins (for example, micronized progesterone) are used in combination with estrogen. Progestins can cause breast tenderness, bloating, agitation, depression, and PMS-like symptoms. These side effects are dependent upon the dose of progestin prescribed. Progestins do not interfere with estrogen's antioxidant activity or its ability to lower LDL cholesterol levels, and increase fibrinolysis. However, they are not without disadvantages, as they lower estrogen's ability to increase HDL cholesterol levels, dilate arteries, and increase cardiac inotrophic activity.

There are largely two combined estrogen and progestin therapies, sequential and continuous. Withdrawal bleeding will occur with sequential estrogen and progestin therapy, but not with continuous therapy. Combined estrogen and progestin therapy is not suitable for women without a uterus; therefore hysterectomized women should be given estrogen only.

## *Therapeutic Effects of Estrogen*

Estrogen has a number of therapeutic effects, including:
- Relief of hot flashes and secondary psychiatric symptoms
- Improvement in genital atrophy
- Improvement of lipoprotein profiles

- Prevention of osteoporosis

Most women see an improvement in vasomotor symptoms such as hot flashes in a matter of weeks. However, it takes several months of treatment before bone mineral density begins to improve. Estrogen has also been thought to reduce the risk of cardiovascular disease and Alzheimer's disease; however, these benefits are controversial at present.

## *Estrogens and the Lipoprotein Profile*

Estrogens exert a number of beneficial effects upon the lipoprotein profile. As well as raising HDL cholesterol levels and lowering LDL cholesterol levels, estrogens may have an anti-arteriosclerotic effect on arteries. They also increase fibrinolysis, enhance the action of vasodilators and antiplatelet aggregation factors, such as nitric oxide or prostacyclin, and have direct inotropic actions on the heart and large blood vessels. They also have antioxidant properties.

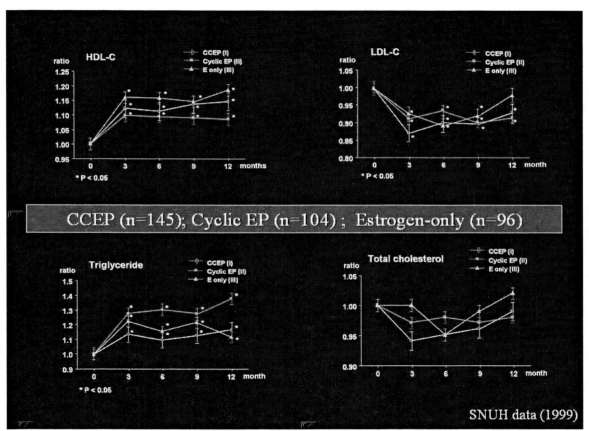

*Figure 4. Effect of 7-12 months of ERT on the lipid profile of postmenopausal women. Data obtained from a study by Lee et al, Seoul National University, South Korea, 1999.*

Figure 4 shows the results of a study conducted at Seoul National University, Korea, in 1999. For the study, the lipid profiles of postmenopausal women were measured before and after 7 to 12 months of estrogen replacement therapy. Three regimens were used: continuous combined estrogen/progestin in 145 women; sequential or cyclic estrogen/progestin in 104 women; and estrogen only therapy in 96 women. Results showed that ET led to a 10% to 20% increase in HDL cholesterol levels, and a decrease in LDL cholesterol levels and total cholesterol levels. However, treatment did slightly increase triglyceride levels.

### Estrogen and Alzheimer's Disease

Research suggests that estrogen has a beneficial effect on the activities of daily living in women with Alzheimer's disease. In a recent Korean randomized controlled trial, Tacrine was given to 26 women, and conjugated equine estrogen (CEE) estrogen to 29 women. The treatment was continued for six months, and the changes before and after treatment were evaluated using a number of tests, including the mini-mental status examination (MMSE), the Hopkins's Verbal Learning Test, instrumental activities of daily living (IADL), and the Boston Naming Test. Interestingly enough, the results were the same for both groups, except that IADL rated more highly in the CEE group. The overall efficacy of estrogen was similar to Tacrine in terms of cognition and mood.

### Contraindications and Complications of Estrogen Therapy

Estrogen replacement should not be started in women with a past history of myocardial infarction or cerebral vascular disease. ET is also contraindicated in women with depressed liver function and acute thromboembolism.

Unfortunately, there are a number of unwanted side effects associated with ET. These include: breast cancer, endometrial hyperplasia, endometrial carcinoma, dysfunctional uterine bleeding, gastrointestinal dysfunction, and thromboembolism.

Recent studies suggest that a significant number of women are quitting ET. A study by *Reynolds et al* revealed that 20% of women quit ET at the end of their first month; 50% at the end of their first year; and 65% at the end of two years. Furthermore, just 20% of women took ET for more than five years. The most common reasons for stopping ET were the unwanted side effects of estrogen and fear of cancer. Interestingly, women who were prescribed ET by a gynecologist were more likely to continue with the treatment. The authors suggested that gynecologists are more likely to prescribe regimens that cause minimal side effects, or they are more able to explain the risks and benefits of estrogen, thus these women are more likely to know what to expect from ET.


## IMPORTANT CLINICAL TRIALS CONCERNED WITH ET

There have been many trials carried out on the efficacy and safety of ET. Here we will discuss the most important of those trials.

### Postmenopausal Estrogen Progestin Intervention (PEPI) Trial

PEPI was one of the first representative studies of ET, and was published in 1995. It was conducted as a randomized, double-blind, placebo-controlled trial, and it lasted for three years. A total of 875 postmenopausal women from seven clinical centers were included in the trial. The regimens included sequential estrogen/progestin using medroxyprogesterone acetate (MPA) or micronized progesterone, continuous combined estrogen/progestin (CCEP) using MPA, estrogen only, and placebo.

Results showed that with regards to increasing HDL cholesterol levels, unopposed estrogen and sequential estrogen/progestin using micronized progesterone were superior to sequential estrogen/progestin using MPA. The decrease in LDL cholesterol levels was similar in all treatment groups. Decreases in fibrinogen levels and a favorable effect on fasting insulin and glucose levels were greater in all treatment groups compared to the placebo group.

### The Women's Health Initiative (WHI) Study and the Heart and Estrogen Replacement Study (HERS)

The Women's Health Initiative (WHI) is a randomized, blind, placebo-controlled multicenter study sponsored by the National Institutes on Health (NIH). It began in 1993. Study subjects were healthy postmenopausal women aged 50 to 79 years. CCEP was prescribed to 16,608 women and unopposed estrogen to 10,739 women. The follow-up period was five years. The CCEP arm of the trial was stopped in July 2002 when it was found that the treatment increased the risk of breast cancer to such an extent that it overweighed the benefits of treatment. The estrogen-only arm of the WHI has been just stopped and is pending its results; however, the results about breast cancer do not seem to be affected by ET.

HERS is another important randomized, blind, placebo-controlled trial. The study involved 2,763 postmenopausal women aged 55 to 79 with documented coronary heart disease. The women were treated with CCEP or an inactive placebo. The total follow-up period was 6.8 years.

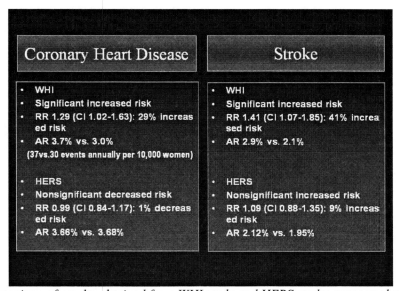

*Figure 5. Comparison of results obtained from WHI study and HERS study; coronary heart disease and stroke.*

Figure 5 shows that the two studies yielded conflicting results when determining the risk of coronary heart disease. The WHI reported that ET led to a 29% increase in relative risk, while HERS found that ET led to a nonsignificant decreased risk. As for stroke, the WHI showed a 41% increase in relative risk while HERS concluded that ET led to a nonsignificant increased risk of stroke. Both studies found that ET increases the risk of thromboembolism by more than 100%. Breast cancer risk was increased by 26% in the WHI study and 27% in HERS, though they were nonsignificant.

As shown in Figure 6, on the positive side, both studies found that estrogen is beneficial when it comes to colon cancer. The relative risk decreased by around 37% in the ERT group of WHI. However, the decrease in this risk was deemed nonsignificant in HERS. As for the risk of osteoporotic fracture, the WHI study showed a 24% decrease in risk, while HERS concluded that ERT led to a nonsignificant increased risk.

Many relevant academic bodies and researchers have questioned the appropriateness of the design of the WHI study. It is an important topic and clearly has to be investigated further.

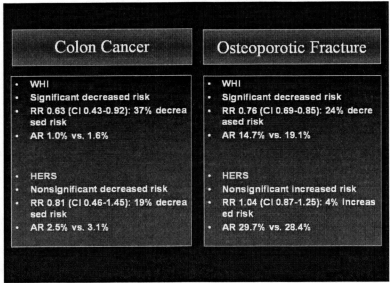

*Figure 6. Comparison of results obtained from WHI study and HERS study: colon cancer and osteoporotic fracture.*

## Recommendations and Regulations Governing ET

The United States Preventive Services Task Force's (USPSTF) recommendations towards a certain service are presented in Figure 7. With regards to ET, the USPSTF recommends against the routine use of estrogen and progestin for the prevention of chronic conditions in postmenopausal women. That is the recommendation "D". Regarding unopposed estrogen, ET was designated as the "I" recommendation.

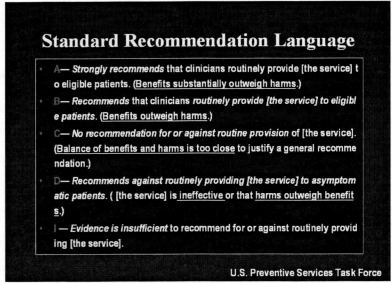

*Figure 7. The United States Preventive Services Task Force (USPSTF) Recommendations*

What about the US Food and Drug Administration (FDA)? Following results obtained in the WHI study, in February 2003 the FDA formulated new guidelines regarding safety warnings for all estrogen and estrogen with progestin products. Specifically, the new warning highlights the increased risks for heart disease, heart attacks, strokes, and breast cancer. It also emphasizes that these products are not approved for heart disease prevention. The FDA also modified the approved indications for Premarin®, Prempro® and Premphase® to clarify that these drugs should be used only when the benefits clearly outweigh the risks.

The three postmenopausal indications for conjugate estrogens are:
1. Treatment of moderate to severe vasomotor symptoms of menopause, such as hot flashes: this indication has not changed.
2. Treatment of moderate to severe symptoms of vulvovaginal atrophy, such as vaginal dryness and irritation: when these products are being prescribed solely for the treatment of vulvovaginal atrophy, topical estrogen should be considered.
3. Prevention of postmenopausal osteoporosis: when estrogens are being prescribed only for the prevention of osteoporosis, non-estrogen treatment should be considered.

The revised contraindications of conjugate estrogens include: undiagnosed vaginal bleeding, known history of breast cancer or estrogen-dependent neoplasm, active deep venous thrombosis, pulmonary embolism, or recent arterial thromboembolic disease such as stroke or myocardial infarction. Cases of known hypersensitivity to the ingredients and known or suspected pregnancy are also contraindications for estrogen use.

The North American Menopause Society's recommendations for ET are shown in Figures 8 and 9.

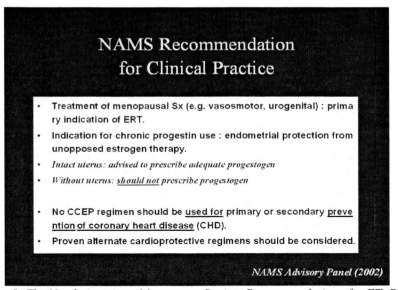

*Figure 8. The North American Menopause Society Recommendations for ET, Part I.*

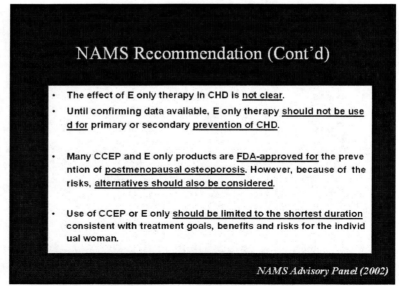

*Figure 9. The North American Menopause Society Recommendations for ET, Part II.*

## Lowering the Dose of Estrogen

Estrogen causes several unwanted side effects. We need to know that ET will still be effective if we lower the dose enough to reduce the side-effects. The Women's Health Osteoporosis Progestin and Estrogen (HOPE) study was a randomized, double-blind, placebo-controlled trial of CEE and MPA. Eight hundred and twenty-two women participated in this study for two years. Participants were given either 0.625, 0.45, 0.3 mg per day of CEE plus either 2.5 or 1.5 mg per day of MPA. After two years of treatment bone density increased, and levels of serum osteocalcin (OC) and urinary crosslinked N-telopeptides of type I collagen (NTx), which are both biochemical markers of bone turnover, decreased in all treatment groups. Doses of less than 0.625 mg per day also effectively increased the BMD. As for the changes in lipid profiles, researchers reported that a lower dose of estrogen induced favorable changes in lipids, lipoproteins and hemostatic factors without affecting carbohydrate metabolism. Vasomotor symptoms and vaginal atrophy can also be treated effectively with a lower dose of estrogen.

## ESTROGEN AND ANTI-AGING

The four major mechanisms for aging are methylation, glycation, inflammation, and oxidative stress. Estrogen may have several anti-aging effects. Here we will consider its homocysteine lowering properties, antioxidant action, and the relationship between ET and oxidative stress.

Increased levels of homocysteine is linked to an increased risk of cardiovascular disease. Methyl donors such as vitamin B-6, vitamin B-12, and folic acid are often used to decrease homocysteine levels. As has been noted, estrogen also has the ability to lower homocysteine levels. Results of one study revealed that 15 months of treatment with 1~2 mg of 17-beta estradiol led to a significant decrease in homocysteine levels. Thus, while homocysteine levels increase after menopause, these levels can be lowered by estrogen treatment.

Estrogen also appears to improve the metabolism of carbohydrates. Results of a study of postmenopausal women with type II diabetes revealed that short-term ET improved insulin resistance. The results also showed that ET led to a significant decrease in glycated hemoglobin and increased suppression of hepatic glucose production by insulin.

With regards to inflammation, we have indirect evidence about the action of estrogen. A randomized, controlled trial by *Hall et al* found that ERT improved the symptoms of rheumatoid arthritis.

50 µg per day of transdermal estradiol was given to 77 patients with rheumatoid arthritis for six months. Results showed that patients treated with the hormone showed significant improvement after six months in articular index and pain score, and a decrease in ESR and morning stiffness.

## *Estrogens and Oxidative Stress*

Estrogen is a cholanthrene ring composed of three 6-carbon rings (A, B, C) and one 5-carbon ring (D). Estrogen is a weak acid and can function as a proton donor or receptor. There is a body of evidence to suggest that estrogen has antioxidant properties. Some research suggests that estrogens may regulate oxidative process in some cells. However, there is also evidence suggesting that one of estrogen's metabolites, catecholestrogen, may be involved in free radical generation.

Endogenous sources of oxidative stress include inflammation, cytokines, and homocysteine. Exogenous sources include ultraviolet light, radiation, and environmental toxins. Exogenous defense against oxidative stress comes from dietary antioxidants, and endogenous defense mechanisms utilize enzymes and coenzymes inside human bodies.

If the body's defense mechanisms are working correctly, it should be able to cope with oxidative stress and homeostasis can be maintained. However, if for some reason homeostasis is not maintained, oxidative damage will result and physiological functions will become impaired, therefore increasing the risk and progression of age-related diseases.

*In vitro* studies conducted on estrogen and oxidative stress, have produced interesting results. A study by *Huh et al* found that the level of malondialdehyde (MDA), which is a marker of oxidative stress, is higher in the liver of the male rat than in the female rat liver. Thus suggesting that the female rat is subjected to lower levels of oxidative stress. This may be due to the female hormonal influence. Meanwhile, a study by *Miura et al* found that estradiol has the ability to inhibit lipid peroxidation. Back in 1993, *Mooradian et al* found that 17 beta-estradiol, 17 alpha-estradiol, and estriol reduced reactive oxygen specious accumulation in an *in vitro* study by 65%; however, estrone did not show any significant antioxidant properties. The authors concluded: "estrogens, especially estriol and 17 beta-estradiol, are naturally occurring antioxidants." In 1998 *Ayers et al* suggested that estradiol's apparent capability to protect against lipid peroxidation could be due to its ability to inhibit the generation of superoxide radicals and prevent further chain propagation.

Relevant *in vivo* studies include one by *Walsh et al* that examined the effect of estradiol on LDL flux in the carotid arteries of ovariectomized rats. The researchers concluded that their findings "support an antioxidant role for estradiol in the protection against LDL accumulation in the artery wall and subsequent progression of atherosclerosis." What about in humans? Myeloperoxidase (MPO) is an enzyme that consumes hydrogen peroxides and decreases ROS (reactive oxygen species) accumulation. It also plays a role in the termination of the whole process of free radical production in granulocytes by the inactivation of the NADPH-oxidase system. This enzyme is present inside granulocytes. *Bekesi et al* evaluated the activity and amount of MPO released at baseline and after some period of ET. Results showed that both increased significantly after treatment. The increased MPO activity and the NADPH-oxidase inactivation seemingly elicited by ET, might have further positive consequences since MPO has an effect on HDL-metabolism and the outflow of cholesterol from "foam cells", and NADPH-oxidase has a suspected role in LDL-oxidation and NADPH is one of the cofactors of NO-synthase (NOS). This Hungarian article did not specify the dose and treatment duration, however it did provide very interesting data that will hopefully be investigated further.

A number of oxidative stress markers are used in anti-aging clinics and laboratories. These molecules help scientists to determine the amount of free radical damage that is occurring in a cell, organ, or organism. The most commonly used markers include alkenals, hydroperoxides, 8-hyroxydeoxyguanosine (8-OHdG), and 8-Epi-prostaglandin F2a (8-epi-PG F2a) or isoprostane. Among these markers, 8-OHdG is widely used in many anti-aging clinics and has a relatively credible index. It is the gold standard for measurement of oxidative damage to chromosomes and DNA. Its measurement reflects the amount of damage that has been caused to the entire body. Results of an unpublished study by *Kang et al.* investigating the effect of HRT on oxidative stress suggest that ET and human growth hormone therapy (hGHT) may help to reduce oxidative stress. Ten postmenopausal women were treated with ET or ET and hGHT for six months. For a control 48 women were not given any form of HRT. Results showed that 8-OHdG levels fell slightly in women receiving ET alone, and significantly in women receiving both ET and hGH treatment. From this pilot result it can be speculated that a possible mechanism for the anti-aging effect of HRT is the fact that it lowers oxidative DNA damage. Many experiments show that long-lived species have lower DNA damage than genetically similar species with a shorter lifespan. Therefore, suggesting that longevity is linked to low levels of DNA damage.

## **ALTERNATIVES TO ESTROGENS**

What can be used instead of estrogens? There are a number of other treatments that can be used to combat the effects of menopause; these include black cohosh, ginseng (Korean), tibolone, and selective estrogen receptor modulators (SERMs) such as raloxifene, alendronate, calcitonin, and vitamin $K_2$.

Women complaining of hot flushes should first change their lifestyles. They should be educated to avoid dressing too heavily, drinking hot beverages or alcohol, and eating spicy food. They should also be educated on how to reduce stress and to breathe deeply when flushes are coming. Sleeping problems are considered to be secondary to hot flushes. Therefore, flush control can resolve these problems. They should be encouraged to try soy foods and black cohosh for more than a few weeks, and if this does not help the use of Effexor, Prozac, and Catapres should be considered.

For vaginal dryness, vaginal lubricants, estrogen creams or tablets, or plastic rings are effective. These agents seldom change the level of estrogen in the blood, therefore they are not effective with hot flushes and, of course, they do not have systemic side effects.

Treatment for the prevention of osteoporosis should be decided based upon the individual woman's bone density. If a woman's risk is not significant, she needs calcium, vitamin D, and exercise. If she has osteoporosis or is at high risk for osteoporosis, medications that help to increase bone mineral content should be prescribed.

As we know, menopausal women are at increased risk of developing heart disease. Therefore, serum cholesterol needs to be regularly measured and controlled. Recommended optimal cholesterol levels can be seen in Figure 10. Blood pressure and blood glucose levels also need to be kept under control. All of these goals can be achieved by adequate counseling, changes in lifestyle, and prescription of adequate medications.

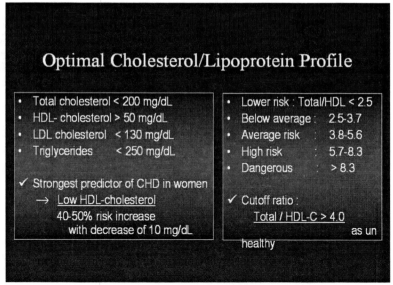

*Figure 10. The optimal cholesterol/lipoprotein profile*

Phytoestrogens are also known to benefit cardiovascular health. Interestingly, they also show an anti-neoplastic effect. In many pre-clinical and clinical studies, they have been shown to lower cholesterol and bone loss, and increase bone mineral density. Genistein, a phytoestrogen present in soy protein, has been found to improve endothelial dysfunction, which is a significant risk factor for heart disease.

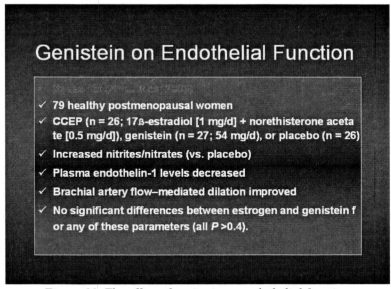

*Figure 11. The effect of genistein on endothelial function.*

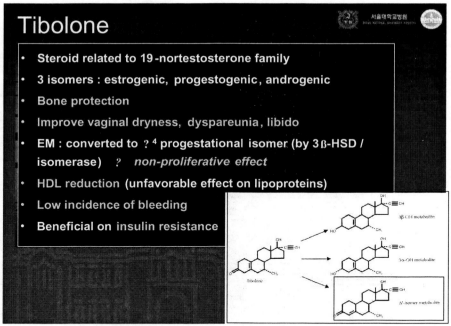

*Figure 12. Benefits associated with use of the steroid tibolone.*

Women who cannot be prescribed estrogen can be treated with tibolone (see Figure 12). If postmenopausal women complain of breast symptoms or experience a change in mammographic density, tibolone can be an alternative to estrogen. Selective estrogen receptor modulator (SERM) (see Figure 13) can also be considered as an alternative to ET.

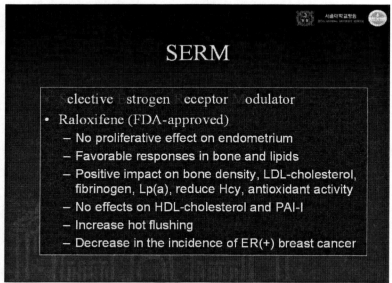

*Figure 13. Benefits associated with Selective Estrogen Receptor Modulator (SERM).*

## CONCLUDING REMARKS

In conclusion, estrogen should be used cautiously after sufficient counseling and appropriate screening tests along with regular checkups. Alternative preparations, such as phytoestrogens, tibolone, SERM, or bisphosphonate should be considered for women with climacteric symptoms or established or increased risk of osteoporosis.

Finally, all postmenopausal women should be encouraged to make certain lifestyle changes, these include stopping smoking, eating a nutritionally balanced diet, controlling body weight, taking adequate exercise, and stress reduction.

## REFERENCES

Brussaard HE, Gevers Leuven JA, Frolich M, Kluft C, Krans HM. Short-term oestrogen replacement therapy improves insulin resistance, lipids and fibrinolysis in postmenopausal women with NIDDM. *Diabetologia*. 1997;40:843-849.

Chlebowski RT, Hendrix SL, Langer RD, *et al*. Influence of estrogen plus progestin on breast cancer and mammography in healthy postmenopausal women: the Women's Health Initiative Randomized Trial. *JAMA*. 2003;289:3243-3253.

Cutler RG, Mattson MP. Measuring oxidative stress and interpreting its clinical relevance for humans. In: Cutler RG, Rodriguez H, eds. *Critical reviews of oxidative stress and aging: Advances in basic science, diagnostics and intervention*. New Jersey: World Scientific; 2003:132-138, 1081-1086.

Hall GM, Daniels M, Huskisson EC, Spector TD. A randomised controlled trial of the effect of hormone replacement therapy on disease activity in postmenopausal rheumatoid arthritis. *Ann Rheum Dis*. 1994;53:112-116.

Harman D. Free radical theory of aging. In: Klatz R, Goldman R, eds. *The science of anti-aging medicine*. Chicago: American Academy of Anti-Aging Medicine; 1996: 15-31.

Lee JY, Choi YM, Ku SY. Effects of Continuous Combined HRT on Lipid Profile. In: Takeshi Aso, Takumi Yanaihara, eds, Seiichiro Fujimoto. *The Menopause at the Millennium*. New York: Parthenon Publishing Group; 2000:441-447.

Lee JY, Ku SY. Healthy aging in the new millennium. In: Schneider HPG, ed. *Menopause - The State of the Art*. New York: Parthenon Publishing Group; 2003:344-347.

The North American Menopause Society. Estrogen and Progestogen Use in Peri- and Postmenopausal Women: September 2003 position statement of The North American Menopause Society. Available at: http://www.menopause.org/HTpositionstatement.pdf.

The US Food and Drug Administration. Estrogen and Estrogen with Progestin Therapies for Postmenopausal Women. Available at http://www.fda.gov/cder/drug/infopage/estrogens_progestins/ default.htm. Date created: January 8, 2003; Date updated: March 2, 2004.

Wassertheil-Smoller S, Hendrix SL, Limacher M, *et al*. Effect of estrogen plus progestin on stroke in postmenopausal women: the Women's Health Initiative: a randomized trial. *JAMA*. 2003;289:2673-2684.

Yoon BK, Kim DK, Kang Y, Kim JW, Shin MH, Na DL. Hormone replacement therapy in postmenopausal women with Alzheimer's disease: a randomized, prospective study. *Fertil Steril*. 2003;79:274-280.

## ABOUT THE AUTHOR

Professor Ku received his Medical Degree in 1991 from Seoul National University (SNU) College of Medicine in Seoul, the top-ranked Medical School in South Korea. He has also received a Master's degree and PhD from SNU Postgraduate School, and continued his education with a fellowship in Reproductive Endocrinology and Infertility. He is currently working for SNU and SNU Hospital as Assistant Professor in the Department of OB/GYN, and has been qualified as NAMS Menopause Practitioner. He also serves as Korean representative of the A4M International Advisory Board and is Director of International Affairs to the Korean Academy of Anti-Aging Medicine (KA3M). He has published numerous articles both in Korea and internationally. He is the co-author of *Anti-Aging Medicine*, the first textbook of its kind in Korea and has been invited as Guest Speaker at A4M, AAWC, APAAC, AOFOG, KSMP meetings, etc. He has also published numerous medical and scientific articles in the field of reproductive endocrinology, both in Korea and internationally.

Chapter 9

# Hypercholesterolemia Treatment: A New Hypothesis or Just an Accident

*Sergey A Dzugan M.D., Ph.D.*
*Principle Consultant Anti-Aging Strategies, North Central Mississippi Regional Cancer Center*

## ABSTRACT

Despite considerable success in the treatment of hypercholesterolemia, atherosclerosis remains the leading cause of death in most Western countries. The treatment of hypercholesterolemia is still a complex and controversial issue. We continue to investigate a new hypothesis concerning the association of hypercholesterolemia and low levels of steroid hormones. The purpose of this paper is to evaluate the importance and effect of multiple steroid hormone restoration to youthful levels in hypercholesterolemia treatment.

**Keywords:** athlerosclerosis; cholesterol; steroidal hormones; hormone deficit; hormonorestorative therapy

## INTRODUCTION

The focus of this paper is hypercholesterolemia and a possible new approach to the correction of this cholesterol disorder. The goals and objectives of the paper are to test a new hypothesis concerning the association of low levels of steroidal hormones and hypercholesterolemia, and to evaluate the importance and effect of restoration of multiple steroid hormones to useful levels in hypercholesterolemia treatment.

Heart disease is still the leading cause of death in the United States. Hypercholesterolemia is a major risk factor for coronary atherosclerosis and myocardial infarction, and most developed countries currently have public health strategies that attempt to lower the level of cholesterol. However, it may be to our advantage if we looked at cholesterol problems from a slightly different point of view. We know that plasma cholesterol levels increase with age, as does the incidence of coronary heart disease. However, the mechanism responsible for age-related hypercholesterolemia is not well understood.

At present, statins play an important role in the treatment of hypercholesterolemia. A number of studies show that although primary prevention is effective, long-term tolerability is still a matter of controversy. Several studies suggest that the reduction of total cholesterol in blood by cholesterol-lowering drugs is accompanied by a decrease in the incidence of coronary heart disease but not in total mortality. Chung *et al* found that 4% to 38% of patients taking cholesterol-lowering drugs experience side effects, which results in dose reduction or discontinuation of treatment. Low, or reduced, serum cholesterol concentration has been shown to increase mortality from hemorrhagic stroke and violent deaths. Adverse events associated with low, or reduced, serum cholesterol concentration include poor quality of life, severe rhabdomyolysis, renal failure, and death. Together, these factors suggest that we need to find better, safer treatment regimens for elevated total cholesterol levels.

## SUGGESTING A NEW HYPOTHESIS FOR HYPERCHOLESTEROLEMIA

Several problems play a key role in the suggestion of a new hypothesis for the cause of hypercholesterolemia; these include:

- Controversial data about the effect of steroidal hormones on hypercholesterolemia.
- Change of serum cholesterol levels during normal pregnancy.
- Diminished concentration of total cholesterol in women with threatened abortion.
- Similarity of symptoms in patients during use of cholesterol-lowering drugs with patients with fibromyalgia and chronic fatigue syndrome.
- The fact that up to 60% of patients with myocardial infarction were found to have "normal" cholesterol levels.
- Significant mortality rate from cancer in young hypercholesterolemic subjects.
- Altered cholesterol level, usually low, in patients with psychiatric disorders such as depression, changed personality, suicidal ideation, impulsive aggressive behavior, and schizophrenia.

What does medical literature say about all these problems? Previously, hormone replacement therapy (HRT) was considered first-line treatment for management of hypercholesterolemia to prevent coronary heart disease in women. Recent studies, however, show no benefit of HRT for secondary prevention of coronary events.

Research by Martin *et al* found that the serum total cholesterol concentration of healthy pregnant women increased progressively throughout pregnancy to a mean of 8.14 mmol/L (314 mg/dL) in the third trimester. The study also found that the level of LDL, or low-density lipoproteins increases dramatically during pregnancy. Erkkola *et al* found that total cholesterol decreases significantly within three months of delivery, and a further significant decrease occurred within the following nine months. Meanwhile, Smolarczyk *et al* found that women with threatened abortion had diminished concentrations of total cholesterol and lower-than-normal LDL levels.

Fibromyalgia is a syndrome characterized by generalized aches, pains, and tender points, fatigue and unrefreshing sleep. In addition, patients complain of vasospastic extremities, irritable bowel syndrome, irritable bladder syndrome, tension headaches, depression, and sexual problems. Similar symptoms are seen quite often in patients using cholesterol-lowering drugs! Fibromyalgia may overlap with symptoms of chronic fatigue syndrome. Fibromyalgia and migraine are two faces of the same mechanism. Because of the clinical similarities between fibromyalgia and chronic fatigue syndrome, it is possible that they share a common pathophysiological mechanism; namely, deficiency and dysbalance of steroidal hormones. Olin suggests that the main cause of fibromyalgia is irreversible disturbance of the neuroimmunoendocrinological system. We partially support this hypothesis, and we believe that fibromyalgia sufferers have a dysfunction of the autonomic nervous system, as a result of hormonal deficiency associated with a loss of sensitivity of the cell membrane to hormonal impulses. We do not agree with Olin that the condition is "irreversible," because fibromyalgia quite often disappears in patients treated with hormonorestorative therapy. For example, a 54-year-old female with a first visit to the hospital in June 2002 had a diagnosis of fibromyalgia, migraine, fatigue, depression, suicidal attempts, insomnia, weight gain, short-term memory problems, sex disorder, and constipation. After conducting a basic hormonal profile and lipid profile it became evident that a few hormones needed to be corrected. We gave the patient hormonorestorative therapy. She came back after that, and in four months she had only one complaint. She had no symptoms of fibromyalgia or any kind of migraine problems, her only complaint was that she was suffering from minimal sleep problems.

All members of the two most popular classes of cholesterol-lowering drugs, the fibrates and the statins, cause cancer in rodents. A study by Umeki revealed that advanced lung cancer patients had significantly lower total cholesterol than healthy participants. Whereas Williams *et al* found that serum cholesterol level was inversely associated with incidence of colon cancer and other cancers in men.

According to Windler *et al*, the mortality of hypercholesterolemic patients is approximately tenfold higher than average, and shows a strong, inverse, linear relationship with cholesterol concentrations. Behar *et al* found that a total cholesterol level of less than 160 mg/dL is associated with higher mortality rates from cancer, liver disease, respiratory disorders, and injuries.

There is plenty of medical literature to suggest that cholesterol levels play an important role in several psychiatric disorders. Atmaca *et al* found that patients with manic episodes and patients with bipolar disorder in full remission had markedly lower cholesterol compared with controls. Meanwhile Cassidy *et al* uncovered a significant statistical correlation between low levels of total cholesterol and suicidal ideation, as well as between low levels of serum total cholesterol and severity of depression. Work by Rabe-Jablonska *et al* found that total cholesterol levels of less than 160 mg/dL and LDL levels of less than 100 mg/dL were observed in persons with suicidal behavior.

## CHOLESTEROL AND THE BODY

Cholesterol is an important part of the story of blocked arteries; however, that is not the whole story of cholesterol. Cholesterol is a major building block from which cell membranes are made, and it is used to make a number of important substances, including: steroid hormones, bile acids and, in conjunction with sunlight, vitamin D3. Neither cholesterol nor triglycerides can be dissolved in blood. They have to be wrapped up in a sphere known as a lipoprotein in order to be transported out of the intestine.

### *Lipoproteins*

In short, lipoproteins provide transport for insoluble cholesterol and triglycerides. Lipoproteins come in many sizes and are classified as follows:
- Chylomicrons: contain approximately 7% cholesterol.
- Very low-density lipoproteins (VLDL): mainly carry triglycerides and 16% to 22% cholesterol.
- Intermediate-density lipoproteins (IDL): contain approximately 30% cholesterol.
- Low-density lipoproteins (LDL): contain approximately 50% cholesterol.
- High-density lipoproteins (HDL): contain approximately 19% cholesterol.

Chylomicrons transport fats and cholesterol from the intestine into the liver. The liver reconstructs the component parts into VLDL and sends them into the bloodstream. VLDL are made in the liver; they transform into IDL particles after they have lost their triglyceride content. IDL are short-lived lipoproteins containing approximately 30% cholesterol, which are converted to LDL in the liver. LDL carries cholesterol from the liver to cells that need it. Any excess cholesterol is reabsorbed by the liver and reused or excreted into the bile. LDL particles are involved in the formation of plaques in the walls of the arteries, which is why LDL is known as "bad cholesterol", even though it is not strictly cholesterol. HDL molecules are made in the intestine and the liver. It helps to remove cholesterol from the artery wall. HDL act as cholesterol "mop", scavenging loose cholesterol and transporting it back to the liver. As such, HDL is known as "good" cholesterol, although like LDL, HDL is not cholesterol.

## HORMONODEFICIT HYPOTHESIS OF HYPERCHOLESTEROLEMIA

The human body is in a state of dynamic equilibrium, or homeostasis. Multiple feedback loop mechanisms play a major role in maintaining homeostasis.

Deterioration of reproductive function, one of the most striking endocrine alterations that the body undergoes throughout life, occurs during aging and is related to a complex interplay factor. A few years ago, we found that some patients who had high cholesterol levels saw their cholesterol levels drop to normal levels after being treated with hormonorestorative therapy. This was not an expected side effect of hormonorestorative therapy, so we began to consider why this had happened.

When the production of hormones starts to decline our body tries to correct this problem by increasing the production of cholesterol. The same thing happens during pregnancy. The woman's body needs more hormones for both herself and her baby, thus cholesterol levels rise significantly. If the woman's body is unable to increase the production of cholesterol, the risk of abortion and miscarriage is increased significantly. A person with low cholesterol levels probably also has low levels of certain hormones: this hormone deficit may contribute to certain problems such as suicide, criminal behavior, depression, attention deficit disorder, and cancer at young age. Every time Dr. R.A. Smith of North Central Regional Mississippi Cancer Center sees people who have cancer before the age of 35, he conducts a blood test. In 95% of cases, these young people have low levels of cholesterol.

When patients take cholesterol-lowering drugs we can surmise that hormonal production will decrease. We suspect that this is why many people who take these drugs experience severe fatigue, fibromyalgia-like pain, depression, weight gain, and impotence. They are also at increased risk of developing cancer and committing suicide.

Normally, our body tries to keep a normal ratio between different hormones. If we have a malfunction in a feedback loop mechanism we start to experience hormone imbalance-related problems, like male or female dominance or estrogen dominance. When the production of hormones starts to decline as a result of aging, or whatever other reasons, the body starts to correct the deficiency of hormones by extra production of cholesterol. Thus suggesting that the elevation of total cholesterol serves as a compensatory mechanism for hormonal deficiency. Considering this, if you restore a useful level of hormones there is no reason for the extra production of cholesterol.

Our proposed hypothesis is called the hormonal deficit hypothesis of hypercholesterolemia. This hypothesis implies that hypercholesterolemia is the reactive consequence of age-related, enzyme-dependent, down-regulation of steroid hormone synthesis and interconversion. In short, we propose that hypercholesterolemia is a compensatory mechanism for age-related decline of steroidal hormone production.

## *Study Methods*

To investigate the hypothesis we analyzed 41 patients, 16 men and 25 women, with hypercholesterolemia. The mean age of participants was 58.2 years. The follow-up period was from two to 68 months. Total cholesterol, HDL, and triglycerides were measured by the enzymatic method developed by Allain *et al* and Roeschlau *et al*. Basic laboratory serum tests for men included: lipid profile, PSA, pregnenolone, DHEA sulfate, testosterone, estradiol, and progesterone. Additional laboratory tests, if needed were: cortisol, free testosterone, DHT, sex hormone binding globulin (SHBG), IGF-1, TSH, T-3, and T-4. Basic laboratory serum tests for women included: lipid profile, pregnenolone, DHEA sulfate, testosterone, total estrogen, and progesterone. Additional laboratory tests, if needed, were: estriol, estradiol, estrone, cortisol, SHBG, IGF-1, TSH, T-3, and T-4. The following basic hormonorestorative therapy for hypercholesterolemia management was used in men: pregnenolone, DHEA, progesterone, and testosterone. Basic hormonorestorative therapy for hypercholesterolemia management in women included: pregnenolone, DHEA, triestrogen, progesterone, and testosterone.

## *Why Hormonorestorative Therapy and Not HRT?*

We use the term hormonorestorative therapy because we feel that the term hormone replacement therapy (HRT) is confusing. The term "HRT" is mainly used in the context of estrogen or combined estrogen/progestin replacement therapy. Secondly, the term "natural HRT" is very unclear. Does this mean natural for human beings, or natural for nature? Natural means not man-made, and thus may refer to phytoestrogens or equine estrogens. Also the term "bio-identical hormones" is ambiguous, however "bio-identical to the human hormone" is acceptable, but only just. In Greek, "bios" means life, and "anthropos" means human. Thus it may be better to say "anthropoidentical hormones."

Anthropoidentical is a more restrictive term than bio-identical. We use the term anthropoidentical restoration when the chemical structure of the hormone employed is identical to the human hormones, and when the normal ratio between hormones of each hormonal group is maintained.

There are additional problems with HRT:
- The majority of studies were performed with only one or two agents.
- No psychological cyclicity.
- Patients are given a "one-size-fits-all" standard dose.
- No anthropoidentical restoration attempted.
- No correlation between dosage and hormone levels.
- Mostly oral route of administration.

## *Optimal Delivery System for Anthropoidentical Steroid Hormones*

The best way of delivering anthropoidentical steroid hormones is both orally and via topical gels. Steroids are highly lipophilic molecules with a low molecular weight, and therefore are very well absorbed through the skin. The topical gels used in the study were:
- Triestrogen (micronized) gel (E3:E2:E1, 90:7:3): strength of 1ml equal to 1.25ml of Premarin.
- Progesterone (micronized) gel 5% (50 mg/mL).
- Testosterone (micronized) gel 5% (50 mg/mL).

Where should these gels be applied? The scrotum or vulva, the neck, forearm, and sides of chest and abdomen are all suitable sites. Approximately 75% of the dose should be applied in the morning, preferably after bathing, and the remaining 25% in the evening.

Oral administration includes capsules for pregnenolone and DHEA, drops for triestrogen (very rare), E3:E2:E1 at 80:10:10; 5 mg/ml (strength of 0.25 ml equal to 1.25 mg of Premarin), and troches or lozenges for progesterone (very rare), 200 mg/troche.

## *Dosage*

Dose recommendations to different patients during hormonorestorative therapy were different and were determined by serum hormonal levels during serial testing. Doses were individually modified during hormonorestorative therapy to produce useful physiological, not normal, serum levels. Doses were titrated to achieve the laboratory-defined hormonal blood levels of young adults between the ages of 20 and 30 for both genders, at which time a good level of all steroid hormones naturally occurs.

Different researchers recommend different ratios between estriol, estradiol, and estrone. For example, in one group of researcher may have found that the normal ratio between estriol, estrone, and estradiol is 70:21:9. However, we found the ratios to be different, and we prefer to use more estriol because we work in a cancer center and we try to make hormonorestorative therapy as safe as possible for patients. And by this way we try to decrease the possibility of cancer. If you look around you will not see many adults who developed cancer before the age of 40.

We must remember that no two people are alike, not everyone thinks alike, and not everyone responds to the same medications.

## *Recommendations for Hormonorestorative Therapy*

To ensure that hormonorestorative is as effective as possible the following recommendations should be followed:
- Hormones used should be anthropoidentical.
- Doses should be individually modified.
- Therapy should be administered in a cyclical manner.
- The larger dose should be taken in the morning.

Mono or bi-hormonal therapy is usually inadequate. Poly or multi-hormonal therapy is optimal. When we talk about administering doses in a cyclical manner we must remember that the production of estrogen and progesterone fluctuates significantly during the menstrual cycle: this is very important if a woman is still menstruating or if she is postmenopausal.

*Study Results*

Study results were promising, as 100% of patients responded to the treatment. The acute morbidity of hormonorestorative therapy is zero. Total cholesterol levels fell significantly in all patients. Overall, total cholesterol levels fell by 25.8%. In men, the average drop in total cholesterol levels was 30.3%, while levels fell in women 22.8% on average. LDL levels were reduced in all patients by an average of 23.9%, in males 42.2%, and in females 15.9%. Triglyceride levels fell in all patients by an average of 54.9%, in males 71.6%, and in females 34.2%. HDL levels decreased overall by 19.6%, 12.4% on average in men; and 21.5% on average in women. We need to stress that HDL levels fell: this result is probably the opposite as to what most people would expect and therefore needs explanation.

Why should elevation of HDL be a good sign during cholesterol-lowering therapy? If you normalize the level of total cholesterol, what reason is there for more HDL to be produced? If there is nothing to transfer back to liver, why produce the extra carrier. By this logic, HDL levels should fall. However, in most studies of cholesterol-lowering treatments HDL levels increase, why? We need to think of the body as having two factories, one that produces cholesterol, and a second that produces hormones. When the production of hormones starts to decline, the body tends to compensate by producing more of the building blocks, in this case cholesterol, that are needed for the production of these hormones. When production of cholesterol increases, and cholesterol is elevated, we need more LDL to deliver the extra cholesterol to the factory that produces the hormones. Then, if you more cholesterol than the hormone factory needs, we need a carrier that can take this extra, or excess, cholesterol back to the liver. This carrier is HDL. But if you normalize hormonal profile, we do not need extra cholesterol. If our cholesterol decreases, LDL levels fall back to normal levels. And when we have no excess of cholesterol, why should HDL levels rise? Therefore, from a logical viewpoint, HDL levels should fall when a person is treated with cholesterol-lowering therapy.

HDL levels fell in all but one of the 41 study participants. In that patient HDL levels increased from 60 mg/dL to 71 mg/dL. This man was a body builder who had abused his body with anabolic steroids; this may at least partially explain why his HDL levels rose, although we cannot give a definite reason as to why his result should differ from all the other participants.

How does hormonorestorative therapy compare with cholesterol-lowering drugs? Comparison of the results of a study of hormonorestorative therapy conducted by Dzugan and Smith at the North Central Mississippi Regional Center with those of a study of cholesterol-lowering drugs by Morimoto *et al* at Osaka University, show that hormonorestorative therapy is as effective as conventional cholesterol-lowering drugs. Total cholesterol at the start of Dzugan and Smith's study was 263.5 mg/dL; by the end of the study, total cholesterol fell to 187.9 mg/dL. Meanwhile, total cholesterol at the start of the study by Morimoto *et al* was 265 mg/dL; at the end of the study, this fell to 216 mg/dL.

## HYPERCHOLESTEROLEMIA, HEART DISEASE, AND MYOCARDIAL INFARCTION

Ladeira *et al* found that 40% to 70% of patients with coronary artery disease had hypercholesterolemia. If this is so, how can we explain Bratus *et al's* discovery that up to 60% of patients with myocardial infarction have normal cholesterol levels?

To explain this is it is important to look at some case studies. Two patients of the same age and a similar medical history had their cholesterol levels measured at 25 and 40 years of age. The first patient had a cholesterol level of 130 mg/dL at age 25, and the second patient 180 mg/dL at 25. Life cycle-related elevation of total cholesterol is 60% in both cases. In the first patient total cholesterol increased to 190 mg/dL by age 40, in the second patient total cholesterol increased to 240 mg/dL. We hypothesize that total cholesterol elevation over time is a critical determinant of the risk for coronary heart disease or myocardial infarction. While, 190 is a normal level according to tradition, 190 is high, maybe too high for arteries that prefer to exist with a total cholesterol level of 130 mg/dL. This is only a theory.

| Effect of Hormonorestorative Therapy on "Normal" Total Serum Cholesterol Levels | | | |
|---|---|---|---|
| SEX | AGE | TOTAL CHOLESTEROL (nl<200 mg/dL) | |
| | | BASELINE | FOLLOW-UP |
| F | 55 | 198 | 168 |
| M | 73 | 202 | 162 |
| M | 63 | 195 | 150 |
| M | 56 | 196 | 113 |
| F | 55 | 189 | 153 |

*Table 1. Effect of Hormonorestorative Therapy on Five Patients with "Normal" Serum Total Cholesterol Levels*

If our hypothesis is correct, would patients who had "normal" cholesterol levels and who started to take hormonorestorative therapy, also see a decrease in their total cholesterol levels? As can be seen in Table 1, hormonorestorative therapy did indeed lower the participants total cholesterol level, even though their cholesterol level before treatment was considered normal.

## HYPO, NORMOCHOLESTEROLEMIA, AND HYPERCHOLESTEROLEMIA

In order to learn more about the important relationship between cholesterol and steroidal hormones it would be useful to consider the cases of three patients with normal, hypo, and hypercholesterolemia.

### Normocholesterolemia Case Study

For the first case, we will consider so-called normocholesterolemia, or relative hypercholesterolemia. Here we have a 24-year-old male, diagnosed with fatigue, major depression, social anxiety disorder, low energy, tiredness, severe depression in spite of Paxil, and erection problems. This young man had been taking antidepressants since the age of 14, and had recently started to take Viagra. Three years ago, at age 21, his cholesterol level was 140 mg/dL. At age 24 his cholesterol had risen to 195 mg/dL, which is still within traditionally "normal" levels. However, this significant increase in cholesterol level indicates that his body is trying to fix a problem. Hormone tests confirmed this. While his testosterone level was fine, his pregnenolone level was very low for his age, as was his level of DHEA-S. Therefore, the man was given pregnenolone and DHEA. After just two months of treatment, he had no health complaints, no depression, and no longer needed to take antidepressants, or Viagra.

*Hypercholesterolemia Case Study*

Here we have a 60-year-old female, complaining of fatigue and depression in spite of her Paxil, hypercholesterolemia, insomnia, arrhythmia, hot flashes, vaginal dryness, no libido, poor sex drive, leg cramps, short-term memory problems, constipation, frequent infections, and poor bladder control. A basic hormonal profile, total cholesterol measurement, and lipid profile, revealed that her total cholesterol was very high, at 278 mg/dL, and her LDL level was high, at 180 mg/dL. After two months of hormonorestorative therapy, total cholesterol dropped from 278 mg/dL to 191 mg/dL and LDL dropped from 180 mg/dL to 130 mg/dL: not bad without cholesterol-lowering drugs. Her HDL level also fell from 74 mg/dL to 48 mg/dl. In addition, her DHEA-S, pregnenolone, and progesterone levels, which had been on the low side also improved significantly. Furthermore, all but one of the woman's complaints, frequent infection, had disappeared.

*Hypocholesterolemia Case Study*

This is the case of a 29-year-old female with hypocholesterolemia. She was diagnosed with major depression, obesity, and menstrual disorder, and complains of fatigue, no energy, depression, anxiety, panic attacks in spite of Zoloft, no libido, poor sex drive, very poor short-term memory, being overweight, and having an irregular menstrual cycle. Tests revealed that her total cholesterol was 130 mg/dL. She weighed 242 pounds and her body fat percentage was 58%. A hormonal profile showed that she also had low DHEA-S, pregnenolone, estrogen, and progesterone levels. She was given hormonorestorative therapy and one-and-a-half years later she has no complaints. Her hormone levels improved dramatically and her memory returned to normal, as did her menstrual cycle, despite the fact that she had never had normal menstrual cycles since she was a teenager. Her old problems with depression, anxiety, fatigue, and lack of energy were also resolved and she started to exercise. Her weight decreased from 242 pounds to 146, and her body fat percentage dropped from 58% to a healthy 18%.

## CONCLUDING REMARKS

In patients with hypercholesterolemia and sub-youthful serum steroidal hormones, broadband steroid hormone restoration was typically associated with a substantial drop in serum total cholesterol. Hormonorestorative therapy is an effective intervention for hypercholesterolemia, and could be a very important and inexpensive treatment for the healthcare system. The elevation of cholesterol is a reflection of a serious problem with steroid formation. Elevation of cholesterol is an excellent aging marker, which can be used to define the time when patients need to begin hormonorestorative therapy.

## REFERENCES

Allain CC, Poon LS, Chan CS, *et al*. Enzymatic determination of total serum cholesterol. *Clin Chem* 1974;20:470-475.

Atmaca M, Kuloglu M, Tezcan E, *et al*. Serum leptin and cholesterol levels in patients with bipolar disorder. *Neuropsychobiology* 2002;46;176-179.

Behar S, Graff E, Reicher-Reiss H, *et al*. Low total cholesterol is associated with high total mortality in patients with coronary heart disease. The Bezafibrate Infarction Prevention (BIP) Study Group. *Eur Heart J* 1997;17:92-99.

Bennet RM. Fibromyalgia: The commonest cause of widespread pain. *Compr Ther* 1995;21:269-275.

Boston PF, Dursun SM, Reveley MA. Cholesterol and mental disorder. *Br J Psychiatry* 1996;169:682-689.

Bratus VV, Talaieva TV, Lomakovs'kyi OM, *et al*. Modified lipoproteins-their types and role in atherogenesis. *Fiziol Zh* 2000;46:73-81.

Cassidy F, Carroll BJ. Hypocholesterolemia during mixed mani episodes. *Eur Arch Psychiatry Clin*

*Neurosci* 2002;252::110-114.

Chung N, Cho SY, Choi DH, *et al*. STATT: a titrate-to-goal study of simvastatin in Asian patients with coronary heart disease. Simvastatin Treats Asians To Target. *Clin Ther* 2001;23:858-870.

Dzugan SA, Smith RA. Broad spectrum restoration in natural steroid hormones as possible treatment for hypercholesterolemia. *Bull Urg Rec Med* 2002;3:278-284.

Dzugan SA, Smith RA. Hypercholesterolemia treatment: a new hypothesis or just an accident. *Med Hypothesis* 2005;59:751-756.

Erkkola R, Viikari J, Irjala K, *et al*. One-year follow-up of lipoprotein metabolism after pregnancy. *Biol Res Pregnancy Perinatol* 1986;7:47-51.

Geiss HC, Parhofer KG, Schwandt P. Atorvastatin compared with simvastatin in patients with severe LDL hypercholesterolaemia treated by regular LDL apheresis. *J Intern Med* 1999;245:47-55.

Ladeia AM, Guimaraes AC, Lima JC. The lipid profile and coronary artery disease. *Arq Bras Cardiol* 1994;63:101-106.

Law MR, Thompson SG, Wald NJ. Assessing possible hazards of reducing serum cholesterol. *BMJ* 1994;308:373-379.

Lee M-LT, Rosner BA, Weiss ST, *et al*. Predictors of cardiovascular death: The Normative Aging Study - 1963-1998. *Clinical Geriatrics* 1999;7.

Martin U, Davies C, Hayavi ST, *et al*. Is normal pregnancy atherogenic? *Clin Sci (Lond)* 1999;96:421-425.

Matsumoto Y. Fibromyalgia syndrome. *Nippon Rinsho* 1999;57:364-369.

Morimoto S, Koh E, Fukuo K, *et al*. Effects of pravastatin administration for 12 months on serum lipid levels in aged patients with hypercholesterolemia. *Nippon Ronen Igakkai Zasshi* 1994;31:310-317.

Mosca LJ. Contemporary management of hyperlipidemia in women. *J Womens Health Gend Based Med* 2002;11:423-432.

Newman TB, Hulley SB. Carcinogenicity of lipid-lowering drugs. *JAMA* 1996;275:55-60.

Nicolodi M, Sicuteri F. Fibromyaliga and migraine, two faces of the same mechanism. Serotonin as the common clue for pathogensis and therapy. *Adv Exp Med Biol* 1996;398:373-379.

Olin R. Fibromyaligia. A neuro-immuno-endocrinologic syndrome? *Lakartidningen* 1995;92:755-758, 761-763.

Oriba HA, Bucks DA, Maibach HI. Percutaneous absorption of hydrocortisone and testosterone on the vulva and forearm: effect of the menopause and site. *Br J Dermatol* 1996;134:229-233.

Rabe-Jablonska J, Poprawska I. Levels of serum total cholesterol and LDL-cholesterol in patients with major depression in acute period transmission. *Med Sci Monit* 2000;6:539-547.

Reiffenberger DH. Fibromyalgia syndrome: a review. *Am Fam Physician* 1996;53:1698-1712.

Roeschlau P, Bernt E, Gruber W. Enzymatic determination of total cholesterol in serum. *Z Klin Chem Klin Biochem* 1974;12:226.

Scheen AJ. Fatal rhabdomyolysis caused by cervistatin. *Rev Med Liege* 2001;56:592-594.

Smith RA, Dzugan SA, Rafique S, *et al*. Peripheral blood natural killer cell increase as a predictor of survival in metastatic cancer patients treated by neuroimmunotherapy with subcutaneous low-dose IL-2 plus melatonin. *Int J Immunotherapy* 1999;15:131-135.

Smith RA, Dzugan SA, Rafique S, *et al*. Covariance of natural killer cells elevation with extended survival during neuroimmunotherapy with subcutaneous low-dose IL-2 and the pineal immunomodulating neurohormone melatonin. *Bull Urg Rec Med* 2001;2:20-23.

Smolarczyk R, Romejoko E, Wojcicka-Jagodzinska J, *et al*. Lipid metabolism in women with threatened abortion. *Ginekol Pol* 1996;67:481-487.

Starfield B. Is US health really the best in the world? *JAMA*. 2000;284:483-485.

Umeki S. Decreases in serum cholesterol levels in advanced lung cancer. *Respiration* 1993;60:178-181.

Wester RC, Noonab PK, Maibach HI. Variations in percutaneous absorption of testosterone in the rhesus monkey due to anatomic site of application and frequency of application. *Arch Dermatol Res* 1980;267:229-235.

Williams RR, Sorlie PD, Feinleib M, *et al*. Cancer incidence by levels of cholesterol, *JAMA* 1981;245:247-252.

Windler E, Weers-Grabow U, Thiery J, *et al*. The prognostic value of hypocholesterolemia in hospitalized patients. *Clin Investig* 1994;72:939-943.

Yang YH, Kao SM, Chan KW. A retrospective drug utilization evaluation of antihyperlipidaemic agents in a medical center in Taiwan. *J Clin Pharm Ther* 1997;22:291-299.

**ABOUT THE AUTHOR**

Dr. Dzugan was formerly Chief of Cardiovascular Surgery at the Donetsk Regional Medical Center in Donetsk, Ukraine. His Ph.D. in cardiovascular surgery was received in 1990. He was Associate Professor of Medical University in Donetsk, Ukraine. His current primary interest is in Anti-Aging Medicine and the biological therapy of cancer, and he participates in patient care in Greenwood, Mississippi. Dr. Dzugan has worked with the Central Mississippi Regional Cancer Center for more than six years and has authored over 100 publications in medical journals.

Chapter 10

# Eye Floaters:
# Causes and Alternative Treatment

*Scott Geller M.D., Board Certified Ophthalmic Surgeon,
Founder & Medical Director, South Florida Eye Clinic*

## ABSTRACT

Vitreous floaters are one of the most common eye findings in people aged 40 and over. In most people they are not problematic, however in very severe cases they can cause intermittent obscuration of vision. The traditional treatment for extremely severe cases is surgical removal of the vitreous gel, however this can lead to further problems. Another approach to treating vitreous floaters, which is highly effective yet scarcely used, is laser treatment. Both of these forms of treatment will be discussed in this paper. We shall also discuss whether or not it is possible to prevent vitreous floaters with lifestyle changes and dietary supplementation.

**Keywords:** hyaluronic acid; free radical toxicity; vitrectomy; Neodymium YAG laser treatment

## INTRODUCTION

Eye floaters are probably one of the few things in medicine, or ophthalmology, which receive virtually no publicity, or research funding, yet can represent a problematic medical condition. Eye floaters are caused by degeneration of the vitreous body, thus the technical name for eye floaters is vitreous floaters. Vitreous floaters are one of the most common eye findings in people aged 40 and over.

## THE ANATOMY OF THE EYE

The eye is really quite a simple structure. The eyeball is approximately 23 mm in diameter. The clear front window of the eye is called the cornea. The cornea is what people put their contact lens on, it is what a surgeon points his laser at for refractive surgery, and it is the structure on which Lasik® is conducted. Behind the cornea is the iris, and the iris of course is a diaphragm, just like the iris in a camera. It opens and closes to let in a greater or lesser degree of light through the pupil. The pupil of the eye is not a physical body. The pupil of the eye, the little black dot that we see, is just a space that we recognize. The ancient Greeks named it "pupil" because the word in Greek means little person, or more precisely, little doll. If you look in somebody's eyes, you see a little reflection of yourself: that little empty spot of the pupil. Within the space behind the iris is the lens of the eye. The lens of the eye is, about 10 mm in diameter. Normally, it is crystal clear. The lens is a living cellular structure. Its cells are constructed in an onion-like structure, with layer after layer after layer being laid down throughout our life. So the older we get, the thicker the lens of the eye becomes. Even if you think you have 20/20 vision, what you think is perfect vision when you're 50 is not the same 20/20 vision that you had when you were 15. Simply because you are looking through more layers, you can see people clearly, but it's not quite the same. The lens is the structure of the eye that is affected by cataract. Now, moving to the back part of the eye. The back part of the eye, the wall of the eye, is the retina. It can be compared to the film in a camera; it works by the same principle. The retina takes the photons from light and changes the electromagnetic radiation energy into an electrical nervous impulse, which travels back to the optic nerve and into the brain. The eyeball really doesn't interpret or do anything. It is more like a transmission device. We see with our brains: actually the back part of the brain, the occipital lobe. The space that occupies the sphere behind the lens of the eye all the way to the retina, the space that is almost clear, is what we call the vitreous; the vitreous body.

## THE VITREOUS

The vitreous is a colloidal gel that occupies approximately 85% of the total volume of the eye, 99% of the vitreous is water. So how is the vitreous constructed? The vitreous is composed of a collagenous, fibrillar framework, which includes some acid glycoproteins. But the main structural constituent is hyaluronic acid, a molecule that has a coil-like appearance and gives the vitreous its gel-like characteristic. Surrounding the vitreous body there is a surface, similar to the surface of a jellyfish. This surface is called the hyaloid membrane. The hyaloid membrane is just a concentration of collagen fibers that encase the whole vitreous body, similar to the way in which a plastic bag would contain a gel.

Normal, healthy vitreous is optically clear. However, it is a complex substance. It is polymorphous in nature. When we look at the vitreous through instruments, such as the slit lamps we use in ophthalmology to shine a fine beam of light, we find that it is actually composed of pseudo membranes that float around. They move like folds and pleats, and they float in front of our view. Thus the vitreous appears to be clear, but it is really not clear. It is very gossamer-like.

The vitreous simply serves as a medium to maintain the shape of the eyeball, and maintain a clear path from the cornea, iris, and lens, back through to the retina. It is normally free from any diffusing or absorbing elements. The lens of the eye actually does absorb light because it is a living structure, its cells have nuclei and mitochondria, and all the other things that a cell would have. The vitreous does not have cells and their accompanying organelles.

## VITREOUS FLOATERS

The vitreous is basically optically clear, but as we age the vitreous changes just like everything else in our bodies. It can undergo liquefaction, opacification, and shrinkage. Ultimately, the gel converts into the gel-sol state, a more liquid, gel-like state, which is slightly contracted. This state can be associated with opacities that are formed from collagen. If this happens the whole framework of the vitreous starts to collapse. When the framework collapses, or when it starts to undergo its degenerative process, we get what we call "floaters," eye floaters. Most people who look up at a clear sky can probably see little hair-like things floating through the blue sky: these are floaters. When the vitreous liquefies (which can occur even at early ages), myopia, or nearsightedness, is a risk factor for vitreous liquefication; we call that vitreous syneresis. Vitreous syneresis occurs when the vitreous framework liquefies somewhat and we get these little spider web-like opacities floating in the gel.

However, vitreous floaters can be very, very severe in some patients. If you get a total collapse of the collagenous framework the vitreous can more or less solidify, or coagulate, into clumps. If this occurs, the vitreous takes on the appearance of a cotton ball. Patients who have this problem can actually have intermittent obscuration of their vision. They can't see past this opacity. The problem in ophthalmology, and the ophthalmic mindset, is that when a patient normally goes in to an ophthalmologist and says they have something floating in their eye, the doctor sees that the patient has 20/20 vision, and looks at the retina and see no retinal tears, he concludes that the patient is fine and tell them not to worry that it is only an intermittent problem. But for some people that can be a big problem, especially if it's bilateral, and especially if they only have one eye. There are many more one-eyed people out there than people think, and when this happens to somebody with one eye they don't have the other eye to compensate, for that person this condition can be very problematic.

There are some other conditions of the vitreous that can cause diffuse degeneration for various reasons. These include asteroid bodies, and calcium salts and soaps. However, these conditions are not the focus of this paper, in which we discuss vitreous collapse and posterior vitreous detachment.

When the vitreous collapses we get what is called a posterior vitreous detachment, which is a complete pulling away of the vitreous from its peripheral attachment: the whole vitreous collapses and we are left with something similar to a bag within a ball. It is like a clear plastic bag that pulls away from the back part of the eye. Sometimes this condition is associated with retinal detachment. As the gel collapses, the collagenous framework within the gel becomes condensed. Some of the hyaluronic acid coagulates and forms dense, dense floaters. When this happens we can get condensation of vitreous opacities. This is when patients really start to get problems, as you have this little membrane floating around inside the sphere of the eye that can really, really cause disturbances in vision.

## PREVENTION OF VITREOUS FLOATERS

Can we prevent or retard the formation of vitreous floaters? At present it is not possible to restore the molecular bonds of the clear vitreous after vitreous collapse. Protein is just a different series of amino acids in a different sequence liked by cross-link bonds. When protein denatures, the end result is a denatured, broken protein molecule. When we have a broken protein molecule, how can we make the molecule go back to its original state? The answer is that we don't know how to put it back together yet. We do know that what causes proteins to break is a lot of free radical damage, and probably several other things that we are not totally aware of.

When a molecule is affected by free radicals, molecular bonds are broken and as far as we know right now, they do not mend themselves. The breaking of protein bonds can be demonstrated very easily. Inside an egg there is the yolk and the white of the egg, which when uncooked is actually clear: the white consists mainly of albumin and a few other protein substances. Once the egg is exposed to high temperature, such as in a frying pan, the clear white of the egg becomes opaque. It becomes opaque because the protein bonds in it have been broken and all of a sudden it doesn't have the structural nature that keeps it clear. It's become cloudy. The same thing happens in our bodies. We are bombarded by ultraviolet rays, cosmic rays, and numerous other things and it takes maybe 50 years for all those environmental insults and whatever else we put in our bodies to do the same to us: denature proteins. If we believe that free radical toxicity is the cause of these protein breakdowns, then it seems logical that anything that is going to decrease free radical toxicity could be beneficial to us.

Recently, the National Eye Institute sponsored the Age-Related Eye Disease Study (AREDS), a study on macular degeneration, in which patients were given antioxidant vitamins in various combinations and forms. The results of the study showed that high levels of antioxidants and zinc significantly reduced the risk of developing advanced age-related macular degeneration (AMD) by approximately 25%. The same nutrients were also found to reduce the risk of vision loss caused by advanced AMD by approximately 19%. Macular degeneration is the leading cause of vision loss in the Western World, thus for people with macular degeneration, or for those at risk of it, the findings of this study are highly significant. However, we don't as yet know if the same nutrients, or a similar cocktail of nutrients, will have the same beneficial effects upon the vitreous. What we can say is that as far as we know at present, taking these vitamins won't hurt you. Although, there is something that we've learned from these types of studies, various manufacturers have come out with what they call a smoker's formula. Several studies suggest that elevated levels of beta-carotene in smokers have been associated with higher levels of lung cancer. So, all these vitamins that we are taking have a two-edged, two-sided point of view. You've got to look at it both ways. It's a double-edge sword.

## TREATING VITREOUS FLOATERS

All we know at present is that the denatured protein cannot be restored to its original state as far as we are aware at this time. Who knows what the future will hold. It seems unlikely that we are going to get nanomachines in there mending broken molecules, so what can we do? Fortunately there are some solutions to this problem.

### *Vitrectomy: Surgical Removal of the Vitreous*

Traditionally, for extremely severe cases, the solution is to surgically remove the vitreous gel. To an ophthalmologist that procedure is known as a vitrectomy. However, most ophthalmologists reserve vitrectomy for either extremely severe cases, in which case the vision is really obscured most of the time from very, very, very severe floaters, or the unusual case where a patient is mentally obsessed by them (there are some patients like that who simply just cannot live with vitreous floaters). However, the main reason why doctors do not do this operation on everybody is because this particular operation does have a negative effect on the eye. It is a positive effect if you have a diabetic hemorrhage and you need to extract all the blood out of your eye, it is a positive effect if you've got membranes growing across your retina. In these cases the risk/benefit ratio is satisfactory. But for an otherwise healthy individual who just has eye floaters, removing the gel sometimes is not the best thing to do because past age 40, with the way the surgery is carried out today, where the gel is simply replaced with the normal aqueous that is secreted within the eye, the patient is almost guaranteed to have a cataract within two or three years, or maybe even sooner than that. So you're looking at a second operation. Therefore, ophthalmologists are very unwilling to take a younger person who has no other eye pathology and actually do something surgically for them.

### *Laser Treatment*

Fortunately, we have another option. We can treat them with lasers. The procedure takes, on average, roughly ten minutes. Most ophthalmologists do not even know that this can be done, nor are they interested. At present there are only two surgeons in the US that are offering laser surgery for floaters, myself and John Karicoff who practices in the Washington DC area. Target a neodymium YAG laser at a floater and it will break it up, and destroy it. Neodymium YAG lasers are commonly used in ophthalmology to open little membranes in the lens after cataract surgery. So how do we avoid hitting the retina? This laser is focused. It is focused to a point of 6 microns, which is about the size of a white blood cell. The beam is focused on the floater, and the pulse of the laser lasts for $10^{-9}$ seconds, or one nanosecond. The energy delivered to the target is approximately 4 millijoules, which is a very small amount of energy, but when you are talking about concentrating those 4 millijoules on a 6-micron spot for $10^{-9}$ seconds you're talking about a relatively tremendous amount of energy.

When energy is targeted at such a small point like this electrons are actually stripped from atoms. It creates a state of matter that we call plasma. The electrons jump up and down a couple of quantums, and when they come back down they release photons, which is light. The photons create a secondary mechanical shockwave, which is similar to a static electricity spark. So it's actually not the stripping of electrons that helps us, it is really the secondary mechanical shockwave. That is what is breaking apart these floaters.

Treatment can take anywhere between two and six hundred shots with the laser, and sometimes it takes more than one treatment to adequately treat the problem. Treating floaters in this way does not always mean that we are dissolving 100% of them. Sometimes we can only remove a floater from the visual access or decrease its density. Since the vitreous is a gel, these opacities are not bouncing off the walls like a ping-pong ball. They are just floating in a general sphere. The floater tends to become problematic for the patient if it happens to be in the visual access. So we break up these opacities.

What is the success rate for this procedure? The success rate depends on the type of floater that is present. Approximately 95% of people with Weiss rings, which are little ring-like opacities, report a high level of success. Whereas, 80% to 90% of patients with what I consider a fibular degenerative plump, rate the procedure as very successful. What about risk? As with any medical procedure, there is a certain amount of risk attached. At the South Florida Eye Clinic, approximately 3,000 to 4,000 patients have been treated with this procedure. Approximately eight patients experienced intraocular pressure rise, and five or six developed small microhemorrhages in the choroid, which is the layer behind the retina, however they all resolved. One or two patients have developed cataracts, which are a potential problem with this type of treatment, however the more experienced the surgeon is, the less of a problem cataract should be. A retinal detachment, which is what most ophthalmologists would consider to be a problem, is not really a problem. In 15 years, just one patient, has reported having a detachment after treatment.

## CONCLUDING REMARKS

Our proteins are being broken down as we speak. We are being bombarded with cosmic rays, x-rays, gamma rays, radio waves, and whatever we ate for breakfast, or drank or smoked last night. We have to say that nutritional and environmental factors do play a part in the development of vitreous floaters, just like they play a part with probably all other degenerative conditions. Certain people might have a predisposition towards certain things through various genetic factors that are unknown to us at this time. Traditional cures can sometimes cause problems that are worse than the disease itself, however as we have learned that laser treatment is a viable alternative to surgery for the treatment of vitreous floaters.

## ABOUT THE AUTHOR

Dr. Geller received his medical degree from Rush University Medical School in Chicago, Illinois. He received additional training at Presbyterian Hospital, San Francisco in medical surgery, Sinai Hospital Kresge Eye Institute in ophthalmology, the Michigan Eye Institute on refractive eye surgery, and Brompton Hospital, London, in the UK. He is a board certified ophthalmic surgeon and founder and medical director of the South Florida Eye Clinic. Dr. Geller was one of the first American eye surgeons to lecture in China and has returned four times to continue his educational work.

# Chapter 11

# Plastic Surgery and Anti-Aging: A Natural Combination

*Robert L Peterson, M.D.*
*Chief of Surgery, Kapiolani Medical Center;*
*Associate Professor of Surgery, University of Hawaii*

## ABSTRACT

The aim of this paper is to discuss plastic surgery and its relationship with anti-aging medicine. We will consider how specific procedures can benefit from anti-aging therapy, and the mechanics of combining a plastic surgery practice with an anti-aging practice.

**Keywords:** internal environment; external appearance; medical practice specialization; professional specialty collaboration

## INTRODUCTION

Anti-aging medicine is designed to optimize the internal environment. It is concerned with medical treatments at the cellular level: antioxidants, mitochondrial health, avoiding the degenerative changes at the cellular/molecular level, and optimizing things from the bottom up: starting with the mitochondria, the cell, the organ, and then the whole body. The treatments are designed to reverse the degenerative changes that are associated with aging. So the role of anti-aging medicine is to optimize the internal environment, with the assumption that this will increase health, vitality, function, and ultimately longevity. This optimization should also help to increase a person's ability to function in a competitive world. This process requires constant fine-tuning. As the body ages, there are natural changes in the hormonal environment and in degenerative changes, requiring changes in the therapies to optimize their internal environment change. This, then, is a lifelong process, with a long-term partnership between the patient and the anti-aging provider. Anti-aging therapy is the ultimate in preventive care. If preventive care were totally effective, then secondary treatments would not be necessary.

What sorts of secondary treatments are there? Well, if anti-aging therapy to prevent heart disease is ineffective, then the patient might need cardiac surgery; for example, coronary artery bypass graft surgery (CABG). If anti-osteoporosis treatment is not effective, then the patient may develop a hip fracture and need orthopedic surgery. If you can't prevent cataracts and degenerative changes in the eye with anti-aging therapies, then eye surgery may be necessary. Many people may need a hearing aid when they get older. A patient may have tooth decay and periodontal disease that requires oral implants. In urology, frequent procedures are performed because of benign prostatic hypertrophy (BPH). In OB-GYN, surgery is performed for incontinence. And finally, there is plastic surgery, which is treating the appearance changes that are related to aging. Ideally, none of these secondary treatments would be necessary, and possibly a hundred years from now we'll look back on them and consider them antiquated.

## PLASTIC SURGERY

Plastic surgery addresses changes in appearance that are due to the effects of gravity, to the loss of elasticity in the skin, to sun damage, and to lifestyle choices such as tobacco and alcohol. Cosmetic surgery is designed to alter the external environment, thereby altering the way in which the person interacts with their social environment. Changing a person's appearance can change the way that the world reacts to the person, creating changes in their social stature. These changes alter the balance of power between patients and the external world, increasing their ability to function in a competitive world. It is astonishing what a simple change in appearance can do to the way people react to the patient; this change then changes the way that they react to the world.

The most popular example of something that makes a huge change in the way that the world interacts with somebody in American society is breast augmentation. It is well accepted that by augmenting a woman's breasts it very much changes the way that the world interacts with the patient, giving her a different power equation in interactions with her environment. This is probably the reason why breast augmentation is so popular. There is no other procedure that can so predictably change the balance of power in such a radical and immediate a way.

Thus, plastic surgery optimizes the external environment of a person. But plastic surgery is episodic and typically does not involve long-term treatment plans. A person comes in, they have surgery, and it is done. It is a single-treatment event that, hopefully, will last for a long time, and not require constant care. Ten years later the patient may come back and ask the surgeon to treat something else, or the surgeon may never see them again. Thus, plastic surgery has a completely different practice philosophy than that of anti-aging medicine.

However, many patients want it all; they want optimal health, appearance, and function. They want to optimize their internal environment and they want to optimize their external environment. So by changing their internal environment with supplements, vitamins, nutritional advice, and various other anti-aging therapies we can hope to help them maintain optimal function. We then optimize their social environment through appropriate cosmetic surgical interventions if those internal changes don't prevent the changes that aging has on appearance.

There is a tendency in the plastic surgery world to try and provide both sets of services within the plastic surgery practice. But the skill sets involved are very, very different and the risks, in terms of medical malpractice and risk to the patient, are very different. Plastic surgeons are surgeons. They think in terms of episodic treatment. They think in terms of a quick fix. They are thus ill suited by temperament and by training to do anti-aging medicine. Nonetheless, there is a strong movement within the plastic surgery community to do anti-aging medicine, and that is because plastic surgery has traditionally been at the top of the mind when people think of anti-aging. The facelift is the canonical, iconographic example of what an anti-aging therapy is, and that is highly associated with plastic surgery. As a consequence, in an attempt to capture this additional business, plastic surgeons are tempted to try anti-aging medicine.

The Plastic Surgery Society gives several anti-aging seminars every year. These seminars cover much of the same information as the American Academy of Anti-Aging Medicine (A4M) meetings and other anti-aging meetings, but with a focus towards bringing it into the specialty of plastic surgery. It is not clear whether this is a sustainable trend or merely a fad.

Combining the skills and knowledge of anti-aging medicine and plastic surgery makes good sense. The problem is that one is a lifelong treatment; the other is an episodic treatment. The training involved in both is very different. As anti-aging medicine continues to develop a core body of expertise that takes time to master, it will become increasing difficult to maintain competence in both fields, and the fields will separate. The presumption, by the patients, by the medical profession, and by the legal profession, is that specialty practice means that you are familiar with the entire corpus of knowledge of that field. Therefore it is better to have two specialists: an anti-aging specialist working with the plastic surgeon, to provide patients access to both and to provide synergies in the way that the care is delivered.

## HOW DO PLASTIC SURGERY AND ANTI-AGING WORK TOGETHER?

How do we make these two very, very different disciplines work together? What areas are the most productive areas of collaboration? How does anti-aging medicine affect plastic surgery?

Plastic surgery deals with the external changes in appearance that come with age: changes in hair distribution, gravitational changes, skin color changes, wrinkles, and the involutional changes, such as loss of fullness in the dorsum of the hands, the face, and the lips, that occur with aging.

However, there are a lot of changes that occur with age that plastic surgery does not really address, such as vein prominence, changes in fat metabolism, voice changes, and nose and ear lengthening. Can these aging things be prevented? Can an active anti-aging therapist come into a plastic surgeon's office and help the surgeon prevent the changes of aging rather than correcting them once they have advanced?

Some things probably can be changed by changes in the cellular environment. Avoiding free radicals is good common sense, and good nutrition and antioxidants seem to help lessen changes due to aging. There are other treatments that change the cellular environment, and these can be modified with anti-aging expertise as well. The classic example of this is the application of retinoids, which are vitamin A derivatives. Retinoids go to the nucleus of the cell, and change the expression of the DNA at the molecular level, and that changes the way that the skin appears. It changes the thickness of the dermis and the thickness of the epidermis. This is the first example of many treatments that we will have in the next 10 to 15 years that are going to change things at the molecular level that will then have expression at the phenotypic level. Most people interested in anti-aging medicine are familiar with hormonal manipulation of fat cells. Testosterone decreases total body fat and increases muscle; so there is the possibility of using hormones to treat fat. As we get more experienced we may be able to target these hormones so that we have involution of fat in areas where we do not want it: around the middle, inner tube area; and preservation of fat in the areas where we wish we had more: like the face and the dorsum of the hands. We can also prevent hair loss. Finasteride is a testosterone-blocking drug that can retard hair loss. Minoxidil is a drug that increases circulation to the scalp, and that can also retard hair loss. We can manipulate fibroblasts using a leukotriene modifier. There are going to be more and more things that we can do in this arena, where we can use supplements or medications to alter the body at the phenotypic level.

Some things, however, cannot be changed. We cannot change the effect of gravity effects unless we move to the moon. The genetic clock: the unraveling of DNA in a programmed manner to cause expression of certain things at certain times in life, such as menopause, and presbyopia; the inability to see close objects clearly as you get into your forties and fifties, this cannot be changed. These things seem to be programmed into us, and at present, we do not have an effective method of changing them. We also cannot currently address the Hayflick phenomenon, which suggests that cells seem to have a predestined number of divisions. This seems to place a limit on regenerative capacity, and wear and tear changes thus accumulate over time.

At present there are some very interesting studies being conducted on elastin in the skin, showing that the accumulation of sun damage in the skin causes irreversible changes in elastin. Elastin is laid down at birth, and the elastin that a person is born with is the elastin that they will die with. The body has a very limited ability to repair elastin. Cigarette smoke damages elastin by triggering the activation of matrix metalloproteins. It is also thought to be damaged by sunlight. So lifestyle choices, such as cigarette smoking, clearly can accelerate the changes of aging.

Thus, it makes sense that we can also minimize these changes by making lifestyle modifications. Does caloric restriction affect aging changes? It does in every animal model that has been studied; thus it stands to reason that this would apply to humans as well, but this is unproven. There are researchers that are trying this experiment right now. Obviously, it is an experiment that will take a long time to yield results. Avoiding smoking is clearly important for maintaining elastin, and elastin is very important not only in the skin but also in the blood vessels, and in helping to keep the blood vessels pliable. If we keep the blood vessels pliable we can help to avoid hypertensive changes and aortic dissections, and things of that only in the skin but also in the blood vessels, and in helping to keep the blood vessels pliable. If we keep the blood vessels pliable we can help to avoid hypertensive changes and aortic dissections, and things of that nature. Exercise is very important. Exactly how much you need, what the least amount you need is, and how much is safe, are still not entirely clear. What is certain is that exercise is clearly beneficial. Dietary supplements and fiber are beneficial as well. Fiber has been under-emphasized by the anti-aging society. There are studies that clearly show an unequivocal benefit to fiber in a variety of different conditions. The problem with fiber is that it's unpalatable. It either doesn't taste good or it causes bloating or gassiness. Developing more palatable fiber supplements would therefore be a very good idea. Other simple lifestyle modifications (e.g. wearing a seatbelt) can also contribute to longevity.

Thus, despite limitations, there are changes that we can make to optimize the internal environment. What about the external appearance? By changing somebody's appearance you can make them more alert and vibrant and more appealing. Surgery can give a cleaner line. The human eye tends to likes things that are smooth so this looks better and also more youthful. By combating or camouflaging the signs of aging, we can reduce the perception that someone is too old to do something: too old to work for them, too old to date, too old to have fun, or any of the other social stigmas attributed to age.

## PLASTIC SURGERY PROCEDURES

People associate certain changes in appearance with aging. These include: wrinkling of the skin, sagging of the skin, a loss of fullness in the lower face, wrinkling around the eye, narrowing of the eye aperture, lengthening of the earlobes and the growth of the scapha in the ears (which continue to grow throughout life), wrinkling in the forehead, descent of the eyebrows, lengthening of the nose, loss of fullness in the lips, and sagging in the neck. These are just some of the clues of aging. Others include male pattern baldness, which usually starts in the twenties and advances through the twenties, thirties, forties and progresses over a lifetime. Graying of the hair is another example.

Can graying of hair be changed? Yes it can to some degree. Chelation therapy has been said to reverse some graying of the hair, and there may be antioxidants or other ways of reducing gray hair. Reducing stress certainly seems to keep it from coming out. Stress reduction would be a nice adjunct to an anti-aging practice in a plastic surgeons office.

Male pattern baldness is due to the action of 5-hydroxytestosterone, which can be blocked by Propecia®, or finasteride. Rogaine® is also used to increase blood supply in the hair areas. If that does not work, then you can resort to hair restoration techniques, such as hair transplantation. The results achievable with hair transplantation are now pretty good. You do not get the cornrow look that was very common in earlier hair transplantation. It is also possible to reduce the size of the bald spot by cutting it out and stretching the other skin over it to cover it. That is called flap surgery. However, flap surgery is much less common now with advent of micrograft hair transplantation techniques.

There is also female pattern hair loss, which isn't balding in a specific area like the top of the head or the back of the head. It is just thinning of the hair all over. Female pattern hair loss is less amenable to surgical treatment because the surgeon would be taking thin hair from one place and putting in as thin hair in another. However, female pattern hair loss does seem to respond quite well to minoxidil. In addition, supplements may considerably improve female and male pattern hair loss.

The forehead is a good area for improving appearance. The forehead widens with age because the brow descends and the hairline recedes. A variety of things can be done to treat this. Changing the hairstyle is probably the most common solution. People will wear bangs to camouflage the fact that their hairline is moving up. Another common thing is for women to pluck the eyebrows and draw, or even tattoo, the eyebrow higher to camouflage the fact that the eyebrow has descended. Surgical options include brow line hair transplantation to lower the hairline, or a browlift to smooth out the wrinkles in the forehead and in the glabella region. A browlift can actually make somebody look brighter and possibly even younger. Few surgical procedures will make a patient look younger because there are so many clues to a person's age, however a browlift actually can make somebody look younger. Forehead wrinkling can also be treated with the most common and most popular treatment now, which is Botox®. Botox® works very well for paralyzing muscle activity in the forehead in the frontalis, in the area of the crow's feet on the side, and in the area of the glabella. Botox® is a very safe procedure. Literally millions of doses of Botox® are given every year in the US, and the incidence of reported complications is very, very low. Chemical peels can also smooth out the skin. This is more effective in areas where the lines are ironed in and are not from muscle activity. Chemical peels can also smooth out sun damage, and this is very beneficial. This is an interesting point because a chemical peel is a plastic surgical anti-aging therapy in the sense that it reverses the signs of sun damage. But it is not a cellular or biological anti-aging therapy. It changes the skin, it causes the top layers of skin to peel off, and then the cells regenerate. But it does not undo the changes themselves. It does it by relying on the body's regenerative capacity. So this is the current paradigm of reversing aging changes by taking away the aging change and letting the body make something new. As we get more sophisticated in our understanding, perhaps we will have ways that can actually reverse the changes, per se.

As we know, multiple changes occur to the eye with age. These include: cataracts, presbyopia, macular degeneration, retinal detachment, pterygium, and dry eye syndrome. Can these be prevented? It has been difficult to demonstrate a very significant effect of antioxidants or supplements so far, but perhaps better ones will be developed or more targeted combinations will be able to show better benefit. There has just been a report that anti-inflammatory medicines may be effective for dry eye syndrome. For cataracts, the lens can be replaced. And patients with stiffening of the lens can wear glasses or contact lenses or undergo Lasik® surgery. The eyes also change in appearance as we age. Making the eyes look brighter tends to make people look brighter, and more awake. Wrinkling and crows feet can be improved with botox or with surgery. Sagging of the eyes generally requires surgical intervention. Looking at the upper eyes, can you prevent excess skin and excess fat on the upper eyelid? Avoiding weight changes is always good advice, although whether that expansion and decrease in the eyelid fat pads causes the skin to stretch out is arguable. Avoiding the sun and tobacco are certainly important. However, from a preventative viewpoint there is not much that can be done. By taking away the extra eyelid skin, which is basically the only way that this problem can be treated, it is possible to make the eyes look brighter and better. Excess skin and fat accumulates on the lower eyelids as well. There may be treatments in the future to dissolve that fat. But at present the only way is to remove it surgically. By doing a forehead lift and eyelid surgery together you can certainly brighten up the area around the eye. Eyelid wrinkling can be treated with Botox® and Retin-A.

A number of methods of preventing and treating facial skin aging are available. Photo-aging is a consequence of UV radiation-induced changes and smoking. It stimulates the matrix metalloproteins, and this affects collagen as well as elastin. Thus, using a sunscreen, and not smoking are simple ways to prevent aging of facial skin. Taking antioxidant supplements may also be of benefit. There is nothing that can really be done to prevent sagging of the skin as it is caused by gravity. The only real treatment for sagging is a facelift: if you take away the extra skin and lift it up, it gives cleaner lines and can improve things. In the lips and in the face, it is possible to take fat from someplace else in the body and move it to the lips or the face. This fat grafting can fill in contours that hollow out with age. We cannot yet manipulate the fat cells themselves *in situ*, but we can move the fat around and that redistribution can help. Wrinkles are caused by either wrinkling the muscle back and forth, or by gravitational changes. These can be improved by botox or by surgery.

Ears continue to grow throughout your life. The reason that they continue to grow is that the cartilaginous structures keep growing. Bony structures fuse. The epiphyses fuse, but the cartilage keeps growing and the ear lobes keep growing. This is why in the Far East long ear lobes are associated with long life. Buddha, who had a very long life, had big ear lobes. It is possible to remedy this surgically.

The nose also continues to grow throughout life. It is the cartilaginous part that keeps on growing, not the bone. Thus, leading to a longer nose and the drooping of the nasal tip, or a "witch's nose." The drooping of the nose can be corrected by surgery.

The lips lose fullness with age. That loss of fullness loses the allure of the young lip as well as causing wrinkling because the lips deflate. Once again, this can be prevented to some degree by avoiding the sun, or using a good sunscreen, and not smoking. It can also be remedied by putting fat, collagen, or a number of other substances, back into the lips to fill them back up. The skin around the lips can also be smoothed out by laser treatment. That does not address the deflation, but at least it smoothes out the wrinkling.

Teeth also change with age. Resorption of bone, periodontal disease, and accumulated trauma, all have a major impact on dentistry. It is possible to prevent some of these changes by practicing good oral hygiene; diet, flossing, fluoride treatments, and they can be treated with a variety of dental treatments. However, if a tooth is broken or lost it is gone for good. It can only be restored or replaced with an artificial alternative.

As we age, the neck skin sags and we get the "turkey gobbler" deformity. Excess fat accumulates, and the skin is damaged by long-term exposure to sunlight. It is possible to try to prevent some of these changes by losing weight and avoiding the sun, or using a sunscreen. One way of treating neck sagging and fat accumulation is liposuction.

In the body, fat distribution changes with aging and we can recontour this with body sculpting techniques, such as liposuction and lipotransplantation. The breasts also change. Men experience breast growth, while women's breasts sag. The breasts can be reduced, augmented, and lifted. Aging is also evident from the hands.

## INTEGRATING PLASTIC SURGERY AND ANTI-AGING MEDICINE

There are several things that can be done to bring together plastic surgery and anti-aging medicine. Fat and muscle ratios can be improved with hormone replacement therapy. With antioxidant therapy, sun damage to the skin can be at least partially prevented and the elasticity of the skin can be retained. Stem cell cybernetics and transplantation may be of help in the future.

In working together, plastic surgeons and anti-aging therapies can try to optimize the environment for the patient. Many people who visit a plastic surgeon are already taking supplements, but they are taking them in an unsupervised manner, or the clerk at the local health foods store gives the impression that s/he is supervising their supplementation. By having a more expert supervision of the supplements that they are already taking, it is possible to get a better result.

Preoperative management is important. The patient needs to be evaluated and medical risks need to be managed. Patients should also be educated about healthy habits. Encourage the patient to sign up for an online medical summary. This is a free product sponsored by the Hawaii version of the American Red Cross. It is a great online service that enables the patient's medical information to be available anywhere to any provider if they are in an emergency situation. It also provides free translation of the information into a variety of languages.

Perioperatively, the hormonal environment can be managed to give better surgical results. Anabolic steroids in the perioperative period can hasten recovery, and there are several vitamins and minerals that may also be of use.

Postoperatively, the surgeon should turn the patient back to the anti-aging practitioner for the lifelong treatment that is necessary. There are limitations. One is financial. Although high-end cosmetic surgery practices are going to be aimed at the type of patients that an anti-aging physician would be interested in looking at, there are also problems of financial exhaustion. The patient that has just paid for a big procedure may not have the money for anti-aging treatments, and vice versa. Another problem is office use. The best time for an anti-aging physician to visit the cosmetic surgery office is when the office is carrying out surgery because then the rest of the office, that is the consulting rooms, is vacant. The anti-aging physician and the surgeon should also discuss treatments and procedures that each will be carrying out. If the anti-aging physician is using a method that becomes the target of bad press, such as hormone replacement therapy has been in the last few months, then that taints both the surgeon and the anti-aging physician.

High-end cosmetic surgery practices typically do a lot of advertising, and they typically have very nice offices that are vacant for significant periods of time. The staff are used to self-pay patients. These patients are typically very demanding. Anti-aging can be added to perioperative follow-ups, and by establishing expertise in this area a practice will become distinguished from other practices that do not have that level of expertise of anti-aging. The periodic evaluations for anti-aging keep the patient in the practice so that when they require their next surgery they are already ready for it, and are more likely to stay with the same surgeon. The surgery can jump-start the lifestyle changes and get the person into the anti-aging practice.

## CONCLUDING REMARKS

Collaboration of plastic surgeons and anti-aging specialists is a natural collaboration. There is a tremendous opportunity to serve patients better, and to use the synergies of the practice environment to the benefit of both.

## ABOUT THE AUTHOR

Dr. Peterson received his undergraduate degree from Williams College in Williamstown, Massachusetts, and completed a masters degree at Rice University, Houston, Texas. He attended Harvard Medical School where he graduated with his medical degree in 1982. As a physician, Dr. Peterson conducted his Plastic Surgery Residence at Baylor College of Medicine in Houston, Texas, and completed Fellowships in Microsurgical Hand Surgery and Pediatric Reconstructive Surgery in China and Japan. Dr. Peterson is fluent in French and Spanish and has comprehension in German, Russian, Chinese, and Japanese. He holds several US patents and is currently Chief of Surgery at Kapiolani Medical Center and is in private practice in Honolulu, Hawaii.

# Chapter 12

# The Impact of Nuclear Energy in Degenerative Disease

*Burton Goldberg, Hon Doctor of Humanities*
*CEO, Alternativemedicine.com & Publisher, Alternative Medicine Magazine*

## ABSTRACT

Nuclear plants release approximately twenty toxins into the environment, you can't see it, smell it, or feel it. The wind blows it downwind. It falls on the grasses, on the water, on the food, and we inhale it. It goes into the animals, into fruits and vegetables, and it goes into our bodies. This paper will discuss the link between Strontium-90 contamination and cancer incidence, and the effect that nuclear power plants have had on cancer rates in the US.

Keywords: toxic contamination; Strontium-90; cancer

## INTRODUCTION

One of the great enemies of longevity is nuclear energy. Nuclear energy emanates from nuclear plants all over the United States. Every nuclear plant spews toxins, and it's measured. Yet the government will not tell you about this, and medicine pays no attention to it. But nuclear energy is one of the greatest deprecators of the immune system.

## NUCLEAR PLANTS AND STRONTIUM-90 CONTAMINATION

Nuclear plants release approximately twenty toxins into the environment, that you cannot see, smell, or feel. Blow downwind, it falls on our everyday environment. Once contaminating the food chain and the air we breathe, it gets into animals, produce, and then into human bodies. The only toxin the government measures is Strontium-90, which can only come from nuclear bombs or nuclear plants. South Florida is one of the greatest purveyors of nuclear energy, with plants at Turkey Point and St. Lucie, and Crystal River.

Once inside the body this radiation is converted to Yttrium-90, which migrates to the various organs and systems in the body. It is insidious. In 1900, 3% of the US population had cancer of any kind. Today, one in two men, that is 50% of men, will develop cancer. American Cancer Society statistics for 1999 revealed that 50% of men and 45% of women developed cancer. These are low numbers. We have an epidemic. Government statistics show that environmental radiation released by nuclear plants has led to increased rates of cancer in children. Cancer rates have risen more significantly in children because children are more susceptible than adults; similarly embryos are more susceptible than toddlers, infants, and teenagers.

It is not only cancer rates that are soaring. Asthma and autism are also on the rise. The incidence of autism in California has risen by hundreds of percent in the last 10 years. Nuclear energy is at least partially responsible for this astounding increase in autism. We know about pesticides and herbicides and heavy metals. You combine these factors together with the toxins being released by nuclear plants, and it spells disaster. Nuclear plants are one of the enemies of longevity medicine.

A study on 19 samples of drinking water in the southeast Florida counties showed that the highest levels of beta radioactivity characteristic of Strontium-90 were found in samples obtained from within five to twenty miles of the Turkey Point and St. Lucie nuclear plants

During 2001 and 2003, the Radiation and Public Health Project (RPHP) carried out a study on the baby teeth of south Florida children. The difference between radiation levels in the teeth of children without cancer ("healthy teeth") and of children with cancer ("cancer teeth") was also studied. Results showed that between 1986-1989 and 1994-1997, there was a 37% increase in the average levels of radioactive Strontium-90 in the baby teeth of children from southeast Florida. This rise reverses a long-term downward trend in Strontium-90 levels that has occurred since the mid 1960's, when the atmospheric testing of nuclear weapons was banned. This temporal trend of increasing levels of radioactive Strontium-90 was found in 485 Florida teeth tested, 95% of which came from six southeast Florida counties. When compared with baby teeth collected from other Florida counties, the highest levels of Strontium-90 were found in the counties closest to the Turkey Point and St. Lucie nuclear plants. The average levels of Strontium-90 found in the 17 cancer teeth were 85% higher than those in the 311 teeth obtained from healthy children born in the same years and in the same counties.

One of the worst areas in this country for Strontium-90 contamination is South Florida. Then comes New York, Chicago, and Philadelphia: the Philadelphia area has nine nuclear plants. The lobsters in Long Island Sound are full of strontium-90. Not in Maine, where the Maine nuclear plant closed many years ago, so Maine lobsters are healthy.

In New Mexico, the Indians eat tortillas with lime: lime blocks the Strontium-90. So one of the most important ways of treating water supplies would be reverse osmosis. A study in the Port St. Lucie area revealed that the water supply contained a tremendous amount of strontium-90. However, when the water was treated by reverse osmosis, the Strontium-90 was removed. It is important to treat both drinking water and shower or bathing water, because the skin is the largest organ in the body, and we get eight times more toxins through the skin via the shower or bath than we do from drinking.

## CONCLUDING REMARKS

The evidence presented shows a clear correlation between Strontium-90 contamination and cancer incidence. The fact that the highest levels of Strontium-90 in water and baby teeth are found in areas close to nuclear power plants, suggests that radiation emissions from these nuclear plants are the predominant cause of these increases, not the fallout from past atmospheric nuclear tests.

## ABOUT THE AUTHOR

Burton Goldberg is a businessman and best-selling author/publisher. He became involved in alternative medicine over 25 years ago when a friend's daughter became ill. Since that time he has traveled to Europe, Russia, China, Mexico, and Israel where he has learned firsthand from alternative practitioners how and why alternative therapies work. The result was the publication in 1994 of a book many refer to as the "Bible of Alternative Medicine," titled *Alternative Medicine The Definitive Guide*. Since that time Mr. Goldberg has begun publishing and distribution of *Alternative Medicine Magazine* and alternativemedicine.com, where he currently serves as Chairman and CEO.

# Chapter 13
# Implications for Medicine: New Energy Biophysics Discoveries

*Eugene Mallove Sc.D.*
*Director, New Energy Research Laboratory*

## ABSTRACT

Our knowledge of biology, medicine, biochemistry, and chemistry is based upon accepted laws of physics. However, if any of this accepted knowledge, the fundamental laws of physics, is flawed, and there is evidence to suggest that three major areas of physics have serious flaws, there are serious repercussions on the other sciences. In this paper, we will consider the existence of such flaws.

Keywords: Aetherometry; cold fusion; hydrogen-derived power

## INTRODUCTION

Physics today in our society, in our technical society, is regarded as the absolute foundation of all other knowledge. And then riding on top of physics, of course, is inorganic chemistry, then organic chemistry, and then above that we have biochemistry, biology, and medicine. That's the way things are set up. Now, if it turns out that there are any flaws in the foundation, and three major areas within physics have serious flaws, there will be a significant effect upon these other sciences.

These areas are cold fusion; the true power of hydrogen (not just the chemical energy as we know it of hydrogen, but the excess energy beyond what we normally thought of as chemistry); and lastly, the area which may, in fact, have most impact on biological systems and our models of the human body and organisms is the new science of Aetherometry, or the Aetherometric Theory of Synchronicity (AtoS).

There is a philosophy spread these days in science that we're nearing the end of science, if you can believe. Nobel Laureate Steven Weinberg encouraged the production of a 53-mile-circumference particle accelerator in the plains of Texas so we could learn the final theory of everything, as he says in his book, *Dreams of a Final Theory*. This man is very uninterested in matters such as cold fusion and so forth. He calls cold fusion a religion. Then we have other people such as Robert Goddard, who launched the world's first liquid fuel rocket. He thought we could go to the moon with such technology and, of course, we eventually did. The *New York Times*, and many silent scientists at the time, was antagonistic to Goddard. The *New York Times* editorialized that we couldn't go to moon because everybody knows that a rocket needs something to push against (which, of course we now know it doesn't) and we couldn't go through space that way. The year 2003 was the 100th anniversary of the Wright Brothers flight on December 17, 1903. Even after they flew on December 17th, there was no major ticker-tape parade for them. In fact, five years went by during which they were flying in broad daylight on Huffman Prairie in Ohio. Flight has been accomplished, controlled heavier-than-air flight, and they were regarded by *Scientific American* and all the Eastern press as frauds. Not too different from what is happening today with respect to these heretical energies.

## THE FLAWS OF PHYSICS

Are the standard biochemical and psychological models of organisms significantly incomplete? The answer is yes. Obviously, we know hormones and amino acids, genetic structure, and the influence of genes on disease. But at the same time we need to know a huge amount more. In addition to the biochemical constituents of the structure of the cell, and of the physiological organization of living organisms is it possible that we've missed something very, very deep and profound that manifests itself in ways that are often regarded as peripheral and unimportant but which may be very fundamental to a lot of the medical issues that we're confronting? So the question is: "What is the evidence of this contention that the main standard model of biochemistry and physiology could be significantly wrong?" The evidence is the efficacy and presumptive mechanisms of some versions of complimentary medicine, or alternative medicine. There is also significant evidence that the foundational paradigms of modern physics and chemistry are either grossly incomplete or seriously flawed. Cold fusion definitely does that. Low-energy nuclear reactions that are occurring at benign conditions without huge high temperatures are very significant pieces of evidence for that contention.

Drs Paulo and Alexandra Correa accidentally discovered excess electrical energy in glass tubes. The pulses that come out of these glass tubes have 10 times the energy of the input power. This finding does not suggest that there is a violation of the conservation of energy occurring here. But it does suggest that there are other sources in the laws of physics of space and time that allow phenomenon like this to occur. You have to take your choice: either this phenomenon is correct and measured properly in the laboratory, or there is some kind of a scam going on here. The Correas have been working on this for 15 years. They have never received any government money. These are the US patents, starting in 1995: patent 5416391, patent 5449989, and patent 5502354. All those patents enable one to build the entire system and reproduce it. Not to use it commercially, of course, but at least to test it out. Since that time, there has been very little interest in anyone doing that.

There was an interesting article about acupuncture in *Newsweek* some time ago. The article talked about some very interesting research using functional MRI with acupuncture. The study the article was concerned about *New Findings of the Correlation between Accupoints and Corresponding Brain Cortices Using Functional MRI* by Jones *et al* was published in the *Proceedings of the National Academy of Sciences* in March 1998. This study was concerned with a point called the BL-67 point on the ankle region of the foot, which is known in Oriental medicine to stimulate the occipital lobe and improve vision. With functional MRI, you can almost instantly see the brain light up and, therefore identify which cortex of the brain is being affected by the stimulus. Jones et al found that, just like a light switch, when they stimulated the BL-67 point it triggered the visual cortex. They did it not only with traditional needles and so forth, which would, of course, allow for a placebo-like effect, unlikely as that is with the on-off feature. They did it with ultrasound so that the subject himself could not even know whether it was being stimulated, and they found the same phenomenon. So here we have an organ system in the body, precisely locating a point, a very specific point, within fractions of a millimeter, that goes from the foot to the brain. There is no wiring set up for that. Worse for modern medicine, and a glib belief that we know everything about biology and physiology, was that the transmission speed from the ankle to the brain was found to be at least 1,000 times the speed of any nerve conduction process. The capture zone of the functional MRI (80 microseconds) is such that it can only determine the transmission speed up to that. It might even be faster. So something is going on in the body that suggests that we still have a lot to learn.

Why was this paper published in the *Proceedings of the National Academy of Sciences* and not in *Nature* or *Science*? The team of physicians, which included people from Tokyo University, tried to take it to *Science* first. It was rejected without review, a standard operating procedure today by the scientific establishment. If something is regarded as preposterous to begin with, it does not get reviewed, period. They took it to *Nature*, and the same thing happened. Five Nobel Laureates in the biological sciences who were very impressed with the paper wrote a letter to *Nature* saying that the study should be published. *Nature* still refused. That's the way the system works. So given that kind of mindset today in the scientific establishment, that something like proof of acupuncture's functionality in a very specific way, what else is being discarded?

Another interesting study by Benveniste *et al* entitled *Human Basophil Degranulation Triggered by Very Dilute Antiserum Against IgE* was published in Nature back in 1988. I won't go into this in a deep way. A very important book was written about this. Jacques Benveniste, a world-famous French immunologist, did this work *in vitro* using basophils that were degranulated to test homeopathic dilutions which, in theory, after thirty-fold X $1/10^{30}$ power dilution, there was the probability of one in a million that there was even one molecule left. Yet, the dilution affected the basophils. *Nature* published this paper, while at the same time saying that while they couldn't find any mistakes they were sure that the findings were wrong. However, other hospitals around the world have reproduced this work. So if there is a functional underlying mechanism, unlikely as it seems: a magnetic tray or whatever you want to call it; a memory of water, we certainly have a major gap in our physiological understanding.

Are there sources of energy, heretofore unrecognized within the framework of conventional, advanced, non-renewable, and renewable energy sources? Something beyond conventional fission even, or hot fusion, which is only being researched today. We have already spent $15 to 17 billion dollars on hot fusion. The Department of Energy actually does not know how much has been spent on it. But we have spent billions and billions of dollars on lasers beaming in and hitting little pellets of heavy hydrogen or tritium. Tokamak reactors using hundreds of millions of degrees at Princeton and MIT are trying to mimic the conditions of the sun to make fusion on earth, but in a controlled fashion, not like in thermonuclear weapons. And we have deuterium, which is heavy water. Deuterium is present in all water; $1/6,000^{th}$ or one $1/6,700^{th}$ of all water has heavy water in it. Now if these two heavy hydrogen nuclei from the heavy hydrogen in water fuse together, as the hot fusion people would like to do it at millions of degrees, they fuse together and make helium. If that happens, you have fusion and a lot of radiation as well. So it is a very large source of energy. In fact, in one gallon of ordinary water, any water, equals 300 gallons of gasoline energy equivalent. That is why so much money has been poured into the hot fusion program, because if we ever do manage to get a football stadium-sized reactor doing hot fusion we have got an infinite energy source. Using hot fusion or cold fusion, all the oil reserves on Earth come from one cubic kilometer of ocean water. So we won't need oil, and we certainly won't need fission nuclear power, if we achieve fusion.

Pons and Fleischmann announced that they had discovered cold fusion in 1989. The data was building up, going positive, but experts in hot fusion at MIT were saying it was negative. These were two exceptional scientists, Martin Fleischmann, Royal Society Member, world-famous electrochemist, and Stanley Pons, head of the chemistry department at the University of Utah. They had a little cell in a bath of unitemperature water. The cell contained heavy water and had a palladium cathode and a platinum anode. They measured the temperatures carefully. They found out that there was an excess heat that they could not explain. Moreover, the excess heat was so large that they said it was nuclear scale. Furthermore, they said they were getting some tritium evidence: radioactive tritium that should not have been there; and they were getting some evidence of neutrons. They also thought that there might also be helium, although they did not measure the helium. This became a gigantic story in the press: *Fusion Illusion - How Two Obscure Chemists Stirred Excitement and Outrage in the World*, *The Race for Fusion - The Scientific Debate - Why the Stakes Are So High*, and *Miracle or Mistake? Fusion in a Bottle*. All of these stories were printed on May 8, 1989.

There are still scientists investigating cold fusion at the Los Alamos National Laboratory, Dr. Tom Claytor and the Tuggle group, who, in a modified cold fusion experiment, repeatedly got radioactive tritium produced in a low-energy system that should never produce it. Just like the cold fusion process. This has all been published. The Electric Power Research Institute funded Dr Michael McKubre and his group at SRI International, a prestigious research firm in Palo Alto, California, to study cold fusion. Their final conclusion, which was reached in 1994, was that their findings confirmed the claims of Fleischmann, Pons, and Hawkins that deuterium-loaded palladium cathodes produce excess heat at levels too large for chemical transformation. They also said that they had nuclear evidence. Dr. McKubre's group used another type of cold fusion in the gas phase, using heavy hydrogen gas, producing helium growing over time. But the helium was consistent with the expected nuclear release, without radiation, for those kinds of reactions that the hot fusion people would say produce helium. NASA confirmed one of the kinds of cold fusion using light water in a NASA report published in February 1996. Then a man from Florida, a former Ph.D. working for Dow Chemical Corporation, Dr. James Patterson, came up with a cell. Another way of doing cold fusion, in which he had little plastic beads coated with nickel and palladium in ordinary water and he got excess heat. They put water through, water came out hotter: 15 degrees centigrade hotter. Motorola tested this type of cell and found that they could turn off the input power and the cell would continue to produce 20 watts continuously for days. The power going into these cells, as measured by current and voltage, was a fraction of a watt.

So why aren't people wanting to invest in cold fusion? Remember the Wright Brothers. They were flying in broad daylight for years, yet *Scientific American* and many other people still called them frauds. In March 1999, *Time* magazine published an article entitled: "The century gave us scientific superstars like Freud and Einstein, but it also produced its share of cranks, villains, and unsung heroes." The cranks and villains this article referred to were Pons and Fleischmann and a man by the name of Wilhelm Reich.

Reich was deemed to be a complete madman. He died in 1957 in federal prison for allegedly selling an anti-cancer device called an orgone accumulator, which is nothing but a Faraday cage covered with layers of dielectric and steel wool. By the way, there is significant anecdotal evidence that the orgone accumulator may be beneficial to some medical conditions. In 1941, Wilhelm Reich asked Albert Einstein to investigate something for him. There ensued a giant correspondence between Reich and Einstein. "Dear Albert, please measure the thermal, the temperature, difference between an air-suspended thermometer in the room, in a dark room; and the thermometer right over a metal Faraday cage. You will find a difference." Einstein, to his credit, found a difference and agreed there was $3/10^{th}$ of a degree Celsius difference. However, Einstein's assistant, Leopold Infeld, interfered and said that the finding could be explained away. Just like the skeptics dismissed cold fusion many years later in 1989. Therefore, the opportunity was missed for Einstein to turn around on the subject of a possible ether that was not encompassed by his Theory of Relativity. By the way, all the equations of Relativity work beautifully, and describe nuclear experiments very well.

So you might ask, "How is it then that cold fusion scientists are seriously suggesting that there might be some flaws in Relativity and other basic theories of physics?" The answer is quite simple. Just because a formula within a theory fits a particular experiment, or many experiments, it does not mean that the experiments describe the right theory. The theory that is true for the universe could be quite different and, in my opinion, probably is.

The Serbian scientist Nikola Tesla was coming close to the proper physics of the universe. Tesla became known for giving exhibitions in his laboratory in which he lighted lamps without wires by allowing electricity to flow through his body. He died a pauper in 1943 in New York, even though all the electrical technology in our civilization today: including radio, for which he did not get credit, although the Supreme Court awarded him credit for it posthumously. Contrary to public belief, Marconi did not invent radio. Marconi made the first transatlantic broadcast, but he was not the inventor of radio. That example shows how even the credit for something, in just a few generations, can disappear, and history can be rewritten.

## CONCLUDING REMARKS

To conclude, there are extreme flaws in the process and structure of contemporary science that have led to many present unsupportable false dogmas. Einstein's Relativity Theory is incontrovertible; no, it is not. The universe is nothing but atoms and space-time. Yes, the universe had a beginning, but the so-called evidence for the Big Bang in unconvincing. The theory of Evolution is obviously true. However, many scientists, for example Lynn Margulis, the famous biologist and former wife of Carl Sagan, and her son, Dorian Sagan, are criticizing one of the key issues in evolution. There is no question that life evolved on earth. But did it evolve in an environmental natural selection process? Of course, there is some of that. No doubt about it. But if you go and check the latest theories of symbiosis and a reconstitution of not the original Lamarckian theory, but other types of Lamarckism, you will find that Darwinism by natural selection is on shaky ground. The second law of thermodynamics is one of the most incontrovertible laws in physics. But in our own laboratory, and in conferences sponsored in the United States by some physics departments and published in a major academic book prestigious scientists are seriously questioning the validity of the second law, that would suggest that we cannot make a machine that uses the heat in the room to run a machine doing work; that is, take a uniform temperature reservoir and make work out of it. But these scientists, signing their names to heretical physics documents and simulations and experiments, are saying, yes, it might happen. A complex ether exists which pervades the universe and which facilitates the creation and destruction of matter continuously. Contemporary physics, for all its apparent effectiveness, is fatally flawed and must be rewritten, and we can extract infinite energy in the form of electrical energy and heat.

## REFERENCES

Cho ZH, Chung SC, Jones JP, Park JB, Park HJ, Lee HJ, Wong EK, Min BI. New findings of the correlation between acupoints and corresponding brain cortices using functional MRI. *Proc Natl Acad Sci U S A*. 1998;95:2670-2673.

Davenas E, Beauvais F, Amara J, Oberbaum M, Robinzon B, Miadonna A, Tedeschi A, Pomeranz B, Fortner P, Belon P, et al. Human basophil degranulation triggered by very dilute antiserum against IgE. *Nature*. 1988;333:816-818.

"The century gave us scientific superstars like Freud and Einstein, but it also produced its share of cranks, villains, and unsung heroes." *Time*. 1999;March 29:111.

## ABOUT THE AUTHOR

Dr. Mallove served as president of the New Energy Institute, a Concord, New Hampshire-based nonprofit organization aimed at educating the world about the possibilities of new energy. He also served as editor-in-chief of its magazine, *Infinite Energy*. Previously, Dr. Mallove worked as an engineer in the private sector, then as chief science writer at the Massachusetts Institute of Technology. Dr. Mallove received his bachelor's and master's degrees in aeronautical and astronautical engineering at MIT, then earned his ScD from Harvard. Dr. Mallove passed away in May 2004.

# Chapter 14
# Towards a Better Vaccine For Alzheimer's Disease

Dr. Kevin A. Da Silva and Dr. Joanne McLaurin
*Centre for Research in Neurodegenerative Diseases & Departments of Laboratory Medicine and Pathobiology, University of Toronto, Toronto, Ontario, Canada*

## ABSTRACT

Alzheimer's disease (AD) is a progressive neurodegenerative disease characterized by two pathological lesions: senile plaques composed of amyloid-ß (Aß) peptide and neurofibrillary tangles consisting of hyperphosphorylated tau protein. Knowledge gained from studies of familial forms of AD led to the generation of transgenic mouse models, in which the first immunization paradigms were tested. Both active and passive immunization strategies reduced AD-like pathology and restored cognitive deficits in transgenic mice. These results were initially met with considerable optimism; however, Phase IIa clinical trials were halted due to a small but significant occurrence of meningoencephalitis. Knowledge gained from studies on Aß immunotherapy will allow optimization of new generation vaccines, targeting highly specific epitopes while reducing undesired side-effects. In harnessing and steering the immune system, an effective response can be generated against what is now believed to be the causative agent of synaptic loss and cognitive decline in AD patients: Aß. If this proves successful, Aß vaccination could provide the first definitive treatment for AD.

Keywords: amyloid-ß (Aß) peptide; hyperphosphorylated tau protein; neurofibrillary tangles; amyloid cascade hypothesis; immunotherapy

## INTRODUCTION

Alzheimer's disease (AD) is the most common cause of age-related cognitive decline, affecting more than 12 million people worldwide (Citron, 2002). Originally described by Alois Alzheimer in 1906, the disease is characterized in its earlier stages by progressive memory impairment and cognitive decline, altered behavior and language deficits. Later, patients present with global amnesia and slowing of motor functions, with death typically occurring within nine years of diagnosis (Davis *et al* 1998; Selkoe, 2001). Current drug therapy aims at slowing cognitive decline and ameliorating the affective and behavioral symptoms associated with disease progression. This however is of little value, as these drugs provide limited symptomatic treatment, without targeting what many scientists believe is the underlying cause of AD; that is, the deposition and neurotoxic effects of amyloid-ß (Aß) peptide. Immunization of AD patients provides a novel means of specifically targeting this protein and will be the topic of this review.

## THE AMYLOID CASCADE HYPOTHESIS

A definitive diagnosis of AD can only be made by postmortem examination of the brain. AD is characterized histopathologically by two classical lesions: extracellular deposits of Aß in senile (neuritic) plaques and intraneuronal neurofibrillary tangles composed of hyperphosphorylated tau; in addition to synaptic and neuronal cell loss (Selkoe, 2001). The former are insoluble deposits typically found in the limbic and association cortices, as well as in cerebral blood vessel walls. Ultrastructurally, these plaques are comprised of a fibrillar amyloid core, surrounded by a dark halo of dystrophic neurites, typically found associated with activated microglia and astrocytes (Selkoe, 2001). The main constituent of amyloid consists of a 40-43 amino acid peptide and is derived from the proteolytic cleavage of a family of ubiquitously expressed membrane-spanning proteins, termed the amyloid precursor proteins (APP) (Li et al, 1999). Under normal conditions, the most abundant species in the brain is the Aß (1-40) peptide (Aß 40), however much of the fibrillar Aß is comprised of the longer, more fibrillogenic Aß 1-42 peptide (Aß 42) (Selkoe, 2001). By way of an unknown mechanism, these normally soluble and innocuous peptides undergo conformational change and polymerize into an aggregated (fibrillar) and toxic form, rich in ß-structure (McLaurin et al, 2000). Initially, Aß 42 is deposited in an immature, diffuse (nonfibrillar) plaque, with little or no detectable neuritic dystrophy. These are thought to represent precursors that act as a seed for further neuritic plaque development (Selkoe, 2001).

Early studies have shown that synthetic fibrillar forms of Aß are toxic to cultured neurons (Pike et al, 1991; Lorenzo and Yankner, 1994; Iversen et al, 1995). Several mechanisms of Aß-induced neurotoxicity have been proposed, including oxidative stress, free-radical formation, disrupted calcium homeostasis, induction of apoptosis, chronic inflammation and activation of complement (Dodel et al, 2003). While it has been shown that increased levels of Aß in the brain correlate with cognitive decline (Näslund et al, 2000), relatively weak correlations exist between fibrillar amyloid plaque density and severity of dementia (Terry et al, 1981; Braak and Braak, 1991; Dickson et al, 1995). Also, amyloid deposits are often found at a distance from neuronal loss and have been found in normal individuals, not diagnosed with AD (Terry, 1999). Recent studies point to other forms of Aß, namely small oligomers and protofibrils as the neurotoxic species (McLean et al, 1999; Klein et al, 2001).

Recent reports using antibodies raised against synthetic Aß oligomers detected a 70-fold increase in oligomeric species in AD patients over control brains, which were also found to attach to cultured hippocampal neurons (Gong et al, 2003). Moreover, Kayed et al (2003) found that soluble oligomers display a common conformation-dependent structure common to all oligomers independent of their sequence, which suggests a shared mechanism of toxicity. Functionally, it has been found that naturally secreted oligomers inhibit hippocampal long-term potentiation *in vivo* (Walsh et al, 2002). Taken together, these results suggest that any strategies aimed at treating amyloid disorders should target at least one pathogenic form of Aß, namely oligomers, protofibrils or fibrils. In doing so, the equilibrium between monomers and higher order aggregates can be disrupted, resulting in neutralization of soluble, toxic species with the potential to affect fibril assemblies.

## FAMILIAL ALZHEIMER'S DISEASE AND TRANSGENIC MOUSE MODELS

Further evidence to support a major role for Aß in the pathogenesis of AD comes from the study of inheritable forms of AD. In approximately 92-96% of all cases, AD manifests itself in a sporadic (idiopathic) form. Familial forms of AD (familial Alzheimer's disease, or FAD) account for approximately 4-8% of all cases, and numerous studies have shown that FAD is caused by autosomal dominant mutations in three separate genes: APP, presenilin 1 (PS1), and presenilin 2 (PS2). Other genetic loci have been linked to predisposition to developing late-onset forms of AD, such as polymorphisms in the ApoE4 gene (Strittmatter *et al*, 1993). However, it should be noted that ApoE4 is a genetic risk factor and not an invariant cause of AD.

The APP gene, located on chromosome 21, is comprised of 18 exons and gives rise to at least 3 alternate splice variants, which encode proteins of 695, 751 and 770 amino acids (Chapman *et al*, 2001). Within and adjacent to the membrane-spanning region of APP are cleavage sites for three secretase enzymes: a, ß and ?. Cleavage of APP within the Aß sequence at the a-secretase site, followed by cleavage by ?-secretase generates the p3 peptides Aß (17-40) and Aß (17-42/43). An alternate cleavage pathway involves cleavage of APP by ß-secretase at the N-terminus of Aß, followed by cleavage within the transmembrane region by ?-secretase generating Aß40 and Aß42 (Li *et al*, 1999). Cleavage by a-secretase precludes formation of pathogenic Aß species; however in FAD, mutations within APP, PS1 or PS2 lead to enhanced production of all Aß peptides (in the case of mutations within APP), or a selective increase in Aß 42 (in the case of PS1 and PS2 mutations; Selkoe, 2001). Interestingly, this results in a phenotype indistinguishable from that of sporadic forms of AD: cerebral amyloidosis, neurofibrillary tangles, synaptic and neuronal loss; which lends additional support to the hypothesis that Aß plays a crucial role in the pathogenesis of AD (Chapman *et al*, 2001).

Further evidence comes from transgenic (Tg) mice, such as TgCRND8, which encode a double mutant form of APP harboring both the Indiana and Swedish FAD-mutations (Chishti *et al*, 2001). These mice produce high-levels of the pathogenic forms of Aß, and develop plaques with neuritic pathology and cognitive deficits, thereby recapitulating human AD pathology and behavior (Janus *et al*, 2000; Chishti *et al*, 2001). Thus, TgCRND8 and other transgenic mouse models of AD overexpressing mutant forms of APP, including PDAPP (Games *et al*, 1995), Tg2576 (Hsiao *et al*, 1996), TgAPP23 (Sturchler, Pierrat *et al*, 1997), J20 (Mucke *et al*, 2000) and 3xTg-AD (Oddo *et al*, 2003) provide a novel means of testing therapeutic strategies aimed at reducing AD pathology and mitigating or reversing cognitive decline. There are several caveats, however. Several factors have been shown to alter both the pathology and behavioral phenotype of Tg mice, including genetic background, the activity of the promoter controlling transgene expression, and the APP mutation itself. Moreover, some mouse models provide incomplete models of human AD, since most mice do not develop neurofibrillary tangles or obvious neuronal cell loss (Dodart *et al*, 2002a). There are, however three exceptions: TgAPP23 mice, which exhibit region-specific neuronal cell loss primarily in the vicinity of plaques (Calhoun et al., 1998); TAPP mice, which exhibit Aß deposits similar to those seen in Tg2576, in addition to neurofibrillary tangle pathology in the limbic system and olfactory cortex (Lewis *et al*, 2001); and triple-transgenic mice (3xTg-AD), harboring PS1, APP and tau mutations, which develop both plaque and tangle pathology reminiscent of human AD (Oddo *et al*, 2003). Notwithstanding, transgenic mice have provided important insights into the etiology and pathogenesis of AD *in vivo*, and in the case of Aß immunotherapy, have proven invaluable in testing novel immunization paradigms.

## IMMUNIZATION AGAINST Aß IN TRANSGENIC MOUSE MODELS OF ALZHEIMER'S DISEASE

Since Schenk *et al* first reported that immunization of PDAPP mice with synthetic, preaggregated Aß 42 reduced the extent and progression of AD pathology, much progress has been made in designing a vaccine appropriate for human use. Several strategies, including active and passive immunization have been explored, which not only hold promise as potential therapeutics, but also provide opportunities to test the amyloid cascade hypothesis *in vivo*.

*Active Immunization*

Monthly immunization of PDAPP mice before the onset of AD neuropathology with synthetic, preaggregated Aß 42 was shown to ostensibly prevent plaque formation and reduce total Aß burden, neuritic dystrophy and astrogliosis (Schenk *et al*, 1999). Follow-up studies sought to investigate whether changes in amyloid burden observed with immunization could rescue cognitive deficits and behavioral impairment in these mice.

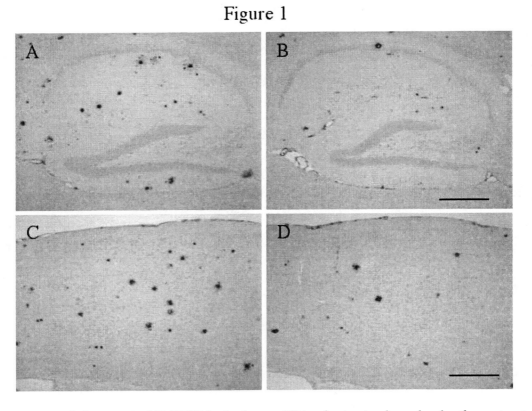

*Figure 1. Aß42-immunized TgCRND8 mice have a 50% reduction in plaque burden than untreated TgCRND8 mice. Representative pictures of the distribution of Aß plaques labeled by Dako 6F/3D anti-Aßantibody in the hippocampus (a,b) and cortex (c,d) of control peptide-immunized (a,c) and Aß42-immunized TgCRND8 mice (b,d). Scale bars, 100 µm.*

In 2000, Janus and colleagues demonstrated a 50% reduction in the number and size of plaques (Figure 1), concomitant with improved performance in the Morris water maze test and a decrease in microglial activation (Figure 2). At the same time, Morgan and colleagues showed that vaccination of two strains of mice (Tg2576 and Tg2576 X PS1 line 5.1) resulted in a modest reduction in Aß deposits, while protecting Tg mice from learning and age-related memory deficits seen in control mice. Many other studies have corroborated these results with several strains of mice using various immunization protocols (Lemere *et al*, 2000; Weiner *et al*, 2000).

## Figure 2

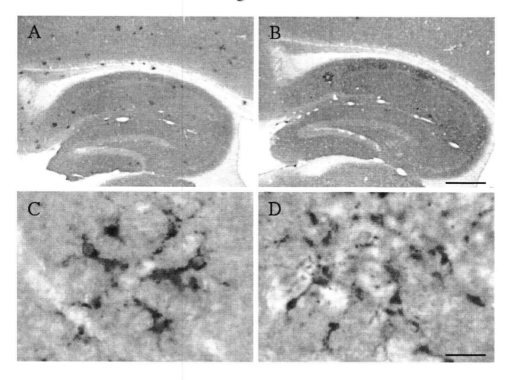

*Figure 2. Aβ42-immnized TgCRND8 mice have reduced microglial activation in comparison to control peptide-immunized TgCRND8 mice. Representative pictures of the distribution of activated microglia as labeled by anti-CD68 IgG in the hippocampus (a,b) of control peptide-immunized (a,c) and Aβ42-immunized TgCRND8 mice (b,d). Higher magnification reviews that activated microglia have similar morphology under both immunization paradigms (c,d). Scale bars, 75 µm (a,b) and 5 µm (c,d).*

It is important to note that these results were obtained using young mice, with little to no established AD-like pathology upon immunization. In 1999, Schenk and colleagues that treatment of older animals resulted in a marked reduction in amyloid burden, while immunohistochemistry revealed that in immunized mice any remaining plaques were decorated with IgG. On the other hand in 2001, Das and colleagues showed that in Tg2576 mice Aβ 42 immunization is more effective in preventing Aβ accumulation (that is, in the earlier stages of the disease), as immunization of older mice with pre-existing plaques revealed no significant difference in plaque load or number as compared to control mice. However, total Aβ levels were significantly decreased with immunization in all treatment groups (young and old), albeit to a lesser degree in older mice. Additionally, no significant differences were found in the maximum antibody titer, kinetics of the immune response or the isotype of antibody produced between age groups, suggesting that the levels of antibody are unlikely to account for differences observed in effectiveness. One suggestion offered by the authors is that other age associated factors, including altered microglial response, may account for the observed outcomes.

### *Passive Immunization*

Promising results obtained from these studies prompted researchers to investigate whether similar results could be obtained by peripheral administration of monoclonal antibodies to Aβ. Prolonged administration of two monoclonal antibodies (10D5 and 3D6) directed against the N-terminus of Aß was sufficient to decrease amyloid burden; despite the fact that only 0.1 % entered the central nervous system (CNS), plaques in the brain were 'decorated' with the antibody (Bard *et al*, 2000). An *ex vivo* assay using unfixed sections from PDAPP and AD brains demonstrated that plaques are cleared by microglia via Fc receptor-mediated phagocytosis, and was found to be a good predictor of *in vivo* efficacy. Additionally, *in vivo* imaging of amyloid deposits in living mice have demonstrated that plaques could be cleared within 3 days, while histochemistry confirmed the involvement of microglia in the process (Bacskai *et al*, 2001). These results stand in contrast to work by DeMattos and colleagues published in 2001, where prolonged peripheral administration of an antibody (m266) directed against the central domain of Aß markedly reduced Aß deposition, without binding to Aß deposits in the brain, suggesting a mechanism independent of central degradation by microglia.

While most of these studies validate the use of immune strategies to decrease plaque burden, several reports have shown that targeting soluble Aß species may prove equieffective. In 2002 Dodart and colleagues (2002b) reported that acute administration of m266 resulted in rapid reversal of memory impairment in PDAPP mice, without any alteration in amyloid burden. Aß/antibody complexes were also found in the cerebrospinal fluid (CSF) and plasma, which suggests that the antibody may sequester toxic, soluble forms of Aß including oligomers and protofibrils. Similar mechanisms are thought to act in other mouse models (Janus *et al*, 2000; Kotilinek *et al*, 2002; McLaurin *et al*, 2002), lending further support to a major role for select soluble Aß species in the pathogenesis of AD (Van Dam *et al*, 2003).

One unexpected finding was the increased incidence of microhemorrhages in APP23 mice following passive Aß immunotherapy (Pfeifer *et al*, 2002). APP23 mice exhibit AD-like pathology including parenchymal Aß deposition, in addition to prominent deposition of Aß within the cerebral vasculature (Sturchler-Pierrat *et al*, 1997; Calhoun *et al*, 1999). This effect was not observed in previous studies, as mouse models used therein do not develop significant cerebral amyloid angiopathy (CAA) (Schenk, 2002). These findings suggest that AD patients may need to be screened for the presence and severity of CAA prior to initiating Aß immunotherapy.

## MECHANISMS OF ACTION

While active and passive immunization strategies have proven efficacious in mouse models of AD, it remains unclear how antibodies elicit this effect. Several hypotheses have been put forth to explain results observed *in vivo* and *in vitro*, but it is important to note that these are not mutually exclusive. Any number of these mechanisms may act under a given set of circumstances, with factors including the epitope, isotype, and amyloid burden likely to influence the primary means of clearance or sequestration.

### *Fc-Receptor Mediated Phagocytosis*

In 2000 Bard and colleagues presented a model whereby peripherally administered antibodies enter the CNS and bind Aß fibrils, with subsequent recruitment of microglia to phagocytose the complex via Fc-receptor ligation. *Ex vivo* assays confirm the presence of internalized Aß within microglia upon incubation with anti-Aß antibodies and tissue sections. Follow-up studies were consistent with these observations, as the most effective antibodies (examined *in vivo* and *ex vivo*) were of the IgG2a isotype, which exhibits high affinity for Fc receptors on microglia (Bard *et al*, 2003). Microglial activation was also found to accompany plaque clearance *in vivo* by active and passive immunization strategies (Bacskai *et al*, 2001; Wilcock *et al*, 2001) or alternatively to decrease activation in active immunization (Figure 2) (McLaurin *et al*, 2002). However, recent reports suggest that multiple clearance mechanisms may act in concert to clear amyloid plaques (Bacskai *et al*, 2002; Das *et al*, 2003). One such possibility involves internalization of Aß/antibody microaggregates by microglia through the type A scavenger receptor (Brazil *et al*, 2000). Indeed, a recent report from Wilcock and colleagues

(2003) suggests a two-phase mechanism of anti- Aß antibody action, both independent and associated with microglial activation.

## Peripheral Sink Hypothesis

An alternate mechanism comes from the observation that long-term peripheral administration of a monoclonal antibody (m266) results in a rapid increase in plasma Aß with subsequent reduction in amyloid burden, without binding of m266 to Aß deposits in the brain (DeMattos *et al*, 2001). The authors suggest that sequestration of plasma Aß disrupts the Aß equilibrium between the CNS and plasma, resulting in increased efflux of Aß out of the brain, into the CSF and ultimately into the periphery where it is degraded. This hypothesis is supported by a number of observations. Aß-peptides have been shown to be transported readily between the CNS and plasma (Ghersi-Egea *et al*, 1996; Poduslo *et al*, 1999; Shibata *et al*, 2000). Moreover, in non-demented patients, intravenous infusion of anti- Aß antibodies led to increased Aß levels in the plasma, with concomitant decreases in Aß within the CSF (Dodel *et al*, 2002). These findings are further supported by Lemere and colleagues in 2003, who observed a 28-fold increase in serum Aß following chronic, active immunization of PSAPP mice. Evidence in support of the contrary include the observation that Aß/antibody immune complexes are taken up by a receptor-mediated process at the blood brain barrier, precluding the absence of Aß antibodies in the CNS of passively immunized animals (Poduslo and Curran, 2001).

## Inhibition of Fibrillogenesis and Cytotoxic Aß Species

Previous work by Solomon and colleagues (Solomon *et al*, 1996; Solomon *et al*, 1997; Frenkel *et al*, 2000a) predicted that antibodies raised against the N-terminus of Aß could inhibit *in vitro* aggregation and could bind to pre-existing Aß fibrils, resulting in disaggregation and protection from their neurotoxic effects. In 2002, McLaurin and colleagues extended this line of evidence *in vivo* by demonstrating that antibodies directed against residues 4-10 of Aß 42 inhibit both fibrillogenesis and cytotoxicity, without eliciting a harmful cytotoxic T-cell response in TgCRND8 mice. Consistent with these results are studies by Bard *et al* demonstrating that plaque clearance is only seen with antibodies directed against the N-terminal region of Aß.

In 2002, McLaurin *et al* also suggested that antibodies induced by immunization of TgCRND8 mice likely target only a subset of Aß, namely soluble species such as protofibrils or oligomers. This seems likely as total Aß brain levels do not decrease following immunization of TgCRND8 mice (Janus *et al*, 2000), and several independent studies have presented similar findings (Lambert *et al*, 2001; Dodart *et al*, 2002; Kotilinek *et al*, 2002).

## Aß VACCINATION IN HUMANS

Following promising preclinical results in several species (mice, rabbits, guinea pigs and monkeys) clinical trials using Aß 42 (AN-1792) in conjunction with the Th1 adjuvant QS-21 were initiated (Schenk, 2002). Although results of Phase I trials showed good tolerability, Phase IIa trials were halted when 18 of 298 patients immunized with AN-1792 presented with symptoms consistent with meningoencephalitis (Senior, 2002; Orgogozo *et al*, 2003). Several reports have since been published regarding the neuropathology and clinical outcome of acute immunization (Hock *et al*, 2002; Nicoll *et al*, 2003; Hock *et al*, 2003; Orgogozo *et al*, 2003), which should prove useful in designing new generation vaccines.

Several findings provide hope for AD patients despite termination of clinical trials. Post-mortem examination of the brain of an AD patient who received five injections of AN-1792 revealed absent or sparse plaques in the neocortex, lacking dystrophic neurites or reactive astrocytes (as compared to unimmunized controls); reactive microglia in association with areas devoid of plaques; and decoration of plaques by IgG and C3 complement. Taken together, these results suggest that an effective immune response was generated, which resulted in clearance of

Aβ from the patient (Nicoll *et al*, 2003). Moreover, in the same year Hock and colleagues showed that patients who generate antibodies exhibit slower rates of cognitive decline; this effect was even observed in patients who experienced transient episodes of meningoencephalitis.

However promising, one must interpret these results alongside the numerous adverse events observed. Neuropathological analysis revealed infiltration of T-lymphocytes, predominantly of the CD4+ type; abnormalities of cerebral white matter, including extensive macrophage infiltration and a reduction in the density of myelinated fibers; and neurofibrillary tangle pathology and CAA similar to unimmunized controls (Nicoll *et al*, 2003). The question remains: could these adverse reactions have been predicted prior to clinical trials, and what changes can be made to prevent their reoccurrence with new generation vaccines?

Although no inflammatory reaction was observed in preclinical trials, a recently published report demonstrates that vaccination of C57BL/6 mice with Aβ and pertussis toxin induces autoimmune encephalomyelitis, with characteristics (inflammatory foci in the CNS containing macrophages, B- and T-cells, circulating anti-Aβ antibodies and a predominantly CD4+-mediated Th1 response) similar to those observed in humans (Furlan *et al*, 2003).

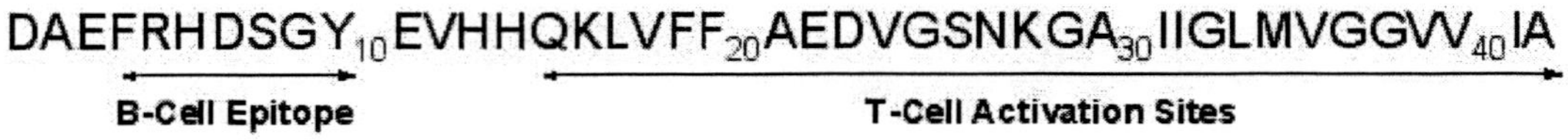

$$\text{DAEFRHDSGY}_{10}\text{EVHHQKLVFF}_{20}\text{AEDVGSNKGA}_{30}\text{IIGLMVGGVV}_{40}\text{IA}$$

**B-Cell Epitope**   **T-Cell Activation Sites**

*Figure 3. The sequence of B- and T-cell epitopes within the Aβ1-42 amino acid sequence as determined by mathematical algorithms.*

Several scientists agree that the inflammatory response observed in human subjects is attributable to a T-cell mediated event (Dodel *et al*, 2003; Weiner and Selkoe, 2002). Infiltration of activated T-cells had been predicted well before commencement of clinical trials (Grubeck-Loebenstein *et al*, 2000). T-cell epitopes have been mapped to the mid-to-carboxy terminal region (residues 15-42) of Aβ (Figure 3) (Monsonego *et al*, 2003a). In 2002, McLaurin and colleagues subsequently showed that antibodies directed toward the N-terminus (residues 4-10) were sufficient to inhibit cytotoxicity and fibrillogenesis, without eliciting an inflammatory response. Thus, immunization with the full-length Aβ 42 peptide, containing both B- and T-cell epitopes would be expected to result in extensive T-cell activation. Recent reports of increased T-cell reactivity in AD patients and older humans, predominantly against amino acids 16-33 of Aβ, seem in line with these predictions; however, these results become difficult to interpret in light of contradictory reports indicating that lymphocytes from AD patients exhibit weak proliferative responses to Aβ and other synthetic peptides corresponding to parts of the APP sequence, as compared to young and aged healthy individuals (Trieb *et al*, 1996). Moreover, APP transgenic mice were found to be hyporesponsive to human Aβ, in terms of humoral and cellular immune responses (Monsonego *et al*, 2001). The authors suggest that increased production of Aβ from such a young age may induce a form of central and peripheral T cell tolerance. As Aβ is also overproduced at a young age in Down's syndrome patients (Selkoe, 2001) one might expect Down's patients to exhibit similar degrees of tolerance, in the form of decreased lymphoproliferative responses to Aβ.

## FUTURE PERSPECTIVES

One issue to come out of the AN-1792 trials is the importance of a directed immune response. Given the distinct location of B- and T-cell epitopes within Aß, new immunogens can be designed which lack the irrelevant C-terminus, while retaining those residues (4-10) required for binding to Aß (McLaurin *et al*, 2002). In 2001, Sigurdsson and colleagues demonstrated that immunization with a synthetic nontoxic/nonfibrillar Aß homologous peptide could reduce AD pathology and potentially offer a safer alternative than immunization with Aß 42.

Immune responses also need to be directed towards a Th2 response, which promotes antibody production, down-regulates pro-inflammatory Th1 responses, and results in the release of anti-inflammatory cytokines that have the potential to mitigate chronic inflammatory conditions already present in AD patients (Neuroinflammation Working Group, 2000). This is particularly important given recent findings that microglia-mediated release of nitric oxide by Aß-reactive Th1 cells can contribute to AD neurotoxicity; Th2 cells however, were found to counterbalance the toxic effects of NO (Monsonego *et al*, 2003b). Nasal immunization paradigms have illustrated the potential to decrease AD pathology while inducing the expression of the anti-inflammatory cytokines IL-4, IL-10 and transforming growth factor beta (TGF-ß) (Lemere *et al*, 2000; Weiner *et al*, 2000). Work by Wyss-Coray and colleagues published in 2001 extended this line of inquiry by demonstrating that modest increases in astroglial production of TGF-ß1 results in a marked reduction in plaque burden and overall Aß load, presumably through promotion of microglia (Wyss-Coray *et al*, 2001). These findings are consistent with the potential for QS-21, a Th1 adjuvant, to exacerbate chronic inflammatory conditions in AD patients upon immunization with AN-1792.

Additionally, elucidation of the precise mechanism(s) whereby anti-Aß antibodies exert their effect could aid in the design of new immunogens or molecular mimics. If it is found that efficient clearance of Aß requires that antibodies enter the CNS, then molecules can be engineered that effectively cross the blood brain barrier. Should the peripheral sink model prove correct, modifications can be made to restrict their entry into the CNS. In 2003 Rangan and colleagues identified recombinant antibody light chain fragments with proteolytic activity, capable of hydrolysing Aß *in vitro*. Although these currently demonstrate broad substrate specificity, they may prove therapeutically useful if the antibody could be engineered to specifically target pathogenic forms of Aß, such as oligomers or protofibrils. Also, Frenkel *et al* suggest a novel approach, where intracellular expression of a site-directed single-chain antibody, which has been shown to inhibit fibrillogenesis and cytotoxicity *in vitro*, could target Aß before it is released from the cell.

## CONCLUDING REMARKS

Insights gained from the pathology, biochemistry and genetics of AD have allowed identification of a target for therapy, Aß, as well as the generation of transgenic mouse models that recapitulate pathological and behavioral aspects of the disease in which to test hypotheses. The first set of evidence that immunization with Aß could reduce AD pathology and restore cognitive deficits in transgenic mice was met with considerable optimism; this however was short-lived, as clinical trials of a vaccine were cancelled due to a small but significant occurrence of meningoencephalitis. Despite numerous adverse events associated with clinical trials of AN-1792, preliminary data demonstrate that vaccination can reduce AD pathology and mitigate progressive cognitive decline associated with the disease. Knowledge gained from studies on Aß immunotherapy will allow optimization of the vaccine in order to avoid side-effects, while generating a highly specific and effective immune response against what is now believed to be the causative agent of synaptic loss and cognitive decline: Aß. If this proves successful, Aß vaccination could provide the first definitive treatment for AD.

## REFERENCES

Alzheimer's Disease Collaborative Group. The structure of the presenilin 1 (S182) gene and identification of six novel mutations in early onset AD families. *Nat Genet.* 1995;11: 219-22.

Bacskai BJ, Kajdasz ST, Christie RH, Carter C, Games D, Seubert P, Schenk D, Hyman BT. Imaging of amyloid-ß deposits in brains of living mice permits direct observation of clearance of plaques with immunotherapy. *Nat Med.* 2001;7:369-372.

Bacskai BJ, Kajdasz ST, McLellan ME, Games D, Seubert P, Schenk D, Hyman BT. Non-Fc-mediated mechanisms are involved in clearance of amyloid-ß *in vivo* by immunotherapy. *J Neurosci.* 2002; 22:7873-7878.

Bard F, Cannon C, Barbour R, Burke R, Games D, Grajeda H, Guido T, Hu K, Huang J. Johnson-Wood K, *et al*. Peripherally administered antibodies against amyloid ß-peptide enter the central nervous system and reduce pathology in a mouse model of Alzheimer disease. *Na. Med.* 2000;6:916-919.

Bard F, Barbour R, Cannon C, Carretto R, Fox M, Games D, Guido T, Hoenow K, Hu K, Johnson-Wood K, *et al*. Epitope and isotype specificities of antibodies to ß-amyloid peptide for protection against Alzheimer's disease-like neuropathology. *Proc Natl Acad Sci USA.* 2003;100:2023-2028.

Braak H, Braak E. Neuropathological staging of Alzheimer-related changes. *Acta Neuropathol.* 1994;82:239-259.

Brazil MI, Chung H, Maxfield FR. Effects of incorporation of immunoglobulin G and complement component C1q on uptake and degradation of Alzheimer's disease amyloid fibrils by microglia. *J Biol Chem.* 2000;275:1694116947.

Calhoun ME, Wiederhold JH, Abramowski D, Phinney AL, Probst A, Sturchler-Pierrat C, Staufenbiel M, Sommer B, Jucker M. Neuron loss in APP transgenic mice [letter]. *Nature* 1998;395:755-756.

Calhoun,ME, Burgermeister P, Phinney AL, Stalder M, Tolnay M, Wiederhold K, Abramowski D., Sturchler-Pierrat C, Sommer B, Staufenbiel M, Jucker M. Neuronal overexpression of mutant amyloid precursor protein results in prominent deposition of cerebrovascular amyloid. *Proc Natl Acad Sci USA.* 1999;96:14088-14093.

Campion D, Flaman JM, Brice A, Hannequin D, Dubois B, Martin C, Moreau V, Charbonnier F, Didierjean O, Tardieu S, et al. Mutations of the presenilin 1 gene in families with early-onset Alzheimer's disease. *Hum Mol Genet.* 1995;4:2373-2377.

Chapman PF, Falinska AM, Knevett SG, Ramsay MF. Genes, models and Alzheimer's disease. *Trends Genet.* 1995;17:254-261.

Chartier-Harlin MC, Crawford F, Houlden H, Warren A, Hughes D, Fidani L, Goate A, Rossor M, Roques P, Hardy J, *et al*. Early-onset Alzheimer's disease caused by mutations at codon 717 of the beta-amyloid precursor protein gene. *Nature.* 1991;353:844-846.

Chishti MA, Yang D, Janus C, Phinney AL, Horne P, Pearson J, Strome R, Zuker N, Joukides J, French J, *et al*. Early-onset amyloid deposition and cognitive deficits in transgenic mice expressing a double mutant form of amyloid precursor protein 695. *J Biol Chem.* 2001;276:21562-21570.

Citron M. Alzheimer's disease: treatments in discovery and development. *Nature Neurosci.* 2002; Suppl. 5:1055-1057.

Cruts M, Backhovens H, Wang SY, Van Gassen G, Theuns J, De Jonghe CD, Wehnert A, De Voecht J, De Winter G, Cras P, *et al*. Molecular genetic analysis of familial early-onset Alzheimer's disease linked to chromosome 14q24.3.*Hum Mol Genet.* 1995;4:2363-2371.

Das P, Murphy MP, Younkin LH, Younkin SG, Golde TE. Reduced effectiveness of Aß1-42 immunization in APP transgenic mice with significant amyloid deposition. *Neurobiol Aging.* 2001;22: 721-727.

Das P, Howard V, Loosbrock N, Dickson D, Murphy MP, Golde, TE. Amyloid-ß immunization effectively reduces amyloid deposition in FcR?-/-knockout mice. *J Neurosci.* 2003;23:8532-8538.

Davis KL, Samuels SC. In: *Pharmacological Management of Neurological and Psychiatric Disorders.* Enna S J, Coyle JT, eds. McGraw-Hill; 1998:267-316.

DeMattos RB, Bales KR, Cummins DJ, Dodart J, Paul SM, Holtzman DM. Peripheral anti-Aß antibody alters CNS and plasma Aß clearance and decreases brain Aß burden in a mouse model of Alzheimer's disease. *Pro. Natl Acad Sci USA.* 2001;98:8850-8855.

Dickson DW, Crystal HA, Bevona C, Honer W, Vincent I, Davies P. Correlations of synaptic and pathological markers with cognition of the elderly. *Neurobiol Aging.* 1995;16:285-298.

Dodart J, Mathis C, Bales KR, Paul SM. Does my mouse have Alzheimer's disease? *Genes, Brain and Behavior* 2002(a);1:142-155.

Dodart J, Bales KR, Gannon KS, Greene SJ, DeMattos RB, Mathis C, DeLong CA, Wu S, Wu X, Holtzman DM, Paul SM. Immunization reverses memory deficits without reducing brain Aß burden in Alzheimer's disease model. *Nat Neurosci.* 2002(b);5:452-457.

Dodel RC, Hampel H, Depboylu C, Lin S, Gao F, Schock S, Jckel S, Wei X, Buerger K, Hoft C, et al. Human antibodies against amyloid beta peptide: a potential treatment for Alzheimer's disease. *Ann Neurol.* 2002;52:253-256.

Dodel RC, Hampel H, Du, Y. Immunotherapy for Alzheimer's disease. *Lancet Neurol.* 2003;2:215-220.

Frenkel D, Katz O, Solomon B. Immunization against Alzheimer's beta -amyloid plaques via EFRH phage administration. *Proc Natl Acad Sci U S A.* 2000(a);97:11455-11459.

Frenkel D, Solomon B, Benhar I. Modulation of Alzheimer's beta-amyloid neurotoxicity by site-directed single-chain antibody. *J Neuroimmunol.* 2000(b);106(1-2):23-31.

Furlan R, Brambilla E, Sanvito F, Roccatagliata L, Olivieri S, Bergami A, Pluchino S, Uccelli A, Comi G, Martino G. Vaccination with amyloid-beta peptide induces autoimmune encephalomyelitis in C57/BL6 mice. *Brain.* 2003;126(Pt 2):285-291.

Games D, Adams D, Alessandrini R, Barbour R, Berthelette P, Blackwell C, Carr T, Clemens J, Donaldson T, Gillespie F, et al. Alzheimer-type neuropathology in transgenic mice overexpressing V717F beta-amyloid precursor protein. *Nature.* 1995;373:523-527.

Gandy S. Molecular basis for anti-amyloid therapy in the prevention and treatment of Alzheimer's disease. *Neurobiol Aging.* 2002;23:1009-1016.

Ghersi-Egea JF, Gorevic PD, Ghiso J, Frangione B, Patlak CS, Fenstermacher JD. Fate of cerebrospinal fluid-borne amyloid beta-peptide: rapid clearance into blood and appreciable accumulation by cerebral arteries. *J Neurochem.* 1996;67:880-883.

Goate A, Chartier-Harlin MC, Mullan M, Brown J, Crawford F, Fidani L, Giuffra L, Haynes A, Irving N, James L, et al. Segregation of a missense mutation in the amyloid precursor protein gene with familial Alzheimer's disease. *Nature.* 1991;349:704-706.

Gong Y, Chang L, Viola KL, Lacor PN, Lambert MP, Finch CE, Krafft GA, Klein WL. Alzheimer's disease-affected brain: presence of oligomeric A beta ligands (ADDLs) suggests a molecular basis for reversible memory loss. *Proc Natl Acad Sci U S A.* 2003;100:10417-10422. Epub 2003 Aug 18.

Gouras GK, Tsai J, Naslund J, Vincent B, Edgar M, Checler F, Greenfield JP, Haroutunian V, Buxbaum JD, Xu H, Greengard P, Relkin NR. Intraneuronal Abeta42 accumulation in human brain. *Am J Pathol.* 2000;156:15-20.

Grubeck-Loebenstein B, Blasko I, Marx F, Trieb K. Immunization with ß-amyloid: could T-cell activation have a harmful effect? *TINS* 2000;23:114.

Hendriks L, van Duijn CM, Cras P, Cruts M, Van Hul W, van Harskamp F, Warren A, McInnis MG, Antonarakis SE, Martin JJ, et al. Presenile dementia and cerebral haemorrhage linked to a mutation at codon 692 of the beta-amyloid precursor protein gene. *Nat Genet.* 1992;1:218-221.

Hsiao K, Chapman P, Nilsen S, Eckman C, Harigaya Y, Younkin S, Yang F, Cole G. Correlative memory deficits, Abeta elevation, and amyloid plaques in transgenic mice. *Science.* 1996;274:99-102.

Hock C, Konietzko U, Papassotiropoulos A, Wollmer A, Streffer J, von Rotz RC, Davey G, Moritz E, Nitsch RM. Generation of antibodies specific for beta-amyloid by vaccination of patients with Alzheimer disease. *Nat Med.* 2002;8:1270-1275. Epub 2002 Oct 15.

Hock C, Konietzko U, Streffer JR, Tracy J, Signorell A, Muller-Tillmanns B, Lemke U, Henke K, Moritz E, Garcia E, *et al.* Antibodies against beta-amyloid slow cognitive decline in Alzheimer's disease. *Neuron.* 2003;38:547-554.

Iversen LL, Mortishire-Sith RJ, Pollack SJ, Shearman MS. The toxicity *in vitro* of beta-amyloid protein. *Biochem J.* 19995;311: 1-16.

Janus C, Pearson J, McLaurin J, Mathews PM, Jiang Y, Schmidt SD, Chishti MA, Horne P, Heslin D, French J, *et al.* A beta peptide immunization reduces behavioral impairment and plaques in a model of Alzheimer's disease. *Nature.* 2000;408:979-982.

Kayed R, Head E, Thompson JL, McIntitre TM, Milton SC, Cotman CW, Glabe CG. Common structure of soluble amyloid oligomers implies common mechanism of pathogenesis. *Science* 2003;300:486-489.

Klein WL, Krafft GA, Finch CE. Targeting small Aß oligomers: the solution to an Alzheimer's disease conundrum? *Trends Neurosci.* 2001;24:219-224.

Kotilinek LA, Bacskai B, Westerman M, Kawarabayashi T, Younkin L, Hyman BT, Younkin S, Ashe KH. Reversible memory loss in a mouse transgenic model of Alzheimer's disease. *J Neurosci.* 2002;22:6331-6335.

Lambert MP, Viola KL, Chromy BA, Chang L, Morgan TE, Yu J, Venton DL, Krafft GA, Finch CE, Klein WL. Vaccination with soluble Abeta oligomers generates toxicity-neutralizing antibodies. *J Neurochem.* 2001;79:595-605.

Lemere CA, Maron R, Spooner ET, Grenfell TJ, Mori C, Desai R, Hancock WW, Weiner HL, Selkoe DJ. Nasal Aß treatment induces anti-Aß antibody production and decreases cerebral amyloid burden in PDAPP mice. *Ann NY Acad Sci,* 2000;920:328-331.

Lemere CA, Spooner ET, LaFrancois J, Malester B, Mori C, Leverone JF, Matsuoka Y, Taylor JW, DeMattos RB, Holtzman DM, *et al.* Evidence for peripheral clearance of cerebral Abeta protein following chronic, active Abeta immunization in PSAPP mice. *Neurobiol Dis.* 2003;14:10-18.

Lewis J, Dickson DW, Lin WL, Chisholm L, Corral A, Jones G, Yen SH, Sahara N, Skipper L, Yager D, *et al.* Enhanced neurofibrillary degeneration in transgenic mice expressing mutant tau and APP. *Science.* 2001;293:1487-1491.

Li Q, Fuller SJ, Beyreuther K, Masters CL. The amyloid precursor protein of Alzheimer disease in human brain and blood. *J Leukoc Biol.* 1999;66:567-574.

Lorenzo A, Yankner BA. Beta-amyloid neurotoxicity requires fibril formation and is inhibited by congo red. *Proc Natl Acad Sci U S A.* 1994;91:12243-12247.

McLaurin J, Yang D, Yip CM, Fraser PE. Modulating factors in amyloid-beta fibril formation. *J Struct Biol. 2000*;130:259-270.

McLaurin J, Cecal R, Kierstead ME, Tian X, Phinney AL, Manea M, French JE, Lambermon MH, Darabie AA, Brown ME, *et al.* Therapeutically effective antibodies against amyloid-beta peptide target amyloid-beta residues 4-10 and inhibit cytotoxicity and fibrillogenesis. *Nat Med.* 2002;8:1263-1269. Epub 2002 Oct 15.

McLean CA, Cherny RA, Fraser FW, Fuller SJ, Smith MJ, Beyreuther K, Bush AI, Masters CL. Soluble pool of Aß amyloid as a determinant of severity of neurodegeneration in Alzheimer's disease. *Ann Neurol.* 1999;46:860-866.

Monsonego A, Maron R, Zota V, Selkoe DJ, Weiner HL. Immune hyporesponsiveness to amyloid beta-peptide in amyloid precursor protein transgenic mice: implications for the pathogenesis and treatment of Alzheimer's disease. *Proc Natl Acad Sci U S A.* 2001;98:10273-10278. Epub 2001 Aug 21.

Monsonego A, Zota V, Karni A, Krieger JI, Bar-Or A, Bitan G, Budson AE, Sperling R, Selkoe DJ, Weiner HL. Increased T cell reactivity to amyloid beta protein in older humans and patients with Alzheimer disease. *J Clin Invest.* 2003;112:415-422.

Monsonego A, Imitola J, Zota V, Oida T, Weiner HL. Microglia-mediated nitric oxide cytotoxicity of T cells following amyloid beta-peptide presentation to Th1 cells. *J Immunol.* 2003(b);171:2216-2224. Erratum in: *J Immunol.* 2004;172:717.

Morgan D, Diamond DM, Gottschall PE, Ugen KE, Dickey C, Hardy J, Duff K, Jantzen P, DiCarlo G, Wilcock D, *et al.* A beta peptide vaccination prevents memory loss in an animal model of Alzheimer's disease. *Nature.* 2000;408:982-985. Erratum in: *Nature* 2001;412:660.

Mucke L, Masliah E, Yu GQ, Mallory M, Rockenstein EM, Tatsuno G, Hu K, Kholodenko D, Johnson-Wood K, McConlogue L. High-level neuronal expression of abeta 1-42 in wild-type human amyloid protein precursor transgenic mice: synaptotoxicity without plaque formation. *J Neurosci.* 2000;20:4050-4058.

Mullan M, Crawford F, Axelman K, Houlden H, Lilius L, Winblad B, Lannfelt L. A pathogenic mutation for probable Alzheimer's disease in the APP gene at the N-terminus of beta-amyloid. *Nat Genet.* 1992;1:345-347.

Murrell J, Farlow M, Ghetti B, Benson MD. A mutation in the amyloid precursor protein associated with hereditary Alzheimer's disease. *Science.* 1991;254:97-99.

Naslund J, Haroutunian V, Mohs R, Davis KL, Davies P, Greengard P, Buxbaum JD. Correlation between elevated levels of amyloid beta-peptide in the brain and cognitive decline. *JAMA.* 2000;283:1571-1577.

Neuroinflammation Working Group. Inflammation and Alzheimer's disease. *Neurobiol Aging.* 2000;21:383-421.

Nicoll JA, Wilkinson D, Holmes C, Steart P, Markham H, Weller RO. Neuropathology of human Alzheimer disease after immunization with amyloid-beta peptide: a case report. *Nat Med.* 2003;9:448-452. Epub 2003 Mar 17.

Oddo S, Caccamo A, Shepherd JD, Murphy MP, Golde TE, Kayed R, Metherate R, Mattson MP, Akbari Y, LaFerla FM. Triple-transgenic model of Alzheimer's disease with plaques and tangles: intracellular Abeta and synaptic dysfunction. *Neuron.* 2003;39:409-421.

Orgogozo JM, Gilman S, Dartigues JF, Laurent B, Puel M, Kirby LC, Jouanny P, Dubois B, Eisner L, Flitman S, *et al.* Subacute meningoencephalitis in a subset of patients with AD after Abeta42 immunization. *Neurology.* 2003;61:46-54.

Pfeifer M, Boncristiano S, Bondolfi L, Stalder A, Deller T, Staufenbiel M, Mathews PM, Jucker M. Cerebral hemorrhage after passive anti-Abeta immunotherapy. *Science.* 2002;298:1379.

Pike CJ, Walencewicz AJ, Glabe CG, Cotman CW. *In vitro* aging of amyloid-beta protein causes peptide aggregation and neurotoxicity. *Brain Res.* 1991;573:311-314.

Poduslo JF, Curran GL, Sanyal B, Selkoe DJ. Receptor-mediated transport of human amyloid-beta protein 1-40 and 1-42 at the blood-brain barrier. *Neurobiol Dis.* 1999;6:190-199.

Poduslo JF, Curran GL. Amyloid ß peptide as a vaccine for Alzheimer's disease involves receptor-mediated transport at the blood-brain barrier. *Neuroreport.* 2001;12:3197-3200.

Rangan SK, Liu R, Brune D, Planque S, Paul S, Sierks MR. Degradation of beta-amyloid by proteolytic antibody light chains. *Biochemistry.* 2003;42:14328-14334.

Rogaev EI, Sherrington R, Rogaeva EA, Levesque G, Ikeda M, Liang Y, Chi H, Lin C, Holman K, Tsuda T, *et al.* Familial Alzheimer's disease in kindreds with missense mutations in a gene on chromosome 1 related to the Alzheimer's disease type 3 gene. *Nature.* 1995;376:775-778.

Schenk D, Barbour R, Dunn W, Gordon G, Grajeda H, Guido T, Hu K, Huang J, Johnson-Wood K, Khan K, *et al.* Immunization with amyloid-beta attenuates Alzheimer-disease-like pathology in the PDAPP mouse. *Nature.* 1999;400:173-177.

Schenk D. Amyloid-ß immunotherapy for Alzheimer's disease: the end of the beginning. *Nature Rev Neurosci.* 2002;3;824-828.

Selkoe D. Alzheimer's disease: genes, proteins, and therapy. *Physiol Rev.* 2001;81:741-766.

Senior K. Dosing in phase II trial of Alzheimer's vaccine suspended. *Lancet Neurol.* 2002;1:3.

Sherrington R, Rogaev EI, Liang Y, Rogaeva EA, Levesque G, Ikeda M, Chi H, Lin C, Li G, Holman K, *et al*. Cloning of a gene bearing missense mutations in early-onset familial Alzheimer's disease. *Nature*. 1995;375:754-760.

Sherrington R, Froelich S, Sorbi S, Campion D, Chi H, Rogaeva EA, Levesque G, Rogaev EI, Lin C, Liang Y, *et al*. Alzheimer's disease associated with mutations in presenilin 2 is rare and variably penetrant. *Hum Mol Genet.* 1996;5:985-988.

Shibata M, Yamada S, Kumar SR, Calero M, Bading J, Frangione B, Holtzman DM, Miller CA, Strickland DK, Ghiso J, *et al*. Clearance of Alzheimer's amyloid-ß (1-40) peptide from brain by LDL-receptor related protein-1 at the blood-brain barrier. *J Clin Invest.* 2000;106:1489-1499.

Sigurdsson EM, Scholtzova H, Mehta PD, Frangione B, Wisniewski T. Immunization with a nontoxic/nonfibrillar amyloid-ß homologous peptide reduces Alzheimer's disease-associated pathology in transgenic mice. *Am J Pathol.* 2001;159:439-447.

Solomon B, Koppel R, Hanan E, Katzav T. Monoclonal antibodies inhibit *in vitro* fibrillar aggregation of the Alzheimer ? -amyloid peptide. *Proc Natl Acad Sci USA.* 1996;93:452-455.

Solomon B, Koppel R, Frankel D, Hanan-Aharon E. Disaggregation of Alzheimer ß-amyloid by site-directed mAb. *Proc. Natl. Acad. Sci. U.S.A.* 1997;94:4109-4112.

St George-Hyslop PH, Tanzi RE, Polinsky RJ, Haines JL, Nee L, Watkins PC, Myers RH, Feldman RG, Pollen D, Drachman D, *et al*. The genetic defect causing familial Alzheimer's disease maps on chromosome 21. *Science* 1987;235:885-890.

Strittmatter WJ, Saunders AM, Schmechel D, Pericak-Vance M, Enghild J, Salvesen GS, Roses AD. Apolipoprtein E: high-avidity binding to ß-amyloid and increased frequence of type 4 allele in late-onset familial Alzheimer's disease. *Proc Nat. Acad Sci USA.* 1993;90:1977-1981.

Sturchler-Pierrat C, Abramowski D, Duke M, Wiederhold KH, Mistl C, Rothacher S, Ledermann B, Burki K, Frey P, Paganetti PA, *et al*. Two amyloid precursor protein transgenic mouse models with Alzheimer disease-like pathology. *Proc Natl Acad Sci USA.* 1997;94:13287-13292.

Terry RD, Peck A, DeTeresa R, Schechter R, Horoupian DS. Some morphometric aspects of the brain in senile dementia of the Alzheimer type. *Ann Neurol.* 1981;10:184-192.

Terry RD, Katzman R, Bick KL, eds. *Alzheimer's Disease*. Lippincott Williams and Wilkins; 1999:187-206.

Trieb K, Ransmayr G, Sgonc R, Lassmann H, Grubeck-Loebenstein B. APP peptides stimulate lymphocyte proliferation in normals, but not in patients with Alzheimer's disease. *Neurobiol. Aging.* 1996;17:541-547.

Van Dam D, D'Hooge R, Staufenbiel M, Van Ginneken C, Van Meir F, De Deyn PP. Age-dependent cognitive decline in the APP23 model precedes amyloid deposition. *Eur J Neurosci.* 2003;17:388-396.

Walsh DN, Klyubin I, Fadeeva JV, Cullen, WK, Anwyl R, Wolfe MS, Rowan MJ, Selkoe DJ. Naturally secreted oligomers of amyloid-ß protein potently inhibit hippocampal long-term potentiation *in vivo*. *Nature*. 2002;416:535-539.

Weiner HL, Lemere CA, Maron R, Spooner ET, Grenfell TJ, Mori C, Issazadeh S, Hancock WW, Selkoe DJ. Nasal administration of amyloid-beta peptide decreases cerebral amyloid burden in a mouse model of Alzheimer's disease. *Ann Neurol.* 2000;48:567-579.

Weiner, H.L. and Selkoe, D.J. (2002) Inflammation and therapeutic vaccination in CNS diseases. Nature 420, 879-884.

Wilcock DM, Gordon MN, Ugen KE, Gottschall PE, DiCarlo G, Dickey C, Boyett KW, Jantzen PT, Connor KE, Melachrino J, *et al*. Number of Aß inoculations in APP+PS1 transgenic mice influences antibody titers, microglial activation, and congophilic plaque levels. *DNA Cell Biol.* 2001;20:731-736.

Wyss-Coray T, Lin C, Yan F, Yu G, Rohde M, McConlogue L, Masliah E, Mucke L. TGF-ß1 promotes microglial amyloid-ß clearance and reduces plaque burden in transgenic mice. *Nat Med.* 2001;7:612-618.

## CORRESPONDING AUTHOR

Dr. McLaurin may be contacted at the Centre for Research in Neurodegenerative Diseases, Tanz Neuroscience Building, 6 Queen's Park Crescent West, Toronto, Ontario, Canada, M5S 3H2 Telephone: (416) 978-1035; fax: (416) 978-1878; e-mail: j.mclaurin@utoronto.ca.

# Chapter 15
# Fine-Tuning Mitochondria to Lose Weight: The Role of CIDE Proteins in the Development of Obesity and Diabetes

*Dr. Peng Li*
*Institute of Molecular and Cell Biology, Singapore*

## ABSTRACT

The thermogenic activity of Brown Adipose tissue (BAT), which is important for adaptive thermogenesis and energy expenditure, is mediated by the mitochondrial uncoupling protein-1 (UCP1) that uncouples ATP generation and dissipates the energy as heat. CIDE-A, a protein sharing sequence similarity with the N-terminal region of DNA fragmentation factor DFF45//40, is expressed at high levels in BAT. CIDE-A$^{-/-}$ mice exhibit increased lipolysis in BAT and higher core body temperature when subjected to cold treatment. Most strikingly, CIDE-A$^{-/-}$ mice are much leaner, with a 64% weight reduction in white adipose tissue (WAT) and are resistant to diet-induce obesity and diabetes. The molecular mechanism of CIDE-A in regulating thermogenesis, lipid metabolism, and obesity will be discussed in detail.

Keywords: thermogenesis; lipid metabolism; brown adipose tissue; white adipose tissue

## INTRODUCTION

The main focus of our work is to study gene function and its role in the development of obesity and diabetes. The thermogenic activity of Brown adipose tissue (BAT), which is important for adaptive thermogenesis and energy expenditure, is mediated by the mitochondrial uncoupling protein-1 (UCP1) that uncouples ATP generation and dissipates the energy as heat. CIDE-A, a protein sharing sequence similarity with the N-terminal region of DNA fragmentation factor DFF45//40, is expressed at high levels in BAT. CIDE-A$^{-/-}$ mice exhibit increased lipolysis in BAT and higher core body temperature when subjected to cold treatment. Most strikingly, CIDE-A$^{-/-}$ mice are much leaner, with a 64% weight reduction in white adipose tissue (WAT) and are resistant to diet-induce obesity and diabetes. The molecular mechanism of CIDE-A in regulating thermogenesis, lipid metabolism, and obesity will be discussed in detail.

## OBESITY

Obesity is not strictly an age-related disease, however it may be correlated very well with aging. Obesity is determined by the body mass index (BMI). If the BMI is larger than 30 a person is classed as obese. Back in 1985, only a few US states had an obesity rate of 10% to 14%, and the rest of the states had obesity rates of less than 10%. Just 10 years later, in 1995, almost half the states in the USA had obesity rates of more than 15% to 19%, and the remainder had obesity rates of about 10% to 14%. This is a dramatic increase within 10 years. However, this is not the end of the story, as just five years after that,

20% to 24% of the population of the majority of US states were classed as being clinically obese. These alarming rises in obesity rates over a relatively short time period has led many people to say that there is an obesity epidemic in the US, and it is causing a huge burden to the society. Some people have even gone as far to predict that the whole of the US population will be obese in the near future.

Obesity is related to a lot of diseases. One of those diseases is diabetes. If you look at the incidence of diabetes, you will find that this has also increased. However, obesity rates have increased much more dramatically than diabetes. What is the cause of obesity? The cause of obesity is quite simple; a person becomes obese when their food intake or energy intake chronically exceeds their energy expenditure. To maintain normal body weight energy intake and energy expenditure must be balanced. We need to consume a certain amount of food in order to perform basic metabolic functions: this is known as the basal metabolic rate (BMR). We also need to consume a certain amount of food for temperature control or adaptive thermogenesis, and to be able to carry out day-to-day physical activities. If a person rests for one day, 50% of their energy intake will be spent on the basal metabolic rate. Of course, if a person is working, the majority of their energy expenditure will be spent on physical activity.

Therefore, if the energy intake is larger than the energy expenditure, the balance tilts to the right, and this leads to energy storage. When this happens lipids will be stored in the white adipose tissue, one of the adipose tissues in the body, and the person will begin to put on weight. The consequence of any excessive energy storage is obesity, which has been associated with many diseases, such as diabetes, hypertension, heart attack, strokes, cancer etc. So the economic or social burden for obesity is not only for obesity itself, but also for all the other diseases that have been caused by obesity. Thus, it is clear why the quest to understand the mechanisms behind obesity, or identifying drugs that specifically regulate body weight or lipid metabolism, has become one of the most important issues in the field.

## ADIPOSE TISSUE

There are two kinds of adipose tissue in the human body. One is brown adipose tissue (BAT). BAT is called this simply because it is brown. The reason why it is brown is because it contains vast numbers of blood vessels and nerves. Each BAT cell has small lipid structures, and contains large numbers of mitochondria. BAT actually performs a function for temperature control, which is called adaptive thermogenesis. It actually consumes energy and stops storing energy. Research has shown that if they ablate the BAT in mice, the mice become extremely obese. This suggests that BAT may have an anti-obesity role. The other type of adipose tissue is white adipose tissue (WAT), which is the fat tissue everyone has. WAT is made up of large cells, and every cell has a single big lipid droplet. The role of WAT is to store excess energy in the form of lipids. WAT makes a severe contribution to the obesity phenotype.

## CIDE PROTEINS

During a study of genes that regulate apoptosis, we discovered a protein. We named this protein CIDE-A (cell death-inducing DFFA-like effector A) because it had a sequence similar to that of one of the cell suicide proteins, DFF45, and when we over-expressed these protein cells, we actually induced cell death. However, the real physiological function of these proteins is really not very clear. One of the clues we had when we worked on this gene is that it has a homologue called SSB-27, which is now called a white fat-specific gene.

Before we go into the gene functions it is important to consider the structure of this protein. CIDE-A has a normal protein-protein interface; it has a hydrophilic residue on the surface and a hydrophobic core. So basically it presented a normal protein-protein interaction.

*The Function of CIDE Proteins*

Unfortunately, learning about the structure of CIDE-A gave us no clues to the function of this protein. However, histology and tissue distribution tests revealed that, very surprisingly, unlike many of the other cell death proteins, this gene is actually expressed in a very specific pattern. During the embryonic stage, embryonic E-15, this gene expressed in a very specific region: the interscapular region around the neck and back. Close examination of this pattern led us to suspect that it is very special; it is not a brain expression, and it is not expressed in any other tissue. So we suspected that this was actually the so-called brown fat. Indeed, when we use another brown fat marker called UCP-1 (uncoupling protein 1) it showed a very, very similar expression pattern. Thus, it appears that CIDE-A is expressed in a very specific and highly regulated region called brown adipose tissue.

Another CIDE protein, called CIDE-B, is expressed in the liver and kidney at quite a high level, and a third protein, SSB-27, is expressed in WAT, skeletal muscle, and BAT. So as a control, UCP1 is expressed very specifically in brown adipose tissue.

We know we express this CIDE-A in cell death, but what is the *in vivo* role of this gene? BAT contains a huge number of mitochondria, and the function of these is to convert chemical energy to heat for thermogenesis. So BAT has a much enriched expression of beta-adrenergic receptors, and these beta-adrenergic receptors activate adenyl cyclase, generating cyclic AMP (cAMP). cAMP in BAT induces phosphorylase protein kinase and induces activity. Activated protein kinase activates one of the hormone-sensitive lipases, and the role of lipase is to degrade the lipids. In BAT this process is activated by the presence of hormones, which activate the beta-adrenergic receptors. Thermogenesis in BAT is triggered by uncoupling proteins. Uncoupling proteins actually have an opposite role from ATPase. ATPase uses these gradients between the inner membrane space and the matrix to generate energy. But UCP1 uses these protein gradients to generate heat. Thus, because of UCP1, the major function of BAT is actually to generate heat.

BAT exists in most mammals. In humans, BAT only exists for about one month, in order to help maintain the temperature of he newborn infant. After one month these interscapular regions disappear. But whether BAT exists among the white fat or not is a debated issue.

To study the physiological function CIDE-A, we generated knockout mice, CIDE-A$^{-/-}$. Thus, CIDE-A is not present in these mice. We know that the CIDE-A gene induces apoptosis. But very little apoptosis occurs in BAT. So we had to check almost everything in the BAT, including development differentiations. In order to check for development differentiations many, many markers needed to be checked. No differences were apparent, which shows that the BAT actually developed normally: all the markers, all the genes, which are expressed in BAT or WAT are there and present in a similar level. Because this gene was suggested to induce apoptosis, we also checked for cell death in adipose tissue. We did not find any differences between wild type and the knockout mice. Therefore, the conclusion is that there is no apoptotic or cell death difference in the BAT. Another factor that needed checking was the temperature of the mice. BAT contributes significantly to the body temperature, especially in a cold climate. The temperature of the mice was measured and the mice were then put in a cold room for 24 hours. The temperature of the mice rose by 0.8 degrees to 1.0 degree Celsius. This is a statistically significant increase of body temperature in both male and female mice. How much does a 0.8 degree or 1.0 degree Celsius temperature difference contribute to the metabolism? This is actually very hard to figure out, but if you have a body temperature increase of 1.0 degree Celsius, the metabolic rate probably has to increase by 8% to 10%.

What is the morphology of BAT? That is the most dramatic data we actually obtained. We cut the BAT from knockout mice and wild type mice that had been kept at room temperature and from those that had been put in the cold room for 24 hours. In the wild type mice there were less lipids in the BAT, which makes sense as lipolysis increases by roughly 25% when you put the mice in cold. But in the knockout mice, we saw a dramatic decrease in the amount of lipids. We did a quantitative examination by looking at the percentage of lipid volume in each tissue. We found that at room temperature both wild and knockout mice have a similar amount of lipids. But when we expose the mice to the cold, the amount of lipids in the knockout mice decreased by 10 to 20-fold. Basically, this suggests that the knockout mice have increased lipolysis, with much less lipid accumulation when we put them in the cold. Even more interesting, when we repeated the experiment with young mice and old mice (remember that young mice are one month old), both groups of animals had a similar amount of lipids. But when we repeated this experiment with old mice and nine-month old mice, the difference was very dramatic. The BAT in the nine-month-olds is similar to WAT. It becomes whitish, not brownish in our mice. There are almost no lipids. If we cut the BAT out and put it into a solution, the BAT taken from the wild type mice actually floats and that from the knockouts sink. This is because the BAT from the knockout mice has much less lipids, and therefore a totally different density to that of the BAT from the wild type mice. Therefore, in the end it was not even necessary to do genotyping to determine which tissue came from the wild type or the knockout mice, because it was so obvious.

We then carried out another study to look at the lipolysis in BAT. To do this we dissected the BAT and sliced it very thinly, about a 20-micron slice. The slice was then put in a culture dish to integrate with the medium. We then treated the dish with hormones. After one hour we collected the medium. Just by looking at the level of glycerol and free fatty acids in the medium it was clear that the BAT from knockout mice had much higher levels of lipolysis compared with the control. This only happens in BAT; not in WAT at all. So our detailed analysis suggests that the BAT of the knockout mice has a dramatic phenotype. When we look at the morphology of the WAT we can see that that of the wild-type mice has big droplets of lipids. That of the knockout mice has much more compact cells with smaller lipid droplets. Even so, the WAT of wild type and knockout mice is similar, and the amount of proteins is also similar. This suggests there is no hypo- or hyperplasia, of the WAT tissue. But, the lipid amount decreased dramatically.

We can now come to some conclusions about the role of CIDE proteins. Firstly, we have shown that deletion of the CIDE-A gene does not lead to defects in development and differentiation and apoptosis. Secondly, we have shown that the BAT of knockout mice shows increased lipolysis and less lipid accumulation. The knockout mice actually show a lymph phenotype, they have a smaller fat pad. It is very obvious when you open the abdomen of the mice that it has much less lipids. If we weigh the mice, dissect all of the WAT from them and weigh them again, we can then work out the adiposity index, the percentage of fat tissue in the mice. In wild type male mice fed a normal diet, there are about 8% to 10% lipids. But in the knockout mice, there are only about 3%. This represents roughly a 70% drop in lipids. If we feed the mice a high-fat diet, as expected the body weight and the adiposity index of the wild type mice increased. However, the adiposity index of the knockout mice actually decreased. This suggests that deleting CIDE-A leads to significantly less lipid accumulation. These mice also showed a resistance to high fat diet-induced diabetics. Usually when we treat mice with a high-fat diet the mice become obese and diabetic. So we checked the glucose levels of the mice fed a high-fat diet. Results showed that glucose levels decreased dramatically in the knockout mice, but increased in the wild type mice. One of the hormones that the WAT secretes is leptin. So the amount of leptin secreted is proportional to the amount of WAT. In this case we saw a dramatic drop of the leptin levels in the knockout mice.

Therefore, the knockout mice have increased lipolysis in the BAT, and decreased fat accumulation of WAT. But we know that WAT and BAT are actually completely different tissues. How do they communicate with each other? There are secondary pathways that contribute to less fat accumulation in the WAT. One of these pathways is likely to be increased lipolysis in BAT. Increased lipolysis in BAT may also have an effect upon other things, for example, metabolic rate.

Metabolic rate can be measured by putting the mice in a metabolic cage and measuring their total oxygen consumption. Results showed that the metabolic rate of the knockout mice was about 10% higher than that of the wild type mice. Such an increase is statistically significant, and correlates very well with the temperature increase.

Another index of use is the IER, which enables us to determine the amount of lipid metabolism and carbohydrate metabolism. A lower IER means that you have a higher amount of lipid metabolism. From this study, we found that the knockout mice had an increased metabolic rate, and an increased rate of lipid metabolism. This may explain why they also had increased lipolysis in BAT, and decreased lipids in the WAT. The raised metabolic rate means that the knockout mice are constantly consuming 10% more energy than wild type mice, thus leading to a decrease of the energy storage. We also looked at the levels of triglycerides and free fatty acids in the plasma. The knockout mice have a dramatically low level of both triglycerides and free fatty acids. These results further confirm that our mice actually have certain increased fatty acid metabolism.

*The Relationship between CIDE Proteins, Obesity and Diabetes*

Why are obese people or obese mice prone to developing diabetes? One of the reasons scientists have suggested is that obese people and obese mice have high levels of free fatty acids, and that free fatty acids could effect beta cell function and change the level of insulin secretion or glucose uptake, and ultimately increase glucose levels. To investigate this we conducted insulin tolerance tests, and glucose tolerance tests. To determine insulin tolerance we injected the mice with insulin and looked at the effect that the insulin had on blood glucose levels. Results showed that there was no difference between the response of the wild type and knockout mice. However, results of the glucose tolerance test showed that the knockout mice were extremely tolerant to high levels of glucose. The wild type mice responded normally: their blood glucose levels increased significantly at first but decreased to normal levels after two hours. However, in the knockout mice there was no initial increase in blood glucose levels. Instead the blood glucose levels of the knockout mice remained at a similar level and within two hours they had dropped to lower-than-normal levels. This suggests that the knockout mice have increased glucose uptake or disposal; we are not sure exactly which mechanism. But nevertheless, the CIDE-A knockout mice are resistant to high fat-induced obesity and diabetes. Thus, we know that deleting the CIDE-A causes the mice to have a high total body metabolic rate, low levels of plasma, triglycerides, and fatty acids, increased glucose disposal or uptake, and are resistant to obesity and diabetes.

Obviously, we want to know how CIDE-A contributes to the anti-obesity and anti-diabetic phenotype. At present we have two possibilities. Firstly, the lipids could contribute to lipid metabolism or could stimulate thermogenesis. If you increase lipid metabolism you could increase body temperature. So lipids and thermogenesis are interconnected. One of the hints we have for the function, or the mechanism, of CIDE-A-regulated obesity is that another CIDE protein, CIDE-D, is localized, specifically in mitochondria. Thus, we checked for CIDE-A in mitochondria. We found that CIDE-A is localized and merged with the mitochondria marker. We also found that CIDE-A is localized to the heavy membrane mitochondria and not in the cytosol. Similarly, UCP1 is also localized to the mitochondria, not in the cytosol. Subsequently, we found out that the CIDE-A proteins interact with UCP1. However, that is another issue. Anyway, CIDE-A does not alter any expression levels of mitochondria proteins. Thus, we have to exclude the possibility that CIDE-A has other functions affecting gene levels. So, we checked for several of the markers in mitochondria, but results did not show any difference in protein levels. Therefore, we have to concentrate on the interactions or the co-localizations. All we found was that CIDE-A specifically interacts with UCP1. It does not interact with any other mitochondrial marker proteins.

As we have established that there is an interaction between CIDE-A and UCP we need also to establish the functional consequence of the interaction. We did this in two ways. Firstly, we actually expressed UCP1 and CIDE-A. Then we looked at the membrane potentials by staining with a specific dye. We found that in the presence of UCP1 delta-3, which is a stronger uncoupling protein compared with the wild type UCP1, there was decreased membrane potential. However, CIDE-A blocks the decrease of the membrane potential caused by UCP1. Thus, CIDE-A plays a role in inhibiting the uncoupling activity of UCP1. We are currently using mice to prove this model.

## CONCLUDING REMARKS

Research suggests that the function of CIDE-A in the development of obesity and diabetes could be due to its activity to inhibit UCP1. CIDE-A exists in the mitochondria, and that interacts with UCP1. UCP1 is also regulated by many factors, for example free fatty acids and nucleotides. Free fatty acids increase the level of UCP1 activity, and nucleotides decrease UCP1 activity. At normal temperatures, BAT does not actually function very well at all because the UCP1 activity is virtually 100% inhibited by the high level of nucleotides. We also think that CIDE-A contributed to the inhibition of UCP1 in this case. In the absence of CIDE-A, UCP1 activity is up-regulated. This up-regulation of UCP1 activity could contribute to the increase of the body temperature and metabolic rate.

Also, we never explored the possibility that CIDE-A may also play a role in other pathways. For example, directly controlling fatty acid metabolism. We have recently obtained some very exciting evidence to show that CIDE-A may indeed have a role in this pathway. We would also like to look at the function of the other CIDE proteins, which are expressed in the liver and also in WAT, to see how they contribute to obesity and the diabetic effect.

So, what is the correlation between obesity, diabetes, and aging? IM mice have an anti-obese phenotype; they actually have an increased rate of metabolism. This goes against the proposal that restricted calorie intake, or lower metabolism, could prolong life. But, there has been talk suggesting that IM mice could actually live longer lives. But there is no hard evidence yet.

# Chapter 16
# Anti-Aging Medicine:
# The Next Generation of Sports Medicine Present and Future Challenges

*Robert Goldman, M.D., D.O., Ph.D.*
*Chairman, American Academy of Anti-Aging Medicine (A4M)*

## INTRODUCTION

The aim of anti-aging medicine is not only to slow down the aging process, but also to keep the body functioning at its optimum level. This paper will discuss the more practical approaches of anti-aging medicine. We will focus on sports medicine, or Olympic medicine, and how anti-aging techniques can be employed to keep the body functioning at its peak.

We all have different capabilities and different levels that we can achieve, and there are different training programs to help us to get there. Today, both men and women are capable of achieving very high levels of muscle mass: lean muscle mass, and that is why many of the world records previously held by men are now being broken by females, and there are very high level female athletes. So weight training, exercise physiology, and biomechanics are applied equally and fairly to both sexes. Thus, in sports medicine and Olympic medicine, men and women are treated as equal and we simply take into account the athlete's prototype, body type, body weight, and potential.

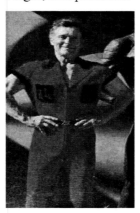

*Figure 1. Jack LaLanne, an example of what was considered to be in excellent physique in the 1930's and 1940's*

Today, the physique shown in Figure 1 is considered to be very, very average. However, in the 1930s and 1940s, having a physique like that in Figure 1 was exceptional. That is because decades ago, we did not have the knowledge in sports medicine, nutrition, resistance training, biomechanics, physiology, and kinesiology that we do today. We have such a wider breadth of how the body functions and what we can do to enhance its capability cosmetically, as well as its capability physiologically.

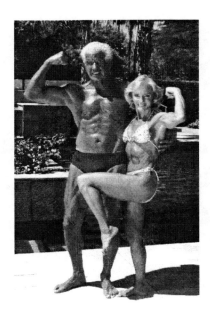

*Figure 2. 74-year-old female weight-training athlete (right), shown with 82 year-old male weight-training athlete (left) [Photo courtesy of Bob Delmontique]*

Figure 2 shows a 74-year-old woman who is a weight-training athlete. At present it is very unusual to see a woman in her mid-70s who has the body of, say, a 25-year-old. However, this will become more commonplace over time.

## BUILDING AN INDIVIUALLY-TAILORED HEALTH AND FITNESS PROGRAM
*Self Perception and Goal Setting*

Many individuals who have let their physique go have allowed their body fat percentage to get very high; have lost the basic muscle mass to fat ratio; and have an out-of-shape cardiovascular system. Yet, these same people perceive themselves as looking far more lean and healthy as in reality. What we have is this perception of what we think we look like. Therefore, we have to take that mind image and put it in a more realistic sense of what are we really dealing with, and what our achievable goals are. If a health practitioner sets a goal that is too hard for the patient, the patient will become frustrated, and s/he will not maintain their treatment program. Thus, it is important to grade these goals so that you gradually move them upwards. When patients start to get some success, such as when they start losing weight, when their muscle mass changes, or when they start having more energy, they will overcome any self-doubt and start to feel like they really can achieve their goals.

Every patient should be treated in the same way as an Olympic athlete. Whether they are 15, 20, 30, 80, or even 90, everyone can have their performance enhanced. It is important to design programs that address realistic and achievable goals that you as a health practitioner can help the patient to achieve.

*Exercise*

Exercise is very important. Exercise is probably the closest thing there is to that elusive magic anti-aging pill. However, you can exercise and you can die anyway, so exercise alone is not the complete program. Exercise cannot override everything. We also need to take into account a patient's diet, laboratory results, and predisposing factors towards disease. It is necessary to have a comprehensive approach so that we know what we are dealing with both on the outside and the inside. A good example of this is women who come into a clinic, seeking cosmetic surgery. They tend to look good on the outside, but they are often very unhealthy on the inside. So we have to be healthy on both the inside and the outside.

People tend to think they exercise far more than in actuality. A lot of guys do curls with beers: they grab their six-pack of cans, put three beers in each hand, and do some curls in front of the television. To exercise properly, one must get off the couch. Another problem is exercise equipment. Where do most people put exercise equipment in the house? The answer is in front of the TV, in the bathroom, or next to the refrigerator. People do this because they visit these parts of the house a lot and figure that seeing their exercise bike or whatever will spur them into action. However, in reality the most common use for an exercise bike in the home is to hang clothes off. Therefore, we need to get away from the habit of not utilizing things properly. When is the right time to start an exercise program? Today. When are you too old to start one? When you are dead. Any time prior , that is, as long as you have a pulse, is time to start a program suited for your particular health needs.

When talking about exercise programs it is important to consider the basic physics of joint motion. We have a range of motion, and whenever you train, you want to go through this full range of motion. A lot of people go those these half-jerky ranges, but by not going through the full range they are not building strength throughout that range of motion. Ensuring that you go through the full range of motion also helps to combat against some of the osteoporotic changes that occur.

In addition to range of motion, we also have balance and symmetry. Training one side unilaterally over the other is very common. Sports like tennis involve unilateral motion. This means that you will get very strong in one arm and not balanced in the other. Thus, it is obviously important to be cognizant of that. Also, some people will work on their abdominal muscles because they want a flat abdomen, but they will forget about their lower back and then they end up with a solar: they become forward-bent and then they cannot function properly. So we must always work towards balance and function.

## *Understanding the Different Types of Muscle Contractions*

There are a few different types of muscle contractions. One is called isometric contraction: "iso" meaning same, "metric" meaning length. Therefore, an isometric muscle contraction is where the muscle remains the same length no matter how much force is put against it. It is like pushing against an immovable force, for example pressing against a solid wall.

We also have isotonic contraction: "iso" meaning same, "tonic" meaning tone. Thus, an isotonic muscle contraction is where the same tone in the muscle is maintained throughout the range of motion. This is the type of muscle contraction that the majority of machines in fitness clubs are designed to produce.

Another type of contraction is isokinetic contraction. Computer-controlled devices that tell us how many foot-pounds of force a person is putting out throughout the range of motion can be used to measure isokinetic contractions. By using these we can tell how much strength someone has at different degrees of motion.

The head is the center of balance in the body. When we move the head we change the whole center of gravity, we change the whole spinal curvature. So you must control the weight and you must control body biomechanics. As an example, there are two ways to lift weights. One is not the right way. The incorrect way is where you throw the weight up. What goes up must come down. If a person lifts a weight in such a way they are dealing with acceleration, gravity, and inertia, and they will have to use their joints and ligaments to stop the weight. That is how people get injured lifting weights. The right way to lift a weight is with slow, controlled movements. Going back to the head as the center of balance in the body, if the head is tilted forwards the spinal curvature will change. A change in the spinal curvature will also affect the shoulders, the hips, and the knees. All of these changes leave a person prone to injury, thus it is vital to be cognizant of head positioning when lifting weights because it does affect the entire spinal column.

## *The Importance of Intensity, Frequency, and Duration*

Today, there are many high-tech devices and different ways of exploring how we can get fit. A number of the machines on the market today have what we call ergometric functions. This means that they are able to tell you how many calories you have burned, and so on. People seem to like them, although they are not of much value.

The three most important things to consider are intensity, frequency, and duration. Intensity simply means how hard a person is training; frequency obviously means how often; and duration means for how long. These three components are the ways that you adjust program. For weight loss and for trimming we would typically recommend lower-intensity exercise for a longer duration. It takes 30 to 45 minutes for the body to begin burning fat during low-intensity exercise; therefore it is necessary to exercise for a little bit longer. Sometimes people do fast aerobic workouts that only last for 10 minutes or so; from a fat-burning point of view, these workouts are pointless.

## *Core Balance Training Programs*

Body biomechanics are extremely important, whether it be in soccer, in baseball, or in basketball. In order to achieve our goals we want to look at some of the basic, easy mechanisms and easy devices that we can use in our practices to create a core, or body, balance training program.

One such device is a balance board. Balance boards are very easy to use and they can even be made at home. All a balance board is simply a piece of plywood with a 2-by-4-inch wood tie underneath. It wobbles, and therefore is also called a wobble board. A balance board trains the tiny muscles in the ankles, the knees, and the hips, to achieve balance. It is extremely important for seniors to maintain or improve their balance because they have a tendency to fall. As well as simply standing on a balance board, patients can also do different exercises on it, all of which will improve balance by training those tiny muscles in the ankles, the knees, and the hips.

There is another device, which can also be made at home, that is actually a variation of the balance board: the beam. The beam is similar to that you see in the Olympic Games where gymnasts perform handstands and the dance effortlessly upon them. It is basically a plank of wood, 4 to 7 inches wide. You train on the beam by walking along it, thereby training the tiny muscles in the knees, the ankles, and the feet. Simple as it sounds, this is actually a highly effective core balance training regimen. Basketball players train by going back and forth across each other on beams. And sometimes two basketball players, opposing each other, will train by crossing their legs back and forth and then they'll start throwing a basketball to one other, going back and forth. The challenges of beam training can become quite complex. We can also put rubber roof tiles under the beams, so the beams wobble when they're going back and forth. All these things can be assembled in the office-based medical practice. The main theme is that all of these regimens are very easy to use, and very effective.

We also have something called a "dog," a device for training the tibialis anterior (the foreleg of the foot). This little device gets people doing dorsiflexion and plantar flexion, and therefore provides us with a way of training tiny muscles in the foreleg and the ankles that we typically would never train. Most people do not train muscles from the knee down. We ignore them. But it is these muscles that are the stabilizing muscles that allow your body to have proper function, so they are quite important.

The Swiss army ball, or exercise ball, has become very popular all through the sports medicine world. People now use this for back training. These balls enable us to do erector spinal training, forward flexion, hyperextension, and back flexion. The Swiss army ball enables us to train the body, and train the tiny muscles by doing things differently. For example, if you do a simple push-up using a Swiss army ball you have to balance the lower torso by using the tiny muscles in the shoulders, elbows, hands, and hips because now a push-up is a more challenging motion and you have to utilize other muscles in order to stabilize. The same thing applies with sit-ups. Add a Swiss army ball to the equation and not only are the abdominal muscles being exercised, but also the stabilizing muscles in the hips and the torso. This is training what we call the core system, the center portion of the body.

There are a variety of ways to address this core system, which we call reverse torso curls and forward torso curls. Now, some people do not have access to a big fitness facility where they can use this heavy type of machinery. So in those particular cases, we employ a device called a power band. Power bands are basically big rubber bands, which make it possible to do something called functional speed training. You are able to go very fast with them, and you don't have inertia of the weight coming back at you. You can do leg extensions, like curls, and virtually almost any other type of exercise with a power band. Another advantage is that they fit in a pocket, thus a lot of athletes bring these on the road with them so that they can do full training programs while travelling.

Let us look more closely at forward torso curls. When doing forward torso curls, patients should not sit all the way up; all that you have to do is curl the torso enough in order to contract the abdominus rectus. We also bend the knee in order to offset the psoas muscle. If you feel like your back goes out and you cannot straighten up, and you feel like you are bent forward or bent to one side, that is because this very powerful muscle called the psoas has gone into contracture. If this happens, it is important to train the hyperextension and the erector muscles to try and straighten the back again. As well as forward torso curls, there are also reverse torso curls. There are a lot of different ways to approach strength training for lower back problems.

## Lower Back Problems

What causes lower back problems? As we get older, we start to get a bit rotund: our body weight increases, and we get a bit of a big belly. This increases the lumbar lordotic curve in the low back and causes the pelvic angle to change. All of these stress factors are being placed on the lower back. People often start walking with what we call a "sway," and then they start to get a spinal orthesis. They get slippage, they get compression of the disks, and before you know it they have serious back problems. Training certain muscles to try and help compensate for that natural weakness that occurs in the joint structure is important for anyone with lower back problems and those at risk of developing them.

Gravity inversion, where people strap boots on their ankles and hang upside down, was very popular in the States in the 1980s. Drs. Goldman and Klatz of the American Academy of Anti-Aging Medicine published the first eight scientific papers on the physiologic changes that occur when somebody inverts. What we found is that intraocular pressure, central retinal arterial pressure, and systemic blood pressure, all skyrocketed. Our bodies are not designed to hang upside down statically. So people were getting petechiae and blackouts and there was concern of stroke.

There are three basic motions for training the back, along the the X, Y, and Z-axes. We have rotation, we have forward flexion, and we have hyperextension. Each of these motions are measured separately. In order to achieve peak function, not everybody wants to go directly to the top level. This is not prudent; rather, our patients should be trained to arrive at the top via gradations. We also must consider what level of function: what level of power, or strength, or muscle mass, we want to achieve. In this age of increased biomechanics and training programs, we now integrate in the ultimate goals of a training program. Do your patients want to trim down? If they want to lose weight, they need to burn more calories than their daily intake. Fad diets do not work. While patients may try these particular diets, the bottom line is that you burn more calories by increasing your internal body thermostat, by training harder. The best way to train is a program on which the patient can remain committed to for an extended period of time, which will likely be a long-duration/low-intensity workout.

## Plastic Surgery

A lot of people are looking for the quick fix. They want to go right in for liposuction. There is nothing wrong with plastic surgery. But it is suggested that you get into the best shape you can first to see really what you need or what you don't need. Many times certain patients are able to get themselves in a good enough shape so that they find that they don't even need the surgical procedure. So instead of going right for the quick fix, it is much better to encourage the patient to thing about the long-term and change their lifestyle and modify their diet so that they end up living longer, healthier lives.

## CONCLUDING REMARKS

Society's attitude to the physique has changed considerably over the decades. A more heavyset physique was considered to be the ideal physique in the 1890s. However, a more trim physique is much more desirable today. There is also a great deal of controversy at present surrounding the use of dietary supplements. However, the general consensus is that sometimes we do need that extra help such as supplements, because we are not getting everything we need from our diet.

As anti-aging physicians we should be concentrating on developing individually-tailored programs that will suit each patient, so much so that the program will become part of their life. To do this it is important to know what a patient is capable of both physically and psychologically, and what their ultimate goal is. Give them blood tests, a full cardiac screen, and an EKG. It is also necessary to do muscle testing: check out your patients' joints and ligaments, making sure that these are all functional.

Invest in balance boards, Swiss army balls, and power bands, and devote an exam room to their use, so that you can begin to develop sports training or stability training programs. You could have a really profound effect on a patient's healthcare simply by integrating these simple devices into your basic healthcare program.

Do not underrate the power of education. Unfortunately, our patients are not well-educated in terms of foodstuffs. They think fast food is good food and, unfortunately, as physicians well know, fast food contains very high levels of fats, cholesterol, and sodium. Tell your patients that fast food is fat food, and start to change their perceptions of food immediately.

In the US we have senior sports organizations. These are for people aged 65 and above who are now competing in Olympic-type sports, such as high jump and pole vaulting. Today, there are close to 300,000 competitive members of these organizations. Then we have the more extreme genetically-gifted athletes. Somebody like Al Oerter, an American Olympian who competed in four Olympic Games, was a multiple gold medal winner, and at the age of 60 tried out for the Olympic team again; he just missed making the team. Individuals like Al Oerter exemplify what it means to have a lifelong health fitness program. Another outstanding example of fitness is John Glenn, the astronaut, who returned to space in his mid-70s.

In summary, it is important for physicians to approach fitness as a comprehensive program. Anti-aging medicine is a comprehensive field. It encompasses the utilization of exercise training, dietary modification, nutritional supplementation, hormone replacement therapy, stress modification, lifestyle modification, and deployment of laboratory blood testing and advanced diagnostic technologies such as full-body spiral CT, MRI, and CAT scans. Our job it to put all these things together into a comprehensive lifelong health and fitness program so that our patients live longer, healthier lives.

## REFERENCES & FOR FURTHER READING

Goldman R and Klatz R. *7 Anti-Aging Secrets for Optimal Digestion and Scientific Weight Loss*, ESM Publications, 1996.

Goldman R and Klatz R. *The New Anti-Aging Revolution: Stopping the Clock for a Younger, Sexier, Happier You,* Basic Health Publications, 2003.

## ABOUT THE AUTHOR

Dr. Robert Goldman is physician co-founder of the anti-aging medical movement and of the American Academy of Anti-Aging Medicine (A4M), a non-profit medical organization dedicated to the advancement of technology to detect, prevent, and treat aging related disease and to promote research into methods to retard and optimize the human aging process.

*Correspondence:* Postal c/o American Academy of Anti-Aging Medicine; 1510 West Montana Street; Chicago, IL 60614 USA.

# Chapter 17
# The Science Behind Growth Hormone

*Dr. Peter E. Lobie*
*Associate Professor and Associate Director, Liggins Institute, Auckland, New Zealand*

## ABSTRACT

Since the isolation of growth hormone (GH) in 1944 it has become increasingly apparent that the GH/insulin-like growth factor-1 (IGF-1) axis (otherwise known as the somatotrophic axis) has a fundamental and obligatory role in regulating normal somatic growth throughout fetal and childhood development. Human GH is used for various clinical purposes including childhood growth retardation and adult senescence-related conditions in a multibillion-dollar and growing worldwide industry. Since GH may be used routinely in the adult population it is vital that the mechanism of GH action be delineated. This paper extracted from a presentation to the Second Asia-Pacific Conference in Singapore will summarize the basic cell and molecular biology of GH and the mechanism by which it affects cellular function. Delineation of the signal transduction mechanism will allow us to understand the specific actions of the hormone that result in its dramatic physiological actions and also to identify possible undesirable actions that may limit its use.

Keywords: growth hormone, signal transduction, kinase JAK2, structure, gene

## INTRODUCTION

Many hormone nutritional factors and related cell regulators contribute to the regulation of mammalian growth and development. However, only growth hormone, or GH, stimulates longitudinal bone growth in a specific and dose-dependent manner. Therefore, in disorders of GH production and secretion we see abnormal growth patterns. Perhaps the best example of this is GH excess occurring before puberty resorting in giantism, a condition not commonly encountered anymore due to effective medical intervention. Conversely, GH deficiency occurring before puberty results in dwarfism, and the dwarfism observed with GH deficiency is a proportionate dwarfism, which can differentiate it from some of the other commonly observed forms of dwarfism, such as achondroplasia. The dramatic growth-promoting effects of GH are not limited to certain mammalian species. Indeed, a large number of organisms use GH to stimulate skeletal growth; from teleost fish to reptiles and amphibians. Most avian and mammalian species also utilize GH for stimulation of longitudinal bone growth.

So how does GH achieve these dramatic effects on longitudinal bone growth? Longitudinal bone growth is achieved at the epiphyseal growth plate. Thus, cell proliferation and differentiation within the epiphyseal growth plate results in a gradual elongation of the length of the long bone, at least until after puberty when the action of the respective sex steroid hormones result in a closure of the epiphysis, therefore preventing further longitudinal bone growth. GH simply stimulates the proliferation of cells within the proliferative layer of the epiphyseal growth plate, and also stimulates the differentiation of these cells to produce bone. This is a very simple explanation as to how GH can stimulate longitudinal bone growth.

Obviously, longitudinal bone growth is not the only effect of GH; otherwise it would not be of great interest to anti-aging physicians. Indeed, the effects of GH are extremely pleiotropic. Medline shows that more than 46-thousand articles detailing more than one thousand effects of GH have been published in the last 50 or so years. It is likely that in the years to come there will be many more effects of growth hormone identified. To emphasize the importance of GH, the majority of cell types in the human body express the GH receptor and are therefore responsive to GH. Therefore, GH exerts a functional effect on all the major organ systems of the human body. Interestingly, GH secretion declines with age. The signs and symptoms of GH-deficiency in adults include decreased bone mineral density, decreased concentration, decreased muscle strength, and thinning of skin and hair.

As you can imagine, GH's role in growth and the purported effects of GH-deficiency in the adult, make hGH big business. A number of multinational corporations share a multibillion a year market for the sale of hGH. In the past, this was predominantly for the treatment of short-stature children, but nowadays GH is being used, or increasingly used, to treat a variety of disorders occurring as a result of GH deficiency in the aging population. Indeed, one would probably be surprised at the number of people that are using GH in an effort to stay young.

The purported, or supposed, effects of GH are very widespread in the popular literature. It is not unusual to be sent e-mails stating that GH will increase strength, stamina and endurance; increase muscle mass and promote fat loss; improve sleep; increase libido and sexual stamina; encourage hair re-growth and a lessening of gray hair; improve skin and strengthen bones; improve vision and hearing; lower blood pressure; and improve memory and cognitive abilities. Thus, it comes as no small surprise that, based on these supposed, or reported, beneficial effects of GH that a rather large and largely unregulated and worrisome market has emerged for the sale of GH and GH-releasing substances.

What is important when we consider all this hype surrounding GH, is for the anti-aging physician to understand the biology of GH and how it functions at a molecular and cellular level to mediate some of its effects on cell and organ physiology.

## WHAT IS GROWTH HORMONE?

GH is a classical pituitary hormone secreted by the anterior pituitary gland, which is situated at the base of the brain. It is secreted by so-called acidophilic cells of the anterior pituitary, which are called somatotropes.

Until recently, GH was thought only to be an endocrine hormone, and only to be secreted from the pituitary gland. However, recently it has become apparent that GH can also function as an autocrine/paracrine growth factor. Therefore, GH synthesis and expression has been detected in a wide variety of tissues at different developmental stages, including the central nervous system; the pineal gland; several reproductive tissues, including the testis, ovary, mammary gland, and placenta; specific cells of the salivary gland; and the lung. It is rather widespread throughout the immune and hematopoietic system, in particular the thymus, the spleen, and the bone marrow. GH is also synthesized in endothelial cells of blood vessels in different locations, and in dermal fibroblasts. Thus, it can be seen that in addition to its endocrine role, GH can also function as a local growth factor in an autocrine/paracrine manner. It is likely that endocrine and hGH share common and possess exclusive effects on cellular function.

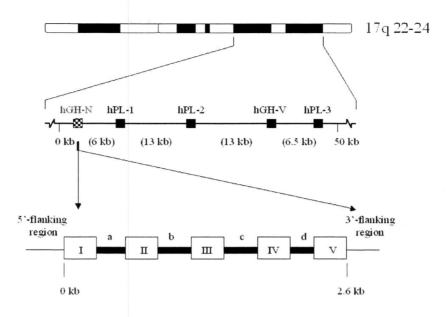

*Figure 1: The hGH-hPL gene cluster.
The five genes comprising approximately 8kb of structural sequences
are spread over 50 kb of DNA in 17q 22-24.*

## The Growth Hormone Gene

The GH gene is contained within a cluster of five structurally and functionally related genes spanning approximately 50 kilobases of the human genome (see Figure 1). Within this cluster of five genes there are two GH genes: the human growth hormone (hGH) normal gene, which is what we think about when we talk about GH; and the hGH-variant gene, which is produced in the placenta and, therefore, obviously, affects half of the population.

The hGH-normal gene is transcribed with five exons and four introns to encode the primarily predominant form of GH that circulates in the blood, the 22-kilodalton isoform of hGH. A 20-kilodalton isoform of hGH also exists, and is identical to the 22-kilodalton isoform except for the deletion of amino acids 32 to 46 by alternative splicing of exon-2.

The hGH gene, at the molecular level, is predominantly regulated by the first 500 base pairs of the hGH gene promoter. This is because the first 500 base pairs contain two DNA binding sites for a transcription factor, a POU-homeodomain transcription factor termed PIT-1.

## The Structure of Growth Hormone

Structurally, hGH is nothing remarkable. It shares many features in common with other cytokine molecules. And like other cytokine molecules, is basically characterized by the presence of four anti-parallel alpha-helices consisting of between 21 and 30 amino acids. Also, GH has, like other cytokines, a hydrophobic core of approximately 20 amino acids.

## Growth Hormone Regulation

At the physiological level, GH is regulated by three major factors. It is primarily regulated by a hormone called growth hormone-releasing hormone (GHRH), which is the target of many of the GH-releasing substances on sale. GHRH binds to somatotrope cells in the anterior pituitary, increases the concentration of the transcription factor PIT-1, and therefore turns on hGH transcription and subsequent secretion. A relatively recent hormone, another growth hormone-releasing hormone, termed ghrelin is released from the stomach and acts directly on somatotropes, again, to increase hGH transcription and secretion. The negative regulatory hormone released from the hypothalamus is somatostatin, and it opposes the effects of these two growth hormone-releasing hormones.

GH secretion from the pituitary is also regulated by some of the end products of hGH action, including insulin-like growth factor-1 (IGF-1), which is the proposed hormonal mediator of the effects of GH on longitudinal bone growth. Therefore, GH binding to liver cells, or hepatocytes, stimulates the production of IGF-1, which then feeds back at different levels to inhibit further hGH production. Some time ago, IGF-1 was postulated to mediate the effects of GH on skeletal growth. Therefore, pituitary GH would stimulate hepatic IGF-1, which would be released to the circulation and mediate the effects of GH on longitudinal bone growth. However, in recent years it has been apparent that both GH and IGF-1 have direct and independent effects on somatic growth.

If we cross one dwarf mouse, which was created by deleting the GH receptor gene, with another dwarf mouse, which was created by deleting the IGF-1 gene, we would produce the second-smallest mammal every known, a 2-gram mouse. The effective decreases in body size are additive. It is therefore obvious that both GH and IGF-1 can have direct and independent effects on longitudinal bone growth.

## *The Growth Hormone Receptor*

The direct effects of GH are mediated by GH binding to the GH receptor, which is located at the cell surface. GH binds to the receptor in a one to two stoichiometry. In other words, one hormone molecule binds to two receptor molecules to induce dimerization of the GH receptor. It is this dimerization of the GH receptor that is thought to initiate signal transduction by GH into the cell.

The GH receptor was the first cloned member of the expanding cytokine receptor super-family. This super-family of receptors includes other important hormones, such as prolactin, which is required for lactation, erythropoietin, which is needed for erythropoiesis or red blood cell production, and the obesity hormone leptin. As well as these hormones, a number of other molecules important for development of the immune and hematopoietic systems are involved: granulocyte colony stimulating factor, granulocyte macrophage colony stimulating factor, and a series of interleukins including interleukins-2 to -7, interleukin-9, and interleukins-11 and -12.

The structural characteristics of cytokine receptors that grouped them into one family are rather limited, but include a few points, for example: a single transmembrane-spanning domain, limit of homology in the extracellular domain running at somewhere between 14 and 44% but including conserved pairs of cystine residues required for the tertiary structure of the molecule and subsequent binding of the ligand. All cytokine receptors have a WSxWS motif required for dimerization of the receptor molecule upon ligand binding, and are characterized by the lack of any intrinsic kinase activity within the intracellular domain of the receptor. Therefore, these cytokine receptors, including the GH receptor, signal via a proline-rich box 1 or box 2, which is the site of association of cytokine receptor-associated kinases.

The GH receptor gene is a single-copy gene spanning a rather large 87 kilobases of the human genome, and is characterized by the presence of at least eight alternative 5' prime untranslated region variances on exon-1. These different variances are differently expressed in different tissues to regulate the tissue or cellular-specific expression of the GH receptor: exons 3 to 7 code for the extracellular hormone-binding domain; exon-8 for the transmembrane domain; and exons 9 and 10 for the intracellular domain of the receptor.

The structure of the GH receptor is obviously very similar to the structure of other cytokine receptors, and includes; conserved pairs of cystine residues in the extracellular domain; a WSxWS-like motif in the GH receptor to mediate dimerization of the receptor; a transmembrane domain; and also a proline-rich box 1 region in the intracellular domain, which is the site of association of the GH receptor associated kinase JAK2.

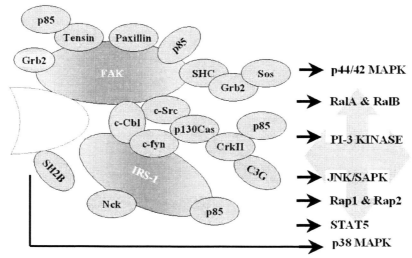

*Figure 2: Diagrammatic representation of the multiprotein signalling complex formed after cellular stimulation with GH.*

## GROWTH HORMONE SIGNAL TRANSDUCTION

At the appropriate GH concentration, GH binding to its receptor will induce heterodimerization, of the GH receptor, resulting in the formation of an active receptor and signal transduction into the cell. At high concentrations of hGH, or with use of a hGH antagonist that has been specifically designed to prevent dimerization of the receptor, no active receptor dimer will be formed and no signaling will occur. Once the receptor is dimerized it activates a kinase called JAK2.

JAK2 is usually associated with the GH receptor, and upon dimerization of the GH receptor is tyrosine phosphorylated and activated. It was thought that activated JAK2 would subsequently mediate all downstream signaling effects of GH. A few years back we, and other groups of researchers, identified a number of dependent pathways, which mediate the effects of GH within the cell. The major pathway is probably the JAK-STAT pathway, and GH utilizes STAT1, STAT3, and STAT5. GH primarily utilizes STAT5, to result in specific patterns of growth such as a male-specific pattern of growth as opposed to a female-specific pattern of growth.

GH also stimulates transcription by use of the classical Ras-MAP kinase pathway, leading to the activation of certain transcription factors. It has also been demonstrated to activate protein kinase C. GH also utilizes components of the insulin-receptor signaling system, especially the insulin-receptor substrate molecules, to mediate certain PI 3-kinase-dependent metabolic effects within the cell, such as glucose uptake. Further work by our team also identified that GH stimulated the formation of a multi-protein signaling complex centered around an adaptor molecule called Crk-II (Figure 2). To cut a long story short, subsequent identification and characterization of all these proteins that were tyrosine phosphorylated in response to GH stimulation of cells, has allowed us provide a diagrammatic representation of the multi-protein signaling complex stimulated by GH.

Thus, GH binding to the receptor induces dimerization of the receptor, phosphorylation and activation of JAK2, and JAK2 then tyrosine phosphorylates and activates another kinase, which is termed focal adhesion kinase (FAK); JAK2 also phosphorylates insulin-receptor substrate 1 and activates its docking function, which is very important for the formation of this multi-protein signaling complex. Many of the major downstream pathways stimulated by GH are dependent on the formation of this multi-protein signaling complex.

For example, p44/42 MAP kinase can be activated within the complex via FAK or directly via Grb2 [associated with FAK]. Another member of the MAP kinase family, JNK/SAPK kinase, can also be activated by GH, via the formation of a CrkII-C3G complex. PI 3-kinase can be activated at multiple points. We observe the p85 regulatory subunit of PI 3-kinase associating with many distinct molecules within this complex, including IRS-1. The regulation of STAT5 activity also comes out of this complex. For example, cCbl is a negative regulator of GH-stimulated STAT5 activity and therefore growth of specific organs such as the mammary gland. What is particularly interesting is the presence in this complex of another non-receptor tyrosine kinase molecule, called c-Src and its association with a number of small, Ras-like GTPases, which are activated by GH.

It has previously been reported that other cytokine receptors could activate c-Src independent of JAK2, and we were therefore very interested to determine the interaction of c-Src and JAK2. What we observed was that GH activation of JAK2 and c-Src were two independent but parallel events. Therefore, dominant negative mutants of c-Src did not affect the ability of GH to activate JAK2, and dominant negative mutants of JAK2 did not affect the ability of GH to activate c-Src. Therefore we can conclude that GH actually initiates its signal transduction by activation of two kinases. One is JAK2 and the other is c-Src.

However, to verify GH activation of c-Src kinase activity was of physiologic importance we needed to demonstrate which pathways were downstream of GH-activated c-Src. To do this we examined GH activation of Ras-like GTPases, since Ras-like GTPases had been demonstrated to be activated by c-Src or in a c-Src-dependent manner by other cytokine molecules. Firstly, we examined the activation of Ras itself. Remember, GH had previously been demonstrated to activate Ras to feed into the p44/42 MAP kinase pathway. We observed, however, that GH activation of Ras was entirely JAK2 dependent. Therefore, dominant negative mutants of JAK2 prevented GH activation of Ras, whereas dominant negative mutants of c-Src did not prevent GH stimulated Ras activation.

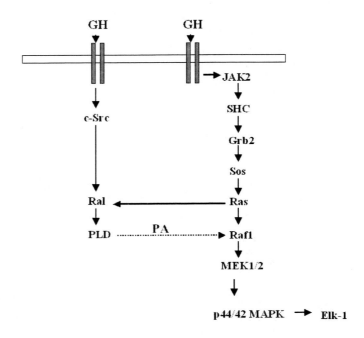

*Figure 3: Diagrammatic summary of JAK2 dependent and c-Scr dependent activation of the p44/42 MAP kinase pathway by GH.*

We were still without a pathway for GH activated c-Src activity. We therefore continued to examine other small Ras-like GTPases. We observed that full activation of RalA and RalB by GH required the combined activities of both kinases. Inhibition of c-Src activity potently inhibited Ral activity and therefore, Ral was a molecule, which is predominantly activated by GH in a c-Src-dependent manner. Activated Ral, subsequently activates another enzyme in the cell, termed phospholipase-D, and GH can activate phospholipase-D in a Ral-dependent manner (Figure 3). Thus we see a rapid increase in phospholipase-D activity within the cell after GH treatment. This increase in phospholipase-D activity stimulated by GH can be prevented with a dominant negative mutant of Ral. Therefore, GH stimulates phospholipase-D activity in a Ral-dependent manner. Once phospholipase-D is activated it catalyses the hydrolysis of phosphatidylcholine within the cell to produce phosphatidic acid. One of the target proteins of phosphatidic acid is Raf kinase, which is involved in the activation of p44/42 MAP kinase. Therefore, if we use Elk-1 mediated transcription as an indicator of p44/42 MAP kinase activity we see that forced expression of Ral-A dramatically enhances the ability of GH to stimulate Elk-1 mediated transcription, whereas a catalytically inactive variant of phospholipase-D prevents both GH stimulation of Elk-1 mediated transcription and the enhanced Elk-1 mediated transcription as a result of forced expression of RalA.

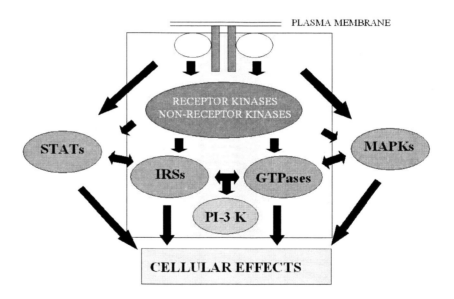

*Figure 4: Simplified diagrammatic representation of the mechanism of GH signal transduction. GH binding to the cell surface receptor induces dimerization of the receptor with subsequent association and activation of JAK2 and c-Src with the GH receptor. JAK2 and c-Src are then responsible for subsequent activation of the various major groups of signalling molecules. These include ; 1) other receptor (EGF receptor) and non-receptor (FAK) kinases, although as in the case of the EGF receptor it may be used simply as an adapter protein ; 2) members of the MAP kinase family including p44/42 MAP kinase, p38 MAP kinase and JNK/SAPK and the respective downstream pathways ; 3) members of the IRS group including IRS-1,2 and 3 which may act as docking proteins for further activation of signaling molecules including phosphatidylinositol-3 kinase ; 4) small Ras-like GTPases and 5) STAT family members including STATs 1,3, 5a and 5b which constitute one major mechanism for transcriptional regulation by GH. The major groups of signalling molecules are not exclusive; for example FAK and c-Src are found in a signalling complex with IRS-1 required for JNK/SAPK activation.*

Therefore, GH binds to its receptor, causing dimerization of the receptor and activation of JAK2, leading to activation of Ras, and subsequent activation of the p44/42 MAP kinase pathway and resultant Elk-1 mediated transcription. At the same time, GH binding to the receptor, causes dimerization of the receptor, resulting in the activation of c-Src. c-Src feeds into the Ral pathway, leading to the activation of phospholipase-D and the production of phosphatidic acid, which positively feeds into the p44/42 MAP kinase pathway to increase the transcriptional effects of GH on this pathway. We can therefore conclude that GH signal transduction is initiated at the cell surface by not one kinase, but it in fact initiated at the cell surface by at least two kinases. This is what we know at present; however it would not be surprising to learn that more than two kinases are involved in initiation of GH signal transduction at the cell surface.

To summarize the mechanism by which GH can affect cellular function: GH binding at the cell surface induces dimerization of the receptor and activation of JAK2 and c-Src independently. These two kinases then feed down further into a number of kinases and the combination of these activated kinases then activate the four major signaling groups of molecules utilized by GH; including members of the STAT family, which are responsible for the growth patterns stimulated by GH: GH utilizes three members of this family: STATs 1, 3, and 5. GH also utilizes three members of the MAP kinase family: p44/42 and p38 MAP kinases and JNK/SAPK. GH also activates a number of Ras-like GTPases and also utilizes components of the insulin receptor signaling system, including insulin-receptive substrates 1 to 3 with subsequent activation of PI 3-kinase. Therefore, the combination of the effects of these major signaling pathways will result in the cellular effects of growth hormone (see Figure 4).

As well as being switched on, it is also important to turn a signal off. GH, like other cytokine molecules that use tyrosine to stimulate or to mediate signal transduction within the cell, also uses specific phosphatase molecules to dephosphorylate the activated molecules, or the molecules that are activated by tyrosine phosphorylation. However, in the case of cytokine receptors and also GH, a more specific negative feedback mechanism exists. This negative feedback mechanism is of immense physiological importance. This mechanism utilizes members of the family of proteins termed SOCS, or suppressors of cytokine signaling, of which there are eight members. These SOCS molecules are transcriptionally activated by the cytokine itself, and then they feed back to act at the level of receptor or kinase to prevent further signaling by the respective cytokine or hormone. These molecules are extremely important physiologically. For example, If one deletes SOCS-2, which is primarily involved in terminating GH signalling, from mice one can generate a giant mouse very similar in phenotype and appearance to what one would see if the mouse transgenic for GH; with a dramatic increase in longitudinal bone growth and an increase in muscle mass.

## CONCLUDING REMARKS

Delineation of the signal transduction mechanisms of GH will allow us to understand the specific actions of the hormone that result in its dramatic physiological actions and also to identify possible undesirable actions that may limit its use.

## REFERENCES

Kopchick JJ, Andry JM. Growth hormone (GH), GH receptor, and signal transduction. *Mol Genet Metab*. 2000;71:293-314.

Lobie PE, Waxman DJ. Growth Hormone. In: Henry HL, Norman AW, eds. *Encyclopedia of Hormones and Related Cell Regulators*. New York, NY: Academic Press; 2003:208-216.

Zhu T, Ling L, Lobie PE. Identification of a JAK2 independent pathway regulating growth hormone (GH) stimulated p44/42 MAP kinase activity. GH activation of Ral and phospholipase D is Src dependent. *J Biol Chem*. 2002;277:45592-45603.

Zhu T, Goh EL, Graichen R, Ling L, Lobie PE. Signal transduction via the growth hormone receptor. *Cell Signal*. 2001;13:599-616

## ABOUT THE AUTHOR

Peter E Lobie obtained a B.Med.Sci. (Distinction) and MBBS (First Class Honours) in 1992 from the University of Queensland in Australia. He was awarded the highest accolade from the University in the form of a University Medal. His postdoctoral work was undertaken at the Karolinska Institute in Sweden where he also obtained a PhD. He has consecutively held faculty positions in Sweden, Singapore and now is Associate Professor and Associate Director of the Liggins Institute in Auckland, New Zealand.

Peter Lobie is author of more than 70 publications mostly in prestigious and high impact international journals and is an international authority on molecular mechanisms of growth hormone action. Recent emphasis in his laboratory has focussed on the oncogenic potential of autocrine human growth hormone in the human mammary epithelial cell.

He is the recipient of multiple local and international awards and is regularly consulted by international journals and funding agencies. Associate Professor Lobie is the inventor on 3 patents and has been associated with industry during his time in Sweden, and in New Zealand is a consultant to Endocrinz Ltd. He has also served on the steering committee for the establishment of the Singapore Tissue Network (S$150 million), and consulted for the Pharmaceutical Department, Ministry of Health in Singapore, Ministry of Education and the Agency for Science, Technology and Research of Singapore.

# Chapter 18
# Update on Nutrient Supplements and Other Types of Treatment for Age Related Macular Degeneration

*Dr. Gerard Chuah*
*The Eye Institute, Tan Tock Seng Hospital, Singapore*

## ABSTRACT

Age-related macular degeneration (ARMD) is a significant cause of visual impairment and blindness among people aged 65 years and older in Singapore, the United States, and other developed countries. Despite advances such as photodynamic therapy, transpupillary thermoplasty, and ablative laser photocoagulation, currently available techniques only reduce the risk of moderate or severe visual acuity loss in some patients with the 'wet' type of ARMD. Surgical means of therapy such as subretinal surgery and macula translocation surgery are under investigation, and each surgical therapy carries risks and specific indications for surgery. Not everyone can and will benefit from surgery.

The latest results from the Age-Related Eye Disease Study (AREDS) show that patients with the 'dry' type of ARMD (extensive intermediate size drusen, at least one druse, non-central geographic atrophy, advanced ARMD, or vision loss due to ARMD in one eye) and without a history of smoking, should consider taking a supplement of antioxidants plus zinc and copper. This has been shown to statistically reduce the risk of progression for the development of advanced ARMD for these patients.

**Keywords:** visual acuity; vision loss; dry ARMD; wet ARMD

## INTRODUCTION

Results of the Age Related Eye Disease Study (AREDS) revealed that Age Related Macular Degeneration (ARMD) is the leading cause of legal blindness in adults aged 65 years and over in North America. There are two main types of ARMD:
- 'Dry' or atrophic ARMD
- 'Wet' or exudative ARMD

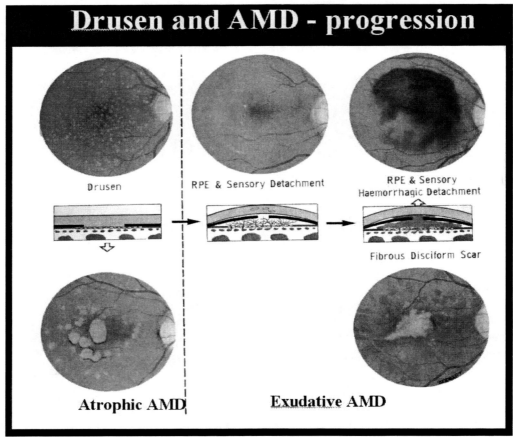

*Figure1: The Progression of Age-Related Macular Degeneration (ARMD) from 'wet' or atrophic ARMD to 'wet' or exudative ARMD*

As can be seen in Figure 1, the dry and wet types of ARMD look very different. The dry variety, which can be divided into the 'atrophic' type and the 'drusenoid' type, is characterized by round deposits called drusen, which are collections of degenerative material and an atrophic retina, which is a retina that is 'thinned out'. Whereas the wet variety is characterized by abnormal blood vessels that grow beneath the retina and bleed or leak. These abnormal blood vessels form what is called a choroidal neovascular membrane (CNVM).

Dry ARMD usually presents with a slow, progressive loss of vision. The vision usually is quite stable and deteriorates slowly to poor levels. In contrast, wet ARMD may present with a rapid onset of drastic loss of vision. This usually occurs when the abnormal blood vessels bleed beneath the retina. The wet type of ARMD is responsible for 90% of legal blindness, yet just 10% of cases of ARMD fall into the wet category.

## THE EYE

In order to understand ARMD, it is important to understand the structure of the eye and the functions of the various parts of the eye. Probably the four most important parts of the eye are: the cornea, which is like the windscreen of a car: it has to be clear otherwise you will not see clearly; the lens, which of is responsible for focusing images on the retina; the pupil, which regulates the amount of light; and finally, the retina. If you compare the eye to a camera, the pupil is like the shutter of the camera, the lens is the lens, and the retina is the film. A camera is useless without a film, and a high-quality camera will not produce a good image if the film is of poor quality.

### *Basic Anatomy of the Eye*

The sclera is the tough outer coat of the eye, which gives structural strength to the eye, and is white in color. Between the retina and the sclera is a vascular layer called the choroid, which is very important. The choroid contains big blood vessels, small blood vessels a membrane called Bruch's membrane, and a fine layer of capillaries called the choriocapillaris. Located just outside the retina and attached to the choroids is the retinal pigment epithelium (RPE); the RPE is separated from the blood vessels of the choroid by Bruch's membrane. Bruch's membrane is one of the key players in the pathology of AMD. Together with the retinal pigment epithelium (RPE), Bruch's membranes are crucial for vision.

The RPE is important for two main reasons; it absorbs stray light, and provides nutrition for the neuroepithelium. Recent research has shown that blue light (light of short wavelength) is actually very toxic to photoreceptors. The RPE contains melanosomes, which absorb ultraviolet radiation. It is also important for nutrition of the neuroepithelium, and is involved in the vitamin-A cycle, and in the regeneration of photoreceptors.

Photoreceptors function on a diurnal basis, that is, they follow a twice-daily cycle. Photoreceptors are either rods or cones, and they regenerate at certain times of the day. Rods are important for night vision and for peripheral vision. They are mainly found outside the central part of the eye: outside the macular. Cones are responsible for color vision and for high-quality vision. The cones are found in the macular region. The RPE is in very close contact with the outer segment of these photoreceptors, and is involved in the regeneration of the outer segment.

The macula is situated in between the temporal, the superior temporal, and the inferior temporal arcade of vessels of the retina, and is bounded by the optic nerve. The macula is where we find the highest concentration of cones, and is therefore responsible for detailed vision. If the macula is damaged you can see around someone, but you may not be able to see his features.

## AGE-RELATED MACULAR DEGENERATION

The diagnosis of ARMD is usually straightforward: the patient is elderly and has the clinical features of ARMD in both eyes. People with ARMD can actually have very good vision, however close inspection of the eye will show that the macula, the central part of the retina, is littered with yellowish deposits called drusens. These yellowish deposits are deposits of lipofuscin, which is actually a degenerative product.

Epidemiological studies have shown that the majority of people with dry ARMD will experience a gradual progression of the disease. They will develop more drusens, and some of them will progress to geographic atrophy, where the RPE starts to die. As we know, the RPE is crucial for vision thus if it dies vision dies with it. Geographic atrophy causes a very slow, progressive loss of vision. The severity of vision loss caused by geographic atrophy all depends on the site of the lesion is. If it is right in the center of the macula, an area called the fovea, a patient's vision is going to be badly affected. However, if the lesion is outside of the fovea the prognosis is not quite as bad. 90% of people with dry ARMD will develop a scotoma, a spot in the central vision that may appear dark, light, or blurred.

Dry ARMD can also progress to wet ARMD, which is considered to be the more serious form of ARMD. Actually, both are just as bad; one is just the lesser evil. The progression of wet ARMD is much faster than that of dry ARMD. 10% of ARMD patients will develop wet ARMD. The wet type presents in a very dramatic fashion. Patients with wet ARMD may come to the doctors and say that they were well yesterday, but when they woke up this morning they couldn't see their wife. The patient may suddenly find that the central spot of their vision has gone: it is black. In such a case, examination of the eye will show bleeding; blood may be present in the vitreous gel of the eye and accumulate underneath the retina. This is called a hemorrhagic pigment epithelial detachment. This bleeding is from abnormal blood vessels that grow underneath the retina and through Bruch's membrane. These abnormal blood vessels come from the choriocapillaris, the fine layer of capillaries located in the choroids, and they are very fragile. They bleed very easily. Eventually the abnormal blood vessels form a scar, which ultimately damages the retina. The end result being that the patient becomes legally blind.

### Risk Factors for Age-Related Macular Degeneration

The incidence of ARMD is increasing. In the West and other developed nations, the incidence of ARMD is quite high, and it is the leading cause of blindness in adults over 65 in these countries. Research studies investigating the risk factors for ARMD have shown that many of the risk factors appear to be oxidative in nature, whereas the protective factors appear to be antioxidative. Smoking is a major risk factor as is having a blue iris.

The color of the iris is related to skin color, which also is related to the concentration of melanosomes in the RPE layer. People with blond hair and blue irises have fewer melanosomes that darker-pigmented people. Melanosomes absorb stray ultraviolet light, thus the more melanosomes a person has the better protected against ultraviolet radiation they are. Therefore, people with light-colored irises are more prone to getting ARMD because they are exposed to more ultraviolet radiation, and therefore have higher levels of oxidative stress.

Several studies determined that certain macular pigments, such as lutein and zeaxanthin, which are found mainly in the macula and screen out blue light, reduce the amount of reactive oxygen species (ROS), or free radicals that are generated by light exposure. Blue light has been identified as a major culprit in damaging photoreceptors. Animal studies have shown that exposure to very high-intensity blue light caused severe damage to the photoreceptors. Vitamin-E and also some of the glutathione antioxidants and amino acid precursors may exert a protective antioxidant effect on photoreceptors.

## TREATMENT OF AGE-RELATED MACULAR DEGENERATION
### Dry Age-Related Macular Degeneration

Unfortunately, there is no proven treatment for the 'atrophic' type of ARMD. However, for certain advanced stages of the 'drusenoid' type of ARMD, the Age Related Eye Diseases Study (AREDS) found that the daily consumption of antioxidants such as Vitamin C and Vitamin E, together with zinc, significantly slowed down the progression of the disease and the subsequent deterioration of vision. Study participants were given vitamin-C 500 mg, vitamin-E 400 IU, vitamin-A 15 mg, zinc 80 mg, copper 2 mg; or an inactive placebo. Subjects were followed for a period of five years. Results showed that the antioxidant, zinc, and copper cocktail reduced the rate of progression of ARMD in high-risk patients by as much as 25%. This discovery is highly significant, because prior to AREDS there was no effective treatment for ARMD.

In addition to taking an antioxidant, copper, and zinc cocktail similar to that used in the AREDS, patients diagnosed with the 'drusenoid' type of ARMD should also be advised to stop smoking as this has been found to be a risk factor in several studies. Whilst not proven, they are also advised to avoid overexposure to ultraviolet radiation by staying out of the sun or wearing protective sunglasses.

Recently, much attention has been focused on the role of carotenoids in the prevention and treatment of ARMD. Carotenoids are plant pigments, and about 700 different types of carotenoids have been discovered so far. Humans cannot synthesize these carotenoids and must obtain them from their diet. Two important carotenoids have been identified for the eye: Zeaxanthin and lutein. Both are fat soluble xanthophylls, which are absorbed in the small intestines and transported to the liver where they are packaged in lipoproteins and transported to the rest of the body. Zeaxanthin is found in mainly yellow, orange and red fruits and vegetables, such as peppers, peaches and corn. Lutein is found mainly in dark green leafy vegetables, such as spinach, collard greens and kale.

Lutein and zeaxanthin have been found in the greatest concentrations in the macula section of the retina. The extremely high concentration of lutein and zeaxanthin in the macula creates a yellow spot, called the "macula lutea," that can easily be seen in a retinal photograph. Most of the xanthophylls reside within Henle's layer, which is a layer of axons found in the inner retinal layer. It was thought by many researchers that by being located within Henle's layer, the xanthophylls are able to filter off the most damaging blue part of the light spectrum before it hits the photoreceptor cells. Research by Bone *et al* revealed that this appears to be the case and that both lutein and zeaxanthin absorb the ultraviolet blue spectrum of light, which is the most damaging to retinal structures.

Research by Thomson *et al* on Japanese quail and other studies on primates seem to bear out the important protective role of lutein and zeaxanthin in preventing ARMD. Evidence from epidemiological studies is also relatively consistent in that high dietary intake of fruits and vegetables rich in xanthophylls reduces the risks of macula degeneration and delays the onset of cataracts. A recent study suggested that a high level of serum zeaxanthin is strongly associated with a reduced risk of advanced ARMD.

The AREDSII trial will begin shortly this year (2003) using lutein and zeaxanthin in addition to the antioxidants studied in the earlier AREDS study. More than 5,000 patients with advanced ARMD have been recruited by the National Eye Institute and National Institutes of Health in the United States.

### *Wet Age-Related Macular Degeneration*

There are treatment options available for the wet type of ARMD. However, the decision to treat the wet type of ARMD depends on the vision of the eye, and the location and the size of the abnormal vessels (CNVM).

Once the diagnosis of a wet type of ARMD is made, in order to determine whether the ARMD should be treated, the patient must be subjected to a test called a fluorescein angiogram (FFA), and if the equipment is available, an indocyanine green angiogram (ICG). The FFA is the 'gold standard' test for ARMD as it provides valuable information about the size and location of the abnormal vessels (CNVM). Many large scale studies done on ARMD were based on FAA findings. The criteria to start treatment are also based on FAA criteria. However, many major eye centers in the world now include the ICG as part of the basic investigations for ARMD, as the ICG gives additional information about the ARMD that may help in treatment.

The FFA involves injecting a dye into the veins of the arm. This dye is unique in that it has the property of fluorescence when blue light shines on it. The dye will enter the circulation and passes into the blood vessels of the eye. Once in the eye, it enters all the blood vessels, including the abnormal blood vessels, and blue light will cause it to fluoresce and the images of the blood vessels can be captured on film or on video. By examining the images captured, one can determine the size and location of the abnormal blood vessels (CNVM). Some patients may be allergic to fluorescein and are not suitable for this test.

The ICG is a test whereby indocyanine green dye is injected into the veins of the arm and special cameras are used to record the images of the blood vessels of the retina and choroid. The ICG test is useful as an adjunct to the FAA as it is able to visualize the abnormal choroidal blood vessels of the CNVM much clearer, even when there is some overlying subretinal blood. For certain types of ARMD such as Idiopathic Polyploidal Choroidovasculopathy (IPCV), the findings on ICG are quite characteristic and are useful if the patient is deemed suitable for laser treatment. If a patient is allergic to iodine or seafood, then ICG is contraindicated.

The only proven treatment for the wet type of ARMD is laser treatment. There are many different types of laser treatment that can now be used to treat wet ARMD, including focal ablation laser treatment, photodynamic therapy (PDT), and transpupillary thermoplasty (TTT).

Focal ablation laser treatment is where a laser is used to destroy the abnormal blood vessels directly by direct heat damage. However, results obtained in a study by the Macula Photocoagulation Study Group showed that focal ablation laser treatment also completely destroys the retina overlying the abnormal blood vessels. Consequently, there will be a drop in vision corresponding to the area of the retina treated, and if this part of the retina is located centrally at the fovea, which is responsible for clear vision, the patient will have an immediate drop in vision after treatment.

PDT is one of the latest treatment modalities. It involves injecting a special light sensitive dye, for example verteporfin, into the veins of the patient's arm. After a short period of time, a laser using a certain wavelength of light is shone into the patient's retina where the abnormal blood vessels are. This special wavelength of laser light activates the dye and causes very localized damage to the blood vessels. PDT does not damage the overlying retina. As a result, the patient's vision is not affected. Results of the Treatment of ARMD with Photodynamic Therapy (TAP) Study showed that PDT was successful in both destroying the abnormal blood vessels in a significant number of patients with certain types of ARMD and preventing further deterioration of their vision.

TTT is one of the latest forms of laser treatment being studied for the treatment of wet ARMD. It basically involves shining a laser light of low intensity and a certain wavelength onto the affected area of the macula. This low intensity laser light does not damage the overlying retina but is postulated to cause damage to the abnormal blood vessels in the underlying ARMD lesion. It does not involve injecting a special dye.

### *Current Research*

The treatment of ARMD has been extensively studied and several large scale trials have published their results recently, these include: the Macula Photocoagulation Study (MPS) and the Treatment ARMD using Photodynamic Therapy Study (TAP). Another study, the Transpupillary Thermoplasty Randomized Treatment Trials (TTRT) is still underway and the results have not been published yet.

As well as the existing developments in laser treatments for ARMD, there are a number of other promising research developments of importance.

### *Antiangiogenesis treatment*

As we have discussed, wet ARMD is characterized by the growth of abnormal blood vessels underneath the retina. If the growth of these abnormal blood vessels can be stopped or retarded, serious vision-threatening complications, such as subretinal hemorrhage and exudates, can be prevented. In 1989, a scientist by the name of Napoleone Ferrara isolated a protein crucial to the growth of new blood vessels called vascular endothelial growth factor (VEGF). By producing a compound which can block VEGF, the growth of abnormal blood vessels can be inhibited or stopped. Recently, several anti-VEGF drugs have undergone patient trials. Macugen, a macula degeneration drug, has just been completed a 1,200 patient drug trial and so far, the results seem promising. The main disadvantage of Macugen is that it has to be injected into the diseased eye monthly for as long as one year and as such treatment with Macugen carries the potential risk of a serious eye infection (endophthalmitis) and of a retinal detachment. Lucentis, another macula degeneration drug, is also in final stage trial testing. Retaane, a third macular degeneration drug,, is a modified steroid that targets enzymes produced by the abnormal blood vessels. It has also completed late stage trial testing.

*Artificial Retina or Retinal Microchip Implants*

The latest research aims to develop an artificial retina that can convert light impulses into microelectrical signals, which can be interpreted by the visual system. A company called Optobionics has developed an Artificial Silicon Retina (ASR) which is surgically implanted in the eye. The ASR microchip is a silicone chip measuring 2mm in diameter and 25 um thick. It contains about 5,000 microscopic solar cells on its surface (called microphotodiodes) that convert light impulses into microelectric impulses. Each of the microscopic solar cells has its own stimulating electrodes and when implanted underneath the retinal surface, they will stimulate the remaining functional retinal cells to produce the sensation of vision.

The ASR microchip is powered solely by light entering the eye and does not rely on external wires or batteries (unlike the other artificial retinas that were developed). As the ASR was designed to interface with a retina that is still functional (with only partial outer retinal degeneration), it is important that the inner part of the retina is undamaged and functional. Hence, the ASR is most suitable for diseases such as ARMD and retinitis pigmentosa. Other diseases that may be suitable for ASR implantation include some forms of chronic retinal detachments, Usher's syndrome, Leber's Congenital Amaurosis, Stargardt's Disease, Choroideremia, Gyrate Atrophy and Best's Disease. Clinical testing for these diseases has not yet begun.

Implantation involves performing a surgery called a vitrectomy with the creation of a hole in the retina (called a retinotomy) through which the ASR is implanted underneath the retina. The vitreous cavity of the eye is then filled with air.

In the ten trial patients who had the ASR implanted, all have shown moderate to significant visual improvement. The risks of the procedure include retinal detachment, infection and inflammation.

## CONCLUDING REMARKS

ARMD is becoming more common. It is a leading cause of blindness, and will result in a significant loss of quality of life. As AREDS showed, there is a way to slow it down or prevent it. People aged 50 and over should be encouraged to see an eye surgeon at least once every two to three years. Regularly visiting an eye surgeon would mean that ARMD, and other diseases such as cataracts and glaucoma, could be caught in their early stages.

Patients diagnosed with ARMD should be told to stop smoking and encouraged to purchase a pair of good quality sunglasses that offer protection against ultraviolet radiation, namely UVA A, B, and C. They should also be given a daily cocktail of antioxidants, copper, and zinc.

## REFERENCES

AREDS Research Group. The Age Related Eye Disease Study (AREDS): A randomized placebo-controlled clinical trial of high-dose supplementation with vitamins C and E, beta carotene and zinc for age-related macula degeneration and vision loss. AREDS Report #8. *Arch Ophthalmol.* 2001;119:1417-1436.

Bone RA, Landrum JT, Guerra LH, Ruiz CA. Lutein and zeaxanthin dietary supplements raise macula pigment density and serum concentrations of these carotenoids in humans. *J Nutr.* 2003;133:992-998.

Falsini B, Piccardi M, Iarossi G, Fadda A, Merendino E, Valentini P. Influence of short-term antioxidant supplementation on macular function in age-related maculopathy: a pilot study including electrophysiologic assessment. *Ophthalmology.* 2003;110:51-60; discussion 61.

Gale CR, Hall NF, Phillips DI, Martyn CN. Lutein and zeaxanthin status and risk of age related macula degeneration. *Invest Ophthalmol Vis Sci.* 2003;44:2461-2465.

Lyle BJ, Mares-Perlman JA, Klein BEK, Klein R, Greger JL. Antioxidant intake and risk of incident age-related nuclear cataracts in the Beaver Dam Eye Study. *Am J Epidemiol.* 1999;149:801-809.

Macula Photocoagulation Study Group: Laser photocoagulation of subfoveal neovascular lesions in age related macula degeneration. Results of a randomized clinical trial. *Arch Ophthalmol. 1991;*109:1220-1231.

Mares-Perlman JA, Fisher AI, Klein R, Palta M, Block G, Millen AE, Wright JD. Lutein and zeaxanthin in the diet and serum and their relation to age-related maculopathy in the third national health and nutrition examination survey. *Am J Epidemiol.* 2001;153:424-432.

Thomson LR, Toyoda Y, Langner A, Delori FC, Garnett KM, Craft N, Nichols CR, Cheng KM, Dorey CK. Elevated retinal zeaxanthin and prevention of light-induced photoreceptor cell death in quail. *Invest Ophthalmol Vis Sci.* 2002;43:3538-3549.

# Chapter 19
# Cartilage Repair with Autologous Chondrocytes and Stem Cells

*Dr. Eng Hin Lee*
*Department of Orthopaedic Surgery, National University of Singapore/National University Hospital*

## ABSTRACT

It is well known that articular cartilage does not respond well to damage, often repairing with fibrocartilage at best. Orthopedic surgeons have over the years used many different techniques to aid or enhance the repair of damaged articular cartilage. These techniques have included drilling the subchondral bone; microfracture; continuous pressure motion; and more recently, transplanting autologous osteochondral plugs (Mosaicplasty).

In the past few years, tissue engineering researchers have advocated the use of autologous cultured chondrocyte transfers to repair chondral defects, especially in the knee joint. Although the early clinical results have been promising, the long tern results in terms of the type of repair tissue formed and the longevity of the new tissue is still questionable.

The Musculoskeletal Tissue Engineering Group at the National University of Singapore has been working on this area for the past several years, and has shown in animal experiments the superior results obtained from the transfer of mesenchymal stem cells derived from periosteum or bone marrow. Controlled studies on articular cartilage healing following drilling, Mosaicplasty, and autologous chondrocyte and mesenchymal stem cell transfers have shown that the repair tissue following mesenchymal stem cell transfer most closely resembles that of articular cartilage.

In the past two years, human clinical trials have been carried out using mesenchymal stem cell transfer in over 30 adults with chondral lesions. The early results are promising. The hope is that with increasing expertise, it may be possible eventually to resurface larger areas of damaged articular cartilage.

**Keywords:** degenerative joint disease; tissue engineering; osteoporosis; osteoarthritis
+

## INTRODUCTION

The focus of this paper is degenerative joint disease and the methods that we have today to treat or manage these problems. Two of the diseases that we face as we age are osteoporosis, which is currently at epidemic proportions, and osteoarthritis. Our focus will be on osteoarthritis, which is basically due to joint degeneration, although there are some chemical, mechanical, and traumatic causes for this problem as well.

There are many ways to treat osteoarthritis. We can modify our life-style, reduce body weight, and do certain exercises (however it is important to remember that some forms of exercise can aggravate osteoarthritis). Medications are available, and nutritional supplements (such as glucosamine) may also be useful. Another treatment option is intraarticular injections, one of those being chorionic acid, which is supposed to be helpful. Some people also choose to wear braces because it helps to alleviate pain. And of course, if all else fails, there is surgery. In some cases of very severe osteoarthritis, for example where the joint is completely destroyed, there is nothing else that can be done to help a patient except surgery to replace the joint.

Joint replacements are typically very successful and have helped elderly people with osteoarthritis live very, very useful lives. However, because they are mechanical they do suffer from wear; and over a period of time they wear out (this is especially true of plastic joint replacements). If that happens, a follow-up operation is necessary to fit another new joint. However, the decision to undergo another surgery really depends on how old the patient is and how fit they are. Sometimes it may not be possible to conduct a revision due to various reasons.

## TREATING OSTEOARTHRITIS

Can we prevent osteoarthritis, or at least slow or halt the progression of disease so that joint replacements will not be needed? Do chondral defects, or lesions in the cartilage, lead to osteoarthritis later on? These are both important questions, which need answering.

The evidence does show to some extent that chondral defects do indeed lead to osteoarthritis later on in life. And I think the evidence does show to some extent that this does happen. So if a patient injures their knee cartilage, is there anything we can do to prevent deterioration and osteoarthritis? A lot depends on the size of the defect, and the extent of involvement; that is, whether it is on the weight-bearing or non-weight-bearing part of the knee. If it is on the non-weight-bearing part, there is obviously less stress to the joint than if the defect were on a weight-bearing part. Another important factor is the depth of the lesion. There is a classification system for grading chondral defects. This varies from just a softening of the cartilage, which we call chondromalacia, to fissuring and larger defects, and then full-thickness defects, which are classified as Grade 4. Other factors also need to be taken into account, for example, the patient's age, their activity level, and their medical history. All of these factors need to be considered before deciding what the best treatment options are for the patient.

A subject of great debate is whether or not cartilage lesions can repair themselves. In most cases, the propensity, or the ability, of cartilage to repair itself is very, very poor. Once cartilage has been injured it almost never heals back to the original type of cartilage, which is hyaline or articular cartilage. At best it repairs itself to fibrocartilage, which is not as good as normal articular cartilage both functionally and biomechanically.

### *Surgical Options for Cartilage Repair*

There are many conventional means that are now being done surgically to repair, or to try to heal, cartilage lesions. These include abrasion, drilling, microfracture, and continuous passive motion (CPM). CPM is a concept that was advanced by Robert Salter, an orthopedic surgeon from Toronto (Ontario, Canada) who found that if you create a lesion in cartilage and then subject the damaged joint to CPM over a period of time, it seems to heal. This seems to suggest that motion is better than immobilization for promoting the healing of cartilage. The repair potential for most of these types of treatment has been to form fibrocartilage. However, there are other methods, for example, trying to resurface the cartilage lesion with grafts taken from either the perichondrium or the periosteum. The problem with these treatment options is that there are problems with the surgery itself; how do you anchor these periosteal grafts? Furthermore, periosteal grafts do form fibrocartilage, and later on they form bone as well, and that is bad because you do not want bone in your joint: you want cartilage.

Then there are types of grafts called osteochondral grafts, which are a combination of cartilage and bone. An example of osteochondral grafts is Mosaicplasty, which involves replacing the patients damaged cartilage with cartilage obtained from a different part of the patients joint. This is also not without problems, as the patient tends to develop problems with the donor site.

Another option is allografts, which mean grafts taken from somebody else (typically a cadaver). This is problematic from the start as the procedure is dependent upon the availability of a joint that is suitable from an immunological viewpoint. It is also vital to endure that the graft did not come from a patient with HIV, hepatitis, or other problems. Furthermore, when you try to transfer cartilage in such huge grafts there is very low viability in the chondrocytes. The short-term results achieved with allografts are not too bad. However, we do not yet know what happens over the long-term.

## Chondrocytes and Stem Cells

More recent developments include autologous cellular implantation, which mainly uses chondrocytes. Autologous chondrocyte implantation created a lot of interest when it was published in the *New England Journal of Medicine* back in 1994. Over the short- term, patients seem to do quite well in terms of symptoms. But of course, we don't know about the long-term viability of these transfers, as well as the mechanical strength of the transfers.

At the National University of Singapore/National University Hospital, we are currently conducting a study on autologous chondrocyte implantation, which is funded by the Ministry of Health from the Health Services Development Program. So far, over the last two years, we have enrolled more than 30 patients, varying between 16 years and 54 years of age. For the study we harvest the cartilage from the non weight-bearing portion of the knee, grow the chondrocytes, and then we re-insert the tissue approximately three or four weeks later. We usually inject about 20- to 40-million cells into that defect, depending on the size of the defect. Seal it off with glue, and the procedure is complete. So how do we assess the success of the procedure? We use various types of questionnaires, including the SF-36 Health Survey and the IKDC (the International Knee Documentation Questionnaire). One of the questions we asked participants deals with stiffness and swelling of the knee. Results showed that preoperatively 72% of participants had stiffness and swelling, whereas postoperatively, just 33% of participants complained of stiffness and swelling. So there was definite improvement in some criteria. The preliminary conclusion from this study is that autologous chondrocyte implantation significantly improves the patient's health.

The most interesting area of research at present is mesenchymal stem cells, and the possibility that they will enable us to repair damaged cartilage. Mesenchymal stem cells are adult stem cells, which give rise to mesenchymal tissues, such as connective tissues, cartilage, bone, tendons, ligaments, and bone marrow. We typically obtain these cells from bone marrow but, in some cases, we derive them from periosteum. They can also be derived from skin and from fat. Animal studies suggest that this technique may give better long-term results. For our experiment we injected stem cells into a defect that we created in the femoral condyle of a group of rabbits. For the experiment we had three groups of rabbits; one without cells that acted as the control group, a second group that were treated with chondrocytes, and a third group that were treated with stem cells. For the stem cell treatment, we injected stem cells into the defect and covered it with a piece of periosteum. Results showed that healing among the control group was not good, as was expected. Chondrocytes performed quite well, however at 36-weeks some degeneration of the cells was apparent, so they don't seem to last very long. The mesenchymal stem cell treatment was the most effective, and 36-weeks after treatment the damaged cartilage looked as if it was very close to normal articular cartilage. So our conclusion from this study was that stem cells appear to be superior to chondrocytes, and probably have great potential in parenchymal application.

## CONCLUDING REMARKS

Our future research will concentrate on autologous stem cells rather than chondrocytes. At the National University of Singapore/National University Hospital, we are investigating the use of different types of scaffolds, constructed from biodegradable polymers, to see whether these can help to heal larger defects. We know that many of these scaffolds can be seeded with cells successfully. So with confocal microscopy, for example, we can see whether cells are seeding into the scaffolds and if they remain alive. Another area of great interest is growth factors, and whether or not these can help us to enhance the healing process.

# Chapter 20
# Modern Management of Diseases of Neurological Deficits

*Dr. Ho King Lee*
*Medical Centre of Gleneagle, Singapore*

## ABSTRACT

Neurodegenerative diseases are progressive disorders that affect nervous system function because of selective cellular loss. Basically, neurodegenerative diseases are a form of accelerated selective neuronal aging. The purpose of this paper is to discuss the characteristics and mechanisms of neurodegenerative disease and consider current management strategies.

**Keywords:** neuronal aging; dementia; Alzheimer's Disease; Parkinson's Disease; acetylcholine esterase inhibitors; nootropics; levodopa; Coenzyme Q10; deep brain stimulation; stem cell therapies

## INTRODUCTION

The purpose of this paper is to discuss the characteristics and mechanisms of neurodegenerative disease and current management strategies. The local epidemiology of neurodegenerative disease in Singapore will also be discussed.

What are neurodegenerative diseases? These are disorders that affect nervous system function because of selective cellular loss. The amazing thing about neurodegenerative diseases is that they do not affect the whole brain all at once. It is not as if you cut off the blood supply to the brain and all of the brain dies. But instead, certain cellular populations within the brain get affected selectively. And, of course, these conditions are progressive. Basically, neurodegenerative diseases are a form of accelerated selective neuronal aging.

What do we know about neurodegenerative disease? Appendicitis is the most common, and is certainly the best understood, of all the programs that lead to cell death, or apoptosis. In short, this is mainly driven by cysteine hepato-proteases, or caspases. Of late, more and more information has come up about the genes and diseases that involve caspase or are involved in caspase substrates. If the caspases work harder, then there is more apoptosis, so this is a fruitful area for molecular research. There are two main types of neurodegenerative conditions. There are those that affect movement, such as Parkinson's disease, motor neuron disease, Kennedy syndrome, and conditions like spinal cerebellar ataxia. And then there are those that are related to memory and cognition, such as Alzheimer's disease, which is probably the most common of all of the neurodegenerative diseases.

How do we define dementia? Well, firstly we say that there is a memory problem. Memory loss is the first and most prominent symptom in Alzheimer's disease or, in fact, in any dementia. But in order to make a diagnosis of dementia, and to distinguish simple memory loss associated with age from true dementia, then we have to look for other features. Firstly, there must be another cognitive problem: a problem with judgement, abstract thought, or problem-solving, and so on and so forth. Secondly, the condition must be chronic. It cannot be reversed. Finally, there is a loss of capacity to handle the activities of daily living.

# DEMENTIA AND ALZHEIMER'S DISEASE

## *Epidemiology*

Research by Kwae E Shok revealed that the prevalence of dementia in Singapore is actually not overwhelmingly high. Studies showed that approximately 2.5% of the Chinese population and 4% of the Malay population of Singapore suffer from dementia. However, if you look at the Western populations, the prevalence of dementia ranges from 3.5% to 14.9%. With respect to Alzheimer's, which is the neurodegenerative form of dementia, or rather the commonest neurodegenerative form of dementia, the rate of Alzheimer's is less than 2% in both Chinese and Malay populations. Singapore has one of the fastest-aging populations in the world. If the government projections on population growth stand, then causing an increase in the Singapore population and an inversion of the age pyramid, the elderly population will increase from 7.2% to 12.9% by 2020, thus meaning that we will have three times more demented people than we would otherwise have today. We know, from local studies again, that about 50% of dementia cases in Singapore are due to Alzheimer's. The bulk of the rest are due to multiple infarct dementia or vascular dementia. So dementia is going to cause Singapore a lot of public health problems. The annual rate of dementia increases almost exponentially with age. With each decade of life, the risk of getting dementia doubles.

## *Diagnosing and Treating Dementia and Alzheimer's Disease*

A study by Silverman *et al* compared the effectiveness of two strategies for assessing whether Alzheimer's disease was responsible for cognitive decline in geriatric patients, and in subsequently managing those patients according to the recommended standards of the American Academy of Neurology (AAN). The first strategy was based on an approach already endorsed by the AAN, which included a general medical and neurological examination, structural imaging and laboratory tests. The second approach was based on many of the same AAN recommendations but additionally incorporated PET (positron emission tomography). Results showed that PET significantly increased diagnostic accuracy. Both false negative (from 8.3% to 3.1%) and false positive (from 23.0% to 11.9%) diagnoses for Alzheimer's were reduced by approximately 50% when PET was used in addition to the conventional strategy. Furthermore, reducing the number of false diagnoses resulted in a 62% decrease in avoidable months of nursing home care, and a 48% decrease in months of unnecessary drug therapy. Currently, PET is a ridiculously expensive investigation, but it is also important to remember that the drugs used to treat Alzheimer's are expensive, as is nursing home care. So by saving money on drug treatment and care, PET becomes a cost-effective procedure. Regardless of cost, it is nice to know that nowadays you can diagnose pre-clinical Alzheimer's.

Up until relatively recently, neurology had quite a bad name as it was seen as a specialty that can diagnose a disease but not do anything about it. Thankfully, that is becoming less and less true because now we have a better understanding of the molecular mechanisms of these diseases, and because there is now a range of drugs available to treat certain neurodegenerative diseases.

At present, there are two classes of drugs that have been shown to be useful in dementia. The first class is acetylcholine esterase inhibitors (ACEIs). Three have been registered in Singapore: donepezil (Aricept®), rivastigmine (Exelon®), and galantamine (Reminyl®). Each one of these has their selling points. Rivastigmine, for instance, is supposed to inhibit not just acetylcholine esterase, but also butylcholine esterase, which is thought to play a more and more important role in the genesis of memory as Alzheimer's disease progresses from time to time. So there's a dual inhibition effect. Galantamine, on the other hand, is a drug derived from daffodil bulbs, and it not only works on acetylcholine esterase, it works through the nicotinic pathway by stimulating nicotinic receptors as well. Unfortunately, there have not been many head-to-head trials of these drugs. However, a study by Wilcock *et al* comparing the long-term efficacy and safety of galantamine versus donepezil, found that galantamine provided superior benefits to donepezil. One other drug that has just been registered in Singapore is memantine (Namenda®). Memantine has been in use in Europe for a long time, and was approved by the FDA for use in the States in October 2003. Memantine is an N-methyl-D-asparate (NMDA) antagonist.

ACEIs enhance anticholinergic transmission, and acetylcholine is probably the most important transmitter involved in memory. In the brains of Alzheimer's disease patients there is a problem with cholinergic loss. So if you cut down the enzyme that destroys acetylcholine then, logically, you should improve neurotransmission. We know that anticholinesterase inhibitors are effective in improving behavior. They improve activities of daily living, and they improve cognition. Now, we also know that to achieve the maximum effect from these drugs they have to be started at as early stage as possible. We also know that they are most effective at higher doses. So there is a clear dose-dependent effect. In fact, the evidence shows that if you start late you never quite catch up in terms of function as opposed to people who start very early on. So you start early and you give the maximum possible dose. Recent evidence also suggests that ACEIs are effective at all levels of disease severity although, the drugs are approved only for mild to moderate Alzheimer's disease. Furthermore, evidence published in 2003 indicates that the drugs are useful not only in Alzheimer's disease but also in vascular dementia. These drugs are probably useful in a wider spectrum of dementias that share a common cholinergic deficit. This means Lewy body dementia, dementia associated with Parkinson's disease, and so on.

Memantine is a derivative of the old drug amantadine, an anti-influenza drug that is now gaining prominence as an anti-Parkinson's drug. This is a moderate-affinity, voltage-dependent, uncompetitive, NMDA receptor antagonist. Memantine is thought to work by blocking background calcium ionic neuronal influx. What is so great about memantine? Well, the first ideas were published in the *New England Journal of Medicine* on moderate to severe Alzheimer's disease. Now, this is a landmark step because never before has a drug been shown to be helpful in moderate to severe Alzheimer's. And generally, as I said, the ACEIs work in mild to moderate disease. However, in a 28-week trial, Reisberg *et al* found that this drug was helpful. So this brought a lot of excitement. The Cochrane Database Systematic Review has helpfully reviewed the whole topic, and they say that a high dose of the drug (20 mg a day for patients with moderate to severe Alzheimer's) leads to significant improvements in cognition and function decline, but not so much in the clinical impression of change. So there are limits to this. Another study, by Wilcock *et al*, showed that patients with mild to moderate vascular dementia. not Alzheimer's, on the same high dose, had less cognitive deterioration at 28 weeks. But, again, this, in fact, was not clinically discernable. In contrast to many NMDA receptor antagonists, which can cause hallucinations and confusion, memantine is well-tolerated. If the dose is increased gradually, it is associated with a very low incidence of side-effects. Post-marketing studies have shown that the drug is safe in combination with ACEIs. But only very recently, in an unpublished abstract presented in the States, has it been shown that when you combine these two classes of drugs, the combination is not only safe, but it provides additional benefit to Alzheimer's patients. Now, this is not surprising because the two drugs work along very different pathways. So, memantine and donepezil work better than donepezil plus placebo.

Nowadays we have a better idea of what the old drugs can do, and it is essential to highlight the importance of two of these: piracetam (Nootropil®) and NSAIDs (non-steroidal anti-inflammatory drugs).

Piracetam is used quite a lot in clinical practice, sometimes because there is nothing better to give. The Cochrane metaanalysis agrees that the global impression of change actually improved with the use of this drug, and this improvement was on the order of three in terms of the odds ratio. But the evidence of effect on cognition and other measures was not conclusive. A more recent study from Belgium looked at 19 other studies, and the metaanalysis again showed that there was an improvement in global impression of change. So, the evidence suggests that piracetam probably does help to some extent.

Another class of drugs is the NSAIDs. The idea of taking aspirin every day to lower dementia risk has become quite popular in recent years. NSAIDs not only appear to lower the risk of vascular dementia, but also Alzheimer's dementia as well. The theory is that if you can cut down inflammatory changes or block inflammatory cascades in the brain, then you will have less neuronal damage. Etminan et al recently reviewed this issue in the British Medical Journal. Everything has been used, from diclofenac to naproxen. What do these studies tell us? Well, firstly, NSAID use is associated with a small but definite benefit in terms of reduction of Alzheimer's risk. We also know that this reduction increases to a maximum, the longer you use the NSAID. In other words, the risk reduction among short-term users (for example, if you take an NSAID daily for less than one month) is practically identical to a non-user. If you use it for less than two years it drops, and if you use it long-term it drops even further, which is compatible with the idea that long-term blockage of an inflammatory-type cascade in the central nervous system is involved in the genesis of Alzheimer's disease. So on epidemiological grounds, then we have the ability to say that NSAIDs are of some value.

## PARKINSON'S DISEASE
### Epidemiology
What about the local epidemiology of Parkinson's? We do not know the local prevalence of Parkinson's disease, simply because no community-based studies have been done. However, in the West, the prevalence of Parkinson's disease is 1 to 2 cases per thousand people. The clinical features of Parkinsonism are: bradykinesia (slowness of movement); rigidity (classically called "lead pipe" rigidity), which means that when you flex somebody's arm the resistance to motion is equal throughout the range of joint movement; this is in contrast to spastic rigidity, where resistance is maximal at the beginning and then it snaps in what is called a clasped-knife kind of rigidity; rest tremor; and finally postural instability.

### Diagnosing and Treating Parkinson's Disease
What can we offer in terms of better management of Parkinson's disease? The first thing is that we can diagnose these diseases at a more early stage so that we can intervene earlier. We have better drugs, and we have better surgical techniques. It is also hoped that advances in genetics and stem cell research will help us diagnose, manage, and possibly even offer us a cure for Parkinson's in the future

Firstly, we have better diagnoses. Traditionally, a diagnosis of Parkinson's disease is not actually confirmed until postmortem, which is a bit late for everybody concerned. At present there is no laboratory test available to confirm Parkinson's disease, so we have to use clinical acumen. These are traditional methods, and they are not particularly reliable. With the advent of MRI (magnetic resonance imaging) scanning you can see the indirect effects of cellular damage in the brain (the brain shrinks at certain portions). But as you can imagine, when you look at structural changes it takes a long time before these structural changes are manifest. So brain structure, although helpful, just doesn't cut it when it comes to early diagnosis. PET scans are wonderful, because as well as showing structure it also shows function. PET scans of people with Parkinson's disease will show that 18-fluoro-deoxyglucose uptake in the basal ganglia is significantly lower than in the normal patient. In the same way, if you look at a PET scan of a person with Alzheimer's disease there is reduced metabolism in the parietal lobes. So new imaging methods now look at brain function. They have the capacity to look at pre-clinical disease and to predict progression to clinical disease later. This opens up vast fields of intervention.

The old mainstay of Parkinson's treatment was, and still is, levodopa. Before the advent of levodopa, people diagnosed with Parkinson's received a death sentence. No other neurodegenerative disease is more treatable than Parkinson's, because you can completely reverse all the symptoms of Parkinson's in a great number of patients when you first start them on levodopa.

Unfortunately, 15% of Parkinson's patients do not respond to levodopa. In fact, these patients may not have typical idiopathic Parkinson's disease. The remaining 85% will get dramatically better, and you have what we call a honeymoon period on first initiating levodopa treatment. Of these 85%, one-third plateau after about three years or so. They do relatively well. These are the lucky ones. One-third drop to where they were before treatment, and one-third deteriorate significantly. So we can see from here that levodopa is not the answer to Parkinson's. It improves the symptoms, but we know it is not neuroprotective. There is even concern that levodopa may be damaging to neurons. So not only is it associated with resumption of all the symptoms of Parkinson's, but levodopa unfortunately also causes dyskinesias. So over time, with the use of levodopa, there is the tendency to develop abnormal, involuntary, socially embarrassing motor movements.

In early Parkinson's disease, there is a big difference in the dose required to relieve the symptoms of Parkinson's and the dose required to induce dyskinesias. Thus, in early Parkinson's there is a large therapeutic window. However, in advanced Parkinson's disease, this therapeutic window narrows dramatically.

In order to understand the role that some of the new Parkinson's drugs have, it is important to have an understanding of the pathway of dopamine metabolism. Dopamine cannot enter from the peripheral to the central compartment of the brain, so it has to be given in the form of levodopa, which does enter. Levodopa is broken down in the peripheries by dopa-decarboxylase as well as catechol-O-methyltransferase (COMT). So there are two pathways of peripheral levodopa breakdown. It makes sense that if you can block these two enzymes, then you will have less peripheral side-effects and more levodopa entering the brain. In fact, this is exactly what we do. Levodopa is always combined with a DDC (dopa-decarboxylase) inhibitor such as carbidopa or benserazide. Of late, however, we've developed COMT inhibitors as well. In the brain, levodopa is also broken down. But dopamine is broken down into dopa by a monoamine oxidase B (MAO B), and this is another fruitful target of drug treatment. Selegiline, is an old drug, however it is still used to cut down the extent of dopamine breakdown in the brain, and selegiline has a modest symptomatic benefit. There are indications that it just might be neuroprotective because it can delay the need for levodopa to be introduced in newly-diagnosed Parkinson's patients.

The only COMT inhibitor currently registered in Singapore is entacapone (Comtan®). A study by Brooks *et al* revealed that entacapone increases the ON time in fluctuating Parkinson's patient, and improves the quality of life in non-fluctuating Parkinson's patients. It also has a good long-term safety and efficacy profile. Despite the cost of this drug, because of the improvements it brings to the quality of life and mobility of Parkinson's patients it is cost-effective, at least in the United States.

Apart from levodopa, there are also drugs that directly act on the dopamine receptor, for example ropinirole (Requip®) and pramipexole (Mirapex®). Ropinirole is another very interesting drug because, in comparison to levodopa, it appears to slow the destruction of the neurons in the basal ganglia. So we do not know from this whether levodopa is neurotoxic, or whether ropinirole is neuroprotective. But there is clear evidence that it does slow down neuronal death compared with the standard methods. Interestingly, despite the slowing down of neuronal degeneration, the symptoms of all these patients who went through the study were still better ameliorated with levodopa. This is, in a sense, rather surprising because it tells us that symptoms do not always correlate with the extent of neuronal loss. But the really nice thing about ropinirole, and the main reason why it is used in younger patients, is that after five years of levodopa versus ropinirole use, 80% of patients on ropinirole or a combination of ropinirole and levodopa remain free of dyskinesias. If you use levodopa alone, that rate drops from 80% to 50%. So 50% of the people on levodopa, in five years, will get motor fluctuations, and this is a dreadful condition; very difficult to treat. We know that ropinirole is safe in high doses in advanced Parkinson's disease where there are dyskinesias, and there is evidence to suggest that it may actually be helpful for dyskinesias. Despite its high cost, Iskedjian and Einarson concluded that ropinirole is cost-effective to society.

Coenzyme Q-10 is found in many health food shops. For a time, it was thought that it was a cure for everything. Now we know that there is at least a role in Parkinson's disease. Now, why is this so? You may have heard the MPTP (1-methyl-4-phenyl-1,2,3,6-tetrahydropyridine) story. MPTP is a contaminant of illicit drugs. Drug addicts began to develop symptoms very much like that of Parkinson's disease, and the cause was eventually found to be MPTP. What was so exciting about MPTP toxicity was that for the first time an environmental toxin was shown to damage selected neuronal populations, thus raising the possibility of an environmental genesis for many neurodegenerative diseases.

So how does MPTP exert its toxicity? It works by inhibiting complex-1 of the mitochondria, the electron transport gene. Which, coincidentally, has its function improved by Coenzyme Q-10, thus raising the possibility that Coenzyme Q-10 might be helpful in ameliorating, or perhaps reversing, the effects of Parkinson's disease. There are two good trials of Coenzyme Q-10. Muller *et al* found that four weeks of treatment with coenzyme Q-10 caused mild symptomatic benefits. Interesting, although not terribly impressive, as four weeks in the life of a Parkinson's patient is a blink of an eye. Meanwhile, Schultz et al treated patients with very early Parkinson's (who had not been given levodopa) with very large doses of Coenzyme Q-10. Three doses of Coenzyme Q-10 were used in the study: 300 mg per day, 600 mg a day, or 1,200 mg a day. In most health food shops Coenzyme Q-10 comes in 30 and 60 mg; it is very hard to find 100 mg or stronger doses. Results showed that Coenzyme Q-10 was superior to placebo, and that there was a clear dose-dependent effect. Thus, suggesting that there is good ground now for us to use Coenzyme Q-10 in Parkinson's. It may also be of benefit to patients who have what we call Parkinson's Plus syndrome, which is similar to Parkinson's but is not typical idiopathic Parkinson's. When levodopa is completely of no benefit, now we have something to offer to people with a more diffuse kind of neurodegenerative condition in the hope that we can do them some good.

We also have better surgical techniques for Parkinson's. There is no surgical technique for Alzheimer's disease. We know that if you can cut the thalamus or the globus pallidus or the subthalamus, then you can relieve excessive movement. There is no surgery that can restore better movement where bradykinesia and rigidity exist. The main concerns about surgery are paralysis, cognitive loss, and development of uncontrollable dyskinesias. Surgery is a destructive operation. Now, apart from destructive operations on the brain, nowadays we can stimulate the parts of the brain that we previously did destructive operations on. With deep brain stimulation (DBS), you can input a low-frequency pulse through a pacemaker-like element that is wired into the brain; this low-frequency pulse basically knocks out the normal function of that particular area. DBS can be very precisely controlled. And best of all, it is non-destructive. If something goes wrong you can pull out the stimulator and the risk of long-term side-effects is far reduced. It also allows you the option of doing a neuroregenerative procedure.

Nowadays, all the talk is about stem cell research. These stem cells can be used to replace dead or dying tissue in the brain or the central nervous system, or you can coax them into forming cells that play a supportive role in order to help all those dead or dying neurons to survive. But do stem cell therapies actually work in Parkinson's disease and Alzheimer's disease?

Stem cell therapies have not reached a stage of development in Alzheimer's worth of reporting here. To-date, no useful study has been published on their use in Alzheimer's disease. In Parkinson's disease, multipotent stem cells harvested from fetuses have been tested. Research has shown that injecting dopamine-rich cells obtained from the nervous tissue of a fetus into the brain of a person with Parkinson's disease does have clinical benefits. However, the clinical benefit is not marked. The cells cannot completely take over the function of the damaged cells of Parkinson's. Thus, there is a delay of many months before any improvement is apparent. This is not surprising because only the minority of cells survive and grow and form new synapses with the surrounding tissue. This can be shown with PET. We know that post donation, more and more dopaminergic neurons do form. This procedure has been around since 1998. The first double-blind study of this treatment was published in 2003. Results showed that the treatment led to mild benefit in four-donor recipients after two years. Unfortunately, dyskinesias developed in 56% of these patients, and this was statistically significant because the placebo group did not develop dyskinesias to this degree. So the promise of this treatment has to be qualified by the fact that although some symptomatic improvement occurs over the long-time, there are significant problems with the procedure.

## CONCLUDING REMARKS

Our understanding of neurodegenerative diseases has grown significantly in recent years; however we are still a long way off understanding them fully. With regards to treatment, there are many, many avenues currently being studied, including drug treatments, surgical procedures, and most recently, stem cell therapy. Unfortunately none of these methods has provided us with a cure for neurodegenerative disease; however with more research we can only hope that a cure, or better ways of slowing the progression or improving the symptoms of these diseases, will be found in the not too distant future.

## REFERENCES

Areosa SA, Sherriff F. Memantine for dementia. *Cochrane Database Syst Rev*. 2003;CD003154.

Brooks DJ, Sagar H; UK-Irish Entacapone Study Group. Entacapone is beneficial in both fluctuating and non-fluctuating patients with Parkinson's disease: a randomised, placebo controlled, double blind, six month study. *J Neurol Neurosurg Psychiatry*. 2003;74:1071-1079.

Etminan M, Gill S, Samii A. Effect of non-steroidal anti-inflammatory drugs on risk of Alzheimer's disease: systematic review and meta-analysis of observational studies. *BMJ* 2003;327:128.

Iskedjian M, Einarson TR. Cost analysis of ropinirole versus levodopa in the treatment of Parkinson's disease. *Pharmacoeconomics* 2003;21:115-127.

Muller T, Buttner T, Gholipour AF, Kuhn W. Coenzyme Q10 supplementation provides mild symptomatic benefit in patients with Parkinson's disease. *Neurosci Lett*. 2003;341:201-204.

Reisberg B., Doody R., Stöffler A., Schmitt F., Ferris S., Möbius H. J., the Memantine Study Group. Memantine in Moderate-to-Severe Alzheimer's Disease. *N Engl J Med* 2003;348:1333-1341.

Shults CW, Oakes D, Kieburtz K, Beal MF, Haas R, Plumb S, Juncos JL, Nutt J, Shoulson I, Carter J, et al. Parkinson Study Group. Effects of coenzyme Q10 in early Parkinson disease: evidence of slowing of the functional decline. *Arch Neurol*. 2002;59:1541-1550.

Silverman DH, Cummings JL, Small GW, Gambhir SS, Chen W, Czernin J, Phelps ME. Added clinical benefit of incorporating 2-deoxy-2-[18F]fluoro-D-glucose with positron emission tomography into the clinical evaluation of patients with cognitive impairment. *Mol Imaging Biol*. 2002;4:283-293.

Wilcock G, Howe I, Coles H, Lilienfeld S, Truyen L, Zhu Y, Bullock R, Kershaw P; GAL-GBR-2 Study Group. A long-term comparison of galantamine and donepezil in the treatment of Alzheimer's disease. *Drugs Aging* 2003;20:777-789.

Wilcock G, Mobius HJ, Stoffler A; MMM 500 group. A double-blind, placebo-controlled multicentre study of memantine in mild to moderate vascular dementia (MMM500). *Int Clin Psychopharmacol*. 2002;17:297-305.

# Chapter 21
# Free Radicals and Antioxidants: Where Are We Now?

*Dr. Barry Halliwell*
*Executive Director, National University of Singapore*
*Graduate School of Integrative Sciences & Engineering;*
*Deputy Director, Office of Life Sciences, National University of Singapore;*
*Head, Department of Biochemistry, National University of Singapore*

## ABSTRACT

Should we take antioxidants and other nutritional supplements? The question has usually been focused on vitamins E and C, but now flavonoids and carotenoids such as lycopene are in the limelight, as well as agents such as lipoic acid and carnitine, and herbal extracts with antioxidant properties. There are two extreme views, namely: (a) eat well and lead a healthy lifestyle and you do not need supplements, as a regular diet will provide the recommended daily allowances of all vitamins and minerals (which are in any case in excess); and (b) maintain optimum health by taking in a "soup of supplements" composed of key vitamins, minerals, flavonoids, antioxidants, and so on. The truth is poised between these two extremes.

We will also discuss the value of Recommended Dietary Allowances (RDAs), including the problems in setting them and the question of individual variation. We will also discuss the threat to human health posed by common substances around us, namely we will review recent studies on how supplements and diet affect free radical damage in the human body and age-related disease. Finally, we will consider the issue of the safety of supplements, in terms of quality control, safety, and toxicity.

Keywords: nutritional supplements; Vitamin E; Vitamin C; flavonoids; recommended dietary allowance

## INTRODUCTION

The focus of this paper is the topic of free radicals and antioxidants. In this field, there are two extreme views, one being that to maintain optimal health you need a "soup of supplements," all the vitamins, minerals, flavonoids, antioxidants, and so on. At the opposite end of the spectrum is the view that if you eat a good diet giving you the recommended daily allowance (RDA), two standard deviations above the estimated average requirement, of all the vitamins and minerals; that is all you need and you're wasting your time and money if you take any supplements. It follows from this second view that supplements are not needed and can do harm. The truth, as ever, is between these two extremes.

For example, it is worth pointing out that many supplements on sale contain excessive amounts of vitamins and minerals: they may contain several hundred times the RDA. So one thing you should look at before you buy supplements, and they have to write this on the label, is the percentage of the RDA that you will be getting if you take these supplements. A number of supplements, particularly things like chromium, may be unsafe if consumed in large amounts because they have never really been studied in people taking large amounts for very long periods.

In defense of supplementation, very few people follow dietary health recommendations. How many people eat five portions of fruits and vegetables every day? It is not even clear what a portion is. Lots of people are on diets. If you go on a diet, your nutrient intake is affected. Illness affects nutrient turnover. One very obvious point that was only realized a couple of years ago is that people in intensive care may effectively have scurvy. Because their plasma vitamin-C levels drop very low, they are not eating, and vitamin-C is not usually added to IV infusion fluids. And as we know vitamin-C plays a key role in wound healing. We also do other things that affect our requirements. If you smoke cigarettes, ideally you should stop smoking cigarettes. But if you cannot do that, or do not want to do that, you should certainly take supplementary vitamin-C. For non-smokers that is a very well established observation. People who drink heavily should drink less, but if they keep on drinking heavily they need more B-vitamins, because alcohol interferes with B-vitamin absorption. And we have all seen recently the evidence that women at risk of becoming pregnant and those trying to become pregnant need more folic acid.

## THE RECOMMENDED DIETARY ALLOWANCE

In order to understand dietary supplementation we need to be aware of the recommended dietary allowance (RDA). What exactly is the RDA? Firstly, what is done is you estimate the average requirements of a nutrient for a population. This will give you the estimated average requirement (EAR). However, some people will need more of that nutrient; some people will need less. And the RDA is set two standard deviations above the EAR. So for most people, the RDA is excessive. It is often presented as the minimum you need. This is not the case. For most people it is excessive. It basically functions as a safety margin. Now, this is fine provided that you estimate the EAR correctly. So if you get the EAR right, your RDA is fine. There will still be a few people who need more of the nutrient. But the huge majority of the population will have more than they need. But can you get the EAR correct? A good example here is vitamin-C. The RDA for vitamin-C in England is 60 mg. In the United States it is now 90 mg. In Singapore, until recently it was 30 mg. So in other words, we have different committees looking at the same body of evidence and arriving at figures that are very different. The second problem is, when you try and work out an EAR what you tend to look at is the amount that will prevent obvious disease. For example, if you don't take vitamin-C you get scurvy, so you look at the intake of vitamin-C that will stop you getting scurvy. That is not necessarily the same as an intake that maintains optimum health. And, indeed, the data set on which the RDAs are derived from is grossly inadequate for most of them. The data is simply not there. What usually happens is a committee of experts meet and one person will suggest an RDA of 200 mg, someone else will dispute that figure saying that it might cause toxicity and suggest an RDA of 30 mg instead. And then after they have argued the matter for several days and got bored and all want to go home, they split the difference and come up with 120 mg. Going back to the example of vitamin-C. Until recently, the RDA in the United States for vitamin-C was 60 mg. How did they arrive at that figure? They did a human experiment, and this was done in the 1960s on five prison volunteers who were placed on a vitamin-C deficient diet until they developed scurvy. The scientists then titrated back to discover how much vitamin-C was needed so that the symptoms of scurvy disappeared. But, in fact, one of the prisoners managed to escape so the RDA was based on data obtained from just four people. That kind of experimentation, we know today, is totally unethical. Yet if you really wanted to determine how much of a vitamin and mineral you needed, it is the experiment that you should do. But you cannot do it. It is totally unethical. And even if you did do it, it does not answer one question. It answers the question of how much you need to prevent overt disease, but it doesn't answer the question of how much you need to maintain optimum health.

The following is a good example of where the requirements of people can vary significantly. As we know, high plasma levels of the amino acid homocysteine are a major risk factor for atherosclerosis: the higher a person's homocysteine level, the greater their risk of developing atherosclerosis. One reason why people can have elevated homocysteine levels is a low activity of the enzyme methylenetetrahydrofolate reductase, which is a genetic polymorphism. If you are one of the 15% or so of the population in Singapore who have this low activity enzyme, you can accelerate its activity and bring homocysteine levels down by raising your intake of folic acid and other B-vitamins. You can compensate for this genetic defect, so this is an example of variation between people.

When talking about supplements, it is important to note that there are different kinds of supplements. High doses of some supplements, for example vitamin-C and vitamin-E, are pretty harmless. However, with some supplements, taking in excess of the RDA can be harmful. Two good examples of this are vitamin-A and selenium. The consumption of high-dose supplements of both of those is contraindicated, and there are others where there is a suggestion of harmful effects. If you take 100 mg of some of the B-vitamins every day you may get minor effects. One piece of information we have about vitamin-C is that men and women are different: in men, you saturate the body pool with vitamin-C by taking 500 mg a day. So if a man takes 500 mg a day he will be completely full of vitamin-C; and it is simply not possible to raise body levels any more. After this was discovered, the Food and Drug Administration (FDA) in the US re-examined the RDA for vitamin-C, and this is an example of a compromise. The original value of 60 mg was based on data obtained from four American prisoners plus a safety factor. One view was that the RDA should be raised to between 200 and 500 because that is the level at which the body saturates it. If you take 10 g vitamin-C a day it will be of no extra benefit, you cannot get any more vitamin-C into the cells and tissues. You produce expensive urine; you absorb it and you excrete it. Thus, if you listened to those arguments you either believe that maybe you should set it at 500 or you should leave it at 60. So as a compromise, the FDA agreed on a new value of 90 mg. That really is an example of how the RDA values are set: the result of informed debate on a very limited database.

## ANTIOXIDANTS

There is a lot of confusion about what supplements people should take. Up until relatively recently, everything was very clear. The belief was that free radicals are bad things and antioxidants are good things; and therefore that if you took vast amounts of antioxidants it would stop you from getting various diseases. We have learned in recent years that the body produces free radicals all the time. Some of them are made accidentally, and we cannot escape that. But some of them are made quite deliberately because they're involved in defense and cell signaling and so on. Another thing we have learnt is that our body's antioxidant defense system does not get rid of all the free radicals. It actually sets up a balance, because some free radicals are useful. The antioxidants keep the level of free radicals down to a useful point. And therefore, free radical damage is inevitable. It is happening to us all the time, and it does relate to the existence of age-related diseases. Thus, to repair this free radical damage is very important in anti-aging. We can maybe give the body a helping hand by taking antioxidant supplements, but the body's own maintenance and repair processes are extremely important.

The interest in antioxidants in health prevention came from a number of areas. Firstly, it was increasingly realized that free radical damage plays a role in human disease. This was first observed in atherosclerosis, with lipid oxidation; in cancer development, with oxidative DNA damage; and more recently we have seen that in neurodegenerative diseases, especially Alzheimer's disease, there is extensive ongoing free radical damage in the brain. In the 1960s and 1970s a large number of epidemiological studies were done which indicated that the higher the blood levels of antioxidants you had the lower the risk of disease. For example, results of a cross-country study in Europe showed that plasma vitamin-E (alpha-tocopherol) and mortality from ischemic heart disease were very nicely negatively correlated. A summary of all those studies indicated that if you have blood levels of vitamin-C above about 50 $\mu$M (micromolar), vitamin-E above about 30 $\mu$M, and beta-carotene of above 0.4 $\mu$M your risk of developing cardiovascular disease and many forms of cancer were significantly decreased. So these were all epidemiological studies. They indicated that if you have these blood levels you are less likely to develop cardiovascular disease and less likely to die of it, and less likely to get any one of a number of cancers.

However, it is important to know how to interpret epidemiology. For example, if you plot the birth rate in the United States against the number of television sets there is a perfect negative correlation. Obviously, people are spending their time watching television instead of making babies. But in fact, as you know, these are both markers of an advanced life-style; as people get richer, the birth rate drops and they spend more time watching television. It does not mean that watching television stops people from having babies. So the next thing you have to do is an intervention trial.

For the sake of example we will use beta-carotene. If you have a high plasma level of beta-carotene, your risk of getting certain kinds of cancer is lower: one of those cancers is lung cancer. So if you are a cigarette smoker who has a high blood level of beta-carotene you are less likely than the average smoker to get lung cancer. But again, you must be careful. Because what exactly does a high plasma level of beta-carotene mean? It means you eat lots of fruits and vegetables. And one of the few things that nutritionists know is that eating lots of fruits and vegetables is good for you and it has an anti-cancer effect. So if you eat lots of fruits and vegetables you will have a high blood level of beta-carotene and you will have a lower risk of getting certain kinds of cancer. This does not mean that beta-carotene itself has an anti-cancer effect. So a number of intervention studies were done. This was the first one: a study that took place in Finland. It focused on people who had smoked for many years, and they were given a high dose of beta-carotene or a placebo. The question the researchers wanted to answer was: Does beta-carotene itself protect against lung cancer development? The answer is no. In fact, for the first two or three years there was very little difference, and then the lines began to diverge. Sadly for the beta-carotene manufacturers, they diverged the wrong way; and the results showed that beta-carotene actually increases your risk of getting lung cancer. This was confirmed by another two or three other studies that got a similar result. So what does this tell us? It tells us that beta-carotene itself in smokers does not protect against lung cancer, but in fact is contraindicated. Similar studies with beta-carotene in non-smokers indicate no effect. It does not protect against cancer and it also does not increase cancer risk. So if you are a cigarette smoker you need more vitamin-C, but you certainly should not be taking supplements of beta-carotene. What this study tells us is that the reason there is a correlation between a high blood level of beta-carotene and a lower risk of cancer is that they are both due to eating diets rich in fruits and vegetables, and that the beta-carotene is a marker of a good diet but is not the protective agent.

What about vitamin-E? Vitamin-E has been used in a whole series of intervention trials to examine its ability to protect against cardiovascular disease. One of those trials, the so-called CHAOS trial (The Cambridge Heart Antioxidant Study) was highly positive. This is often the case in science: the first time you do an experiment it works beautifully, but you can never repeat it. The more trials that have been done; the less positive the results have been. For example, the HOPE (Heart Outcomes Prevention Evaluation) trial found no protective effect of vitamin-E at all, and results of the Italian trial GISSI were questionable. The recent Medical Research Council and British Heart Foundation (MRC/BHF) trial, a very large trial, showed, for example, that lowering cholesterol was tremendously protective against cardiovascular disease; but found no effect of vitamin-E at all. But at least the vitamin-E was better than the beta-carotene in that it wasn't toxic.

So what does this mean? Are we barking up the wrong tree, or should we actually forget about antioxidants as protective agents? Let's go back to why we think antioxidants might be beneficial in the treatment of human disease. There is good evidence that ongoing free radical damage to DNA contributes significantly to cancer development, from both human and animal studies. Things that increase risk, like cigarette smoking and chronic inflammation, increase cancer development. Things that lower it decrease cancer development. Similarly, free radical damage to lipids contributes to cardiovascular disease. These were our starting assumptions. Therefore, if we decrease this we should get less cancer eventually, and if we decrease this we should get less cardiovascular disease. This was the idea between the various clinical trials that were done; to give an antioxidant like beta-carotene to lower DNA damage and get less cancer, but that certainly didn't work; and to give vitamin-E to lower lipid oxidation and get less cardiovascular disease. Equivocal results. So what is going on?

The first thing is that most of the studies that were done with vitamin-E asked the wrong question. The original hypothesis was that lipid oxidation contributes to the development of atherosclerosis. Most, not all, but most, of the studies that were done looked at something different. They looked at people who already had extensive atherosclerosis and had had one cardiovascular event, and asked the question: If we give them vitamin-E can we stop a second cardiovascular event? And the general answer is, no, you can't. But this is not the same as your starting hypothesis. And, indeed, more recent studies that examine atherosclerosis progression are giving more positive results, although, again, more confusion. For example, results of the ASAP (Antioxidant Supplementation in Atherosclerosis Prevention) trial have recently been released. For this trial hypercholesterolemic men and women were given a combination of vitamin-E and vitamin-C, in order to see what effect it had on the progression of carotid atherosclerosis. Results showed that supplementation had a very significant reduction effect in men, but was much less significant in women, we don't know why. Similarly, the Harvard IVUS (Intravascular Ultrasound) studied the effect of vitamin-C and E supplementation on the progression of atherosclerosis after heart transplantation. One of the problems of cardiac transplantation is that, of course, the new heart, the coronary vessels, can develop atherosclerosis. This again showed a significant decrease in transplant-associated atherosclerosis. So lots of studies appear to be looking at the wrong parameters.

The second area is that we made an assumption in those original studies. We assumed that we decreased oxidative damage. So the idea was: give an antioxidant, get less DNA damage, and get less cancer. You give beta-carotene, you get more cancer; clearly something is wrong. You give vitamin-E, you decrease lipid oxidation; you should get less cardiovascular disease. That theory did not work very well either.

But the big flaw in all of these studies was that they never tested the basic assumption. In other words, did you actually decrease oxidative damage in the subject? Now, an analogy here would be that you wanted to test an anti-hypertensive drug to see if it would decrease stroke incidence. The first thing you would do is you would actually examine the effect of the drug on blood pressure, because if you gave a dose that did not lower blood pressure, you would not expect any effect on stroke. On the other hand if you gave a dose that lowered blood pressure too much, you might actually have negative effects. This was never done. It was assumed that when you give an antioxidant you decrease oxidative damage.

Several years ago in England we began to examine this question with human volunteers. We took a group of healthy human volunteers and we supplemented them with either a placebo or a mixture of vitamin-E, vitamin-C, and beta-carotene, and we measured levels of oxidative DNA damage. This was a randomized placebo-controlled study; the subjects did not know what they were getting. We asked the question: Are levels of oxidative DNA damage decreased by giving this supplement? The surprising answer was, no, they are not. As expected no change occurred in the placebo group. However, in the people receiving the supplement, there was a rise in oxidative DNA damage, which then disappeared, surprisingly, even though we continued the supplementation. We did this study three times and got quite similar results. There was never any decrease in oxidative DNA damage with beta-carotene. Therefore, you would not expect it to have an anti-cancer effect, and it didn't. We did this work in collaboration with the Department of Nutrition; so they persuaded us to do an experiment that scientists don't really like, which is to change diets. So we took the same group of human volunteers and we made them stick to their normal diet, but we made them eat 300 g of tomatoes. Now, the reason scientists and pharmaceutical companies do not like this kind of study is that you cannot do a double-blind, placebo-controlled trial, simply because people know whether they have eaten tomatoes or not. Therefore this kind of study is intrinsically messy, and therefore a lot of people will not do them. What you have to do is a crossover study. And what we found is that these volunteers, who really did not respond to supplements, responded beautifully in all except one case: the levels of oxidative DNA damage decreased significantly between 24 and 48 hours of consuming 300 g of tomatoes. Measurement of oxidative DNA damage is extremely difficult. There are endless conferences held to discuss the methodology. Therefore the best thing to do is not believe anything unless it is confirmed in different laboratories using different techniques. As we were publishing this data, exactly that happened. Prieme *et al* were measuring oxidative DNA damage by different methods. We were measuring it directly in extracted DNA; they were measuring it as end products of damage coming out in the urine. They found the same thing as we did: no effect. In fact, their data actually revealed a trend to an increase in oxidative DNA damage, although this was not significant. So in other words, we did not really change oxidative DNA damage in the subjects we gave vitamin-E, C, and beta-carotene. In fact, we tended to increase it. If we made them eat more fruits and vegetables, the levels dropped. And this is exactly what we know: vegetables decrease cancer risk.

So, one of the reasons behind this cancer-lowering effect could be that they decrease oxidative DNA damage. There may be other reasons as well. It also means that the agents in fruits and vegetables that have those effects are not what we commonly suppose: they are not beta-carotene or vitamin-E or vitamin-C.

Similarly, a number of studies have been published recently looking at the effects of vitamin-E on lipid peroxidation in healthy persons. What these studies found was that the effects are quite minimal. So high-dose vitamin-E does not change levels of lipid peroxidation in healthy people very much. However, what has been found in some recent papers is that lowering cholesterol does decrease lipid peroxidation. People with high blood cholesterol have high lipid peroxidation levels. If you bring down the cholesterol, those levels drop. This is probably because the more lipid you have circulating, the longer it hangs around and the more oxidized it gets. Losing weight: very surprisingly, losing weight decreases lipid peroxidation. One or two studies, probably not enough to be definitive, have also shown that consuming more fruits and vegetables decreases lipid peroxidation. Therefore, things that we know decrease the risk of heart disease also decrease lipid peroxidation.

What scientists have basically done is they have picked out compounds, like Vitamin-E and Vitamin-C, and decided that they are responsible for the beneficial effects gained from eating a diet rich in fruits and vegetables. However, that is clearly not the case. The fruits and vegetables have physiological effects that we cannot reproduce with the compounds that have been tested. Thus, other compounds are obviously responsible. Fruits and vegetables contain a very wide range of phenolic compounds, including: other tocopherols and tocotrienols; flavonoids; fiber; phase II inducers; anti and pro-apoptotic agents; and other compounds that may cause inhibition or upregulation of cytochrome p450 enzymes. So really this is an example of misinterpretation of epidemiology.

Plasma levels of vitamin-E, vitamin-C, and beta-carotene in people who are not taking supplements could be surrogate markers for a whole range of different things that can affect cancer and cardiovascular disease. Maybe if it is not the vitamin-E or vitamin-C or beta-carotene, it might be the flavonoids.

## *Flavonoids*

There has been a lot of talk about flavonoids in the last few years. They first came to light when it was shown that red wine has very powerful antioxidant properties in a test tube; much more so than vitamin-E or vitamin-C. Then scientists began to refer to the so-called French Paradox: the fact that, in general, the French, despite higher rates of cigarette smoking and hypercholesterolemia and hypertension, have relatively low rates of cardiovascular disease. And again, the extrapolation was that it's because they drink a lot of red wine. However, red wine is not the only source of flavonoids. You can get them from fruits and vegetables, and green and black tea (black tea is almost as good a source as green tea). People are focused on flavonoids because of their antioxidant properties. And, again, in the test tube they have excellent antioxidant properties.

To investigate this we decided to do an experiment in which we switched people between high- and low-flavonoid diets. This, again, is a messy nutritional experiment, and it is not easy to do because if you give people fruits and vegetables you modulate oxidative DNA damage. So what we had to give them instead was black tea and onions. We switched people between these two diets. The study was published in the *American Journal of Clinical Nutrition*, which is rated as the world's best nutrition journal. In this case, we found that flavonoids generally have no effect on rates of lipid oxidation. A number of studies on this have been published. Some people say red wine has an effect and some say green tea does; but we could not find an effect on lipid oxidation. In fact, as far as wine is concerned there is, in Caucasian populations, a demonstrated effect of taking moderate amounts of alcoholic drinks on incidence of cardiovascular disease. But whether that is the alcohol or something else is not clear. But taking one or two drinks a day appears good for you. If you are a Caucasian, going above four or five is certainly not good for you. But alcohol itself seems to raise HDL levels, and it may positively influence the vascular endothelium up to a point. So you may not need red wine. You may be able to drink whiskey or beer instead.

Flavonoids are also very complex molecules. In fact, our research has shown that they are not only antioxidants but that they also inhibit certain enzymes, including COX-1, COX-2, and lipoxigenase. More recently, we suddenly realized that we are probably missing something. Flavonoids are not that well absorbed. So when you eat a flavonoid-rich diet, the plasma level of flavonoid is quite low. It's 1 or 2 $\mu$M, so it is very difficult to imagine it having a direct antioxidant effect. This would explain our data showing that they do not have much of an antioxidant effect. But then we suddenly realized that the levels of these compounds in the GI tract are huge. If you drink your glass of red wine, and eat a few vegetables, you have millimolar (mM) levels of flavonoids in the stomach. And these pass all the way through the GI tract. Some of them are absorbed; most of them are metabolized in colon. So we actually think that flavonoids are beneficial; that they do protect against gastric cancer, and possibly against colon cancer, but that they are doing it by direct actions in the GI tract.

For example, it is known that many colon cancers are COX-2 dependent. This is why taking aspirin can sometimes decrease the risk. Many flavonoids inhibit COX-2. Thus suggesting that there are several mechanisms that can help us explain why flavonoids appear to offer some degree of protection against tumors of the GI tract. So going back to the original question: Is the anti-cancer effect of fruits and vegetables due to antioxidants? The answer is possibly, because fruits and vegetables decrease DNA damage. But if so, which ones are responsible? The answer is we don't know. So in other words the foods decrease oxidative damage, but we cannot repeat that effect by using vitamin-E, vitamin-C, and beta-carotene.

Therefore, what we should do, and what we should have done from the beginning, is start with the food and work backwards, assuming we can do that, and that we are not looking at a synergistic effect of components. For example, we have recently been busy looking at Asian foods for powerful antioxidant activity. This is a pure test tube measurement of antioxidant activity. On this scale, vitamin-E is 1. A good red wine is 12 to 24, much more powerful than vitamin-E or vitamin-C. However, dark soy sauce gave us some very impressive results. Different brands of fermented dark soy sauce scored 128 and 148 on the same scale. Thus there is clearly something in dark soy sauce that has very powerful antioxidant activity. In fact, it is very similar, if not identical, to a compound that is generated in the colon by fermentation of soy products. So we now have good evidence what the compound is. It may, in fact, be a useful antioxidant. However, all this data is derived from test tube studies. Human studies to see if dark soy sauce really works are due to start soon.

## CONCLUDING REMARKS

The vast majority of people do not follow the dietary recommendations and they probably never will. But the RDA values are approximations, and everybody would benefit by taking a multivitamin that contains the RDA of all the vitamins and minerals. What is not advisable is taking very high doses of any one particular supplement, and certainly not of things like vitamin-A and selenium. A lot of people may benefit by doubling their intake of folic acid. But if it contains 500 or 1,000 times the RDA, that is almost a pharmaceutical dose and it may do unexpected things if taken for a long enough period and we do not have the evidence to support that.

## ABOUT THE AUTHOR

Professor Halliwell holds BA (first class honours) and PhD degrees from the University of Oxford and a Doctor of Science degree from the University of London. Before coming to Singapore, he was Professor of Medical Biochemistry at Kings College, University of London and co-director of both the Antioxidant and Neurodegenerative Disease Research Centres. He was formerly Research Professor on Internal Medicine and Biochemistry at the University of California and a Lister Institute Research Fellow in biomedical sciences.

The Institute for Scientific Information (publishers of the Science Citation Index) has identified Professor Halliwell as one of the 112 most influential scientists worldwide in Biology and Biochemistry. His current research interests include molecular nutrition, especially the role of antioxidants in the human diet, and the mechanism of neuronal cell loss in the major neurodegenerative diseases. He has published over 300 scientific journals in top journals, is editor of two journals, and on the board of several others. His textbook *Free Radicals in Biology and Medicine* published by Oxford University Press is regarded as the authoritative reference text in the field.

# Chapter 22
# Growing a New Pancreas

*Sir Roy Calne*
*Department of Anatomy, University of Cambridge, United Kingdom*

## ABSTRACT

Scientists are currently striving to develop various methods of treating diabetes, primarily Type I diabetes but possibly also Type II diabetes, by means of cell transplant. This paper will review possible approaches to cell transplantation for diabetes, including islet cell transplantation, and the use of duct progenitor cells and both embryonic and non-embryonic stem cells to produce insulin-producing beta cells.

Keywords: diabetes; insulin-producing beta cells; pancreas transplantation; islet cell transplantation; duct progenitor cells; stem cells

## INTRODUCTION

The almost-epidemic aspect of the increase of diabetes, particularly Type II diabetes worldwide is significantly shortening peoples' lives. Scientists are currently striving to develop various methods of treating diabetes, primarily Type I diabetes but possibly also Type II diabetes, by means of cell transplant. This paper will review possible approaches to cell transplantation for diabetes. This is not quite the same as growing a new pancreas, although that is one of the approaches that some people have looked at. If we take into consideration the severity, the cost in human suffering, and also the financial cost of diabetes, this is a very worthwhile cause. Whether it can be successfully accomplished in a reasonable period of time is another matter.

## PANCREAS TRANSPLANTATION

Pancreas transplantation has become fairly commonplace, and usually it is a transplant that is performed at the same time as a kidney transplant. In Singapore, the commonest cause of kidney failure is diabetic nephropathy and that story is repeated in many parts of the world. Diabetic nephropathy is a very important cause of renal failure. Of course, by the time that a patient needs a kidney graft for diabetic nephropathy they may have quite severe complications of diabetes. Many have got severe impairment of vision, some are totally blind, and many have lost limbs and have had myocardial infarcts. So, although it is a bit late in the day, it is still possible to get very good results.

A kidney and pancreas transplantation is a big operation. The kidney is put on one side, and the kidney transplant and the pancreas from the same donor placed on the other side. They are vascularized transplants. Some surgeons carry out the transplant in such a way that the pancreatic juice drains into the bladder, which means that the exocrine function of the pancreas can be monitored but it is not very physiological. However, more and more centers are now returning to draining the pancreatic juice into the gastrointestinal tract.

The results of pancreatic transplants, certainly in America, are approximately the same as with kidney transplants. Immunosuppression has been improved. The use of high-doses of steroids, which were much feared because of their diabetogenic effect and also their impairment of wound healing, is on the decrease. And we have even got a protocol with an immunosuppressant called Campath®, which is an antibody, that permits us to avoid steroids altogether in many transplant patients.

When we started doing pancreas transplants in Cambridge, England, approximately 18 years ago we only used half a pancreas. We used the half vascularized on the splenic vessels because of the surgical ease of using just two anastomoses. And we found that when the operation was done satisfactorily the patients had perfectly good glucose control just with half a pancreas. Half a pancreas has quite enough islets of Langerhans to keep somebody in very good, normal glucose homeostasis. However, nowadays techniques have changed and the whole pancreas is used, although half a pancreas was enough.

A patient whose life has been dominated by diabetes and the requirements of insulin and a controlled diet, and who has then suffered the unfortunate side-effects of diabetes, of renal failure, and subsequently had to be on dialysis with restrictions of fluid and dialysis three times a week, has had an utterly terrible quality of life. Therefore those patients' who have been lucky enough to be given a successful combined kidney and pancreas transplant have had their way of life completely transformed in one operative procedure.

## ISLET CELL TRANSPLANTATION

The idea of using islets of Langerhans as a source of cell transplants to avoid an operation is an interesting one that we are currently trying to develop. So what about using just the islets? This has been a dream and an objective of many research centers over the last 25 years or so. Islets can be extracted, although it is not an easy procedure. However, isolation techniques have improved. We do not know the best site for transplantation at present, but it can be done without an operation, with a needle injected via the liver into the portal vein. Since 1990 there have been 267 attempts at islet implantation, but only 8.29% of the patients maintained insulin dependence at a year. Therefore islet transplantation was a pretty depressing field until Shapiro *et al* published significantly better results in the *New England Journal of Medicine*. They used no steroids. Steroids, of course, are diabetogenic and interfere with healing. They used an antibody against IL-2, and tacrolimus and sirolimus. Tacrolimus is also a diabetogenic drug, so it was used in the lowest dose possible. Shapiro *et al* also used a large number of donor islets, two to three cadaveric pancreases for each patient, which equates to between 10 and 14-thousand islets per kilogram of body weight. This raises the question that if half a pancreas contains enough islets to maintain glucose homeostatis, why did Shapiro *et al* need to use two to three total pancreases to get reasonable results?

The reason why Shapiro *et al* needed to use two to three cadaveric pancreases is that they chose patients who had not got renal failure, but had brittle diabetes. So the study used patients who had potentially fatal complications of diabetes, but not renal failure or cardiac disease or peripheral vascular disease. Therefore, these patients were a different cohort from those studied previously and the results have been quite good. More than 80% of participants required no exogenous insulin at a year. However, this falls to about 75% at two years, and there is a gradual attrition. We do not know exactly why there is attrition, whether it is caused by chronic rejection, exhaustion of the islets, or simply that the islets do not have enough progenitor cells to make up for those that are dying naturally from apoptosis.

When carrying out islet transplantation the islets are injected very slowly into the portal vein. These islets apparently live quite happily in the liver producing insulin. So it is possible to get good results and at least to get a temporary cure; possibly even a prolonged cure in some patients. But, of course, the patient switches from needing insulin to needing immunosuppressant drugs. A lot of work is being done at the moment to try and decrease the toxicity and the side-effects of immunosuppressant drugs.

The site of implementation is critical, and initially the injected islets have to survive just on diffusion. So they get their nourishment and removal of toxic products just by diffusion. They are very delicate and very vulnerable. And, as has been mentioned, some of the drugs that we give are toxic to them. Once they get revascularized, the islets are far more robust and then they really become part of the patient. The portal vein is currently considered to be the optimal site for islet transplantation. Normally, insulin has its first passage into the liver and that is where it is metabolized and glycogen is produced. Thus, transplanting the islets into the portal vein maintains the correct physiological route of insulin. It is possible to get an intraportal drainage of islets by putting them into an omental pouch, the spleen, or the pancreas itself; or under the capsule of the liver, or under the submucus layer of the gut, the rectum, the small bowel, or the stomach. Alternatively, one can use the site that gives drainage into the inferior vena cava. When we do clinical pancreas transplants the drainage is typically into the cava, although it can be into the portal vein. In rodents, the subcapsule of the kidney is considered to be the optimum place for putting islets. There is also the possibility of combining islets under the kidney capsule with a kidney allograft. Subcutaneous is another possibility. Thus, we do not know the best place to put the islets. All we know is, at present, the best place for them is the portal vein.

Why are so many islets needed for transplantation and how can we get more islets, or insulin-producing glucosensitive cells, to treat our patients? Camilo Recordi in Miami is one of the world's pioneers of methodology of extracting islets. It is a complicated process that requires great skill and five people to be available at any time of day or night to do the procedure when a cadaver pancreas happens to become available. It takes these five highly-skilled people between five and six hours to extract the islets. To do this a cannula is put in the pancreatic duct and librase, a purified collagenase, is injected into it. The chunks of partially digested pancreas that are obtained are then further digested in a Recordi chamber. The digested pancreas tissue is then put into a differential fical separation centrifuge, and the islets are separated. Throughout this process the islets have to be tested repeatedly to find out whether they are alive, whether they are contaminated, and whether they are getting clean. If an experienced team is carrying out the procedure, the end result will be 2 or 3 cc of islets, which are then diluted to 10 mL and injected into the portal vein. It does not matter how experienced or how careful the team are, only some of the islets will be removed intact, many will be damaged, and a lot will be missed. Moreover, when the islets are inserted into the bloodstream some of them will cause activation of complement and fibrinogen. This may lead to clumps of islets, which are much too big to become viable insulin-producing islets, and may actually damage the liver. Therefore, it is not surprising that more islets are needed than one would expect in a nice vascularized, intact pancreas.

## DUCT PROGENITOR CELLS AND STEM CELLS

Beta cells are highly specialized. They produce large amounts of specialized protein in response to the glucose ambience, and they produce it at the right time at the right level. It is no use having cells that just produce insulin without any control because they either produce too much and kill the patient or too little and have no effect.

Would it be possible to de-differentiate beta cells to get them to grow rapidly, proliferate, and then reverse them back to increase the beta cell mass? So far we have no way of doing that. Could precursor beta cells be differentiated to provide proliferating beta cell culture? Well, there has been some success with that. Susan Bonner-Weir and colleagues at the Joslin Diabetes Center in Boston have taken the "rubbish" after removing the islets out of the pancreas, which is mainly duct and exocrine tissue, and cultured it to produce a growth of cells that eventually became beta cells. Unfortunately, nobody as yet has been able to produce enough cells to be of use in the therapeutic sense.

In embryonic development, all of us have grown pancreases starting, of course, with embryonic stem cells within the fertilized egg. But can it be possible to repeat this miracle of nature in the laboratory? A group in Paris have shown a rather remarkable progression of human fetal pancreatic primordia injected under the capsule of a kidney of a skid mouse, which was unable to mount an immune reaction. In the course of six months, the number of insulin-producing cells increased by 5-thousand-fold. Of course, we are not skid mice, and it is not at the moment feasible to think in terms of getting human pancreatic primordia. But at least outside of the normal embryonic environment, in fact a very abnormal environment, a skid mouse, it is possible for human cells to develop and grow and produce potentially metabolically active cells that could, in theory, work in a different host.

Could we guide embryonic stem cells into beta cell differentiation, or what about insulin synthesis in response to glucose sensor, which is what we need? Could we get this by genetic engineering? There has been a lot of talk in the literature about using adult stem cells or stem cells from newborn babies from the umbilical cord blood or peripheral blood after growth factor stimulation. There are stem cells in hepatocytes in the liver. There are stem cells in the fat. There are K cells in the small bowel, which already have the glucose sensor. And then there are mesenchymal stem cells. Can we really change these cells and persuade them to produce insulin? There has been a lot of debate and argument, and some of the claims have been disproved. It has been shown that some of these adult stem cells in fact fuse with recipient cells and they are not truly functioning on their own. But nevertheless, there is a lot of interest in stem cells, both embryonic and non-embryonic.

Could you put a pancreatic remnant, blood stem cells, hepatic stem cells, or mesenchymal stem cells in a culture medium containing growth factors that would cause differentiation into beta cells? There have been some techniques in the laboratory using that approach, which have looked quite encouraging. Maybe one could use foetal cells, also putting them in similar culture medium. Almost all attempts at using stem cells have required specialized differentiation factors. The great difficulty is the move from an undifferentiated stem cell, which can turn into anything in the body, to a very specific cell that will produce insulin in response to glucose. There may be very many different stages, maybe even hundreds of stages where critical factors at different concentrations are required. Our knowledge of these processes at present is very fragmentary. We just know a few of these stages.

## CONCLUDING REMARKS

Therefore, for the treatment of diabetes we can consider the vascularized pancreas. This, of course, has been remarkably successful, usually in late cases with renal failure. Clinical islets have been successful in Edmonton. The longest survivor with function is now about four years, so the proof of principle has been shown. But there will never be enough cadaver islets to treat patients with diabetes, which is such a common disease.

If we could use islets from animal sources, particularly the pig, we would have a limitless source of islets. We already know that porcine insulin works in man. It has a similar sensing mechanism, and the glucose levels in the pig are about the same as in man. There has been suggestion that specially-bred pigs, transgenic pigs and knockout pigs, might have tissues that would be compatible to man. It seems extremely irritating that the pig could provide all the islets that we need, but unfortunately every protein made by the pig is chemically different from the similar protein in man. Even insulin is different. We do not know how to prevent rejection of pig tissue in man.

Of course, if the islets are revascularized with the recipient's blood cells they would become "chimeric", in that they would have blood vessels of recipient type and insulin-producing cells of the pig type that might make it easier to control. But to get to that stage has yet to be demonstrated clearly in scientific methodology.

It has been shown that duct progenitor cells can be cultured and coaxed to transform into beta cells, but that technique does not, at present, produce enough cells to be used therapeutically. What about engineering adult stem cells, or non-pancreatic cells, for example liver and intestine, or even naked DNA constructs injected into the muscle or the liver? DNA is difficult to introduce. With time, it tends to fade, sometimes very quickly. If a virus is used, there is a danger of the virus itself causing infection and malignant change. Professor Kon Oi Lian at the Cancer Research Centre in Singapore is conducting pioneering work in this area and has made considerable progress. But this is still a long way from the clinic.

Bernat Soria, Dennis Wang, and Allan Coleman are working on human embryonic stem cells. And we hope that eventually beta cells, or even conglomerates of beta cells, like a real mini organ, may be produced. That again is likely to be a long way off, as we don't even know if it is possible at present. However, Soria has been successful in doing this with mouse embryonic stem cells. So if it can be done with a mouse, it is difficult to argue that it would be impossible in man, although it may be very difficult.

Another possibility is autotransplantation. To do this, one would have to take a stem cell from a patient, engineer it to remove the diabetic target which is currently unknown change it by culturing with growth differentiating factors to produce autologous beta cells, then inject these cells, which would be the "autotransplant", into the patient. No immunosuppression would be needed, and one would have got rid of the target for autoimmune diabetes. While this technique has not yet been used for the treatment of diabetes, a group in Boston has used it in an attempt to treat hemophilia. What they did was to take a piece of skin from a patient, grow fibroblasts from the patient's own skin, and introduce factor 8 for the treatment of hemophilia and then inject these fibrocytes into the muscle of the patient. Results showed that it produced a considerable amelioration of the hemophilia and bleeding tendency, but unfortunately the effect did not last very long. Thus, while this type of genetic engineering may look very attractive, it has been rather disappointing in terms of good, long-lasting effects.

Chapter 23

# A Lifestyle Plan for Long Lasting Weight Loss

*Shari Lieberman Ph.D.*
*Faculty, University of Bridgeport, School of Human Nutrition Graduate Program;*
*Board Member, Certification Board for Nutrition Specialists;*
*President, American Association for Health Freedom;*
*Fellow American College of Nutrition*

## ABSTRACT

Preserving muscle mass and losing weight predominantly as body fat is the key to improve metabolic control. Here we will discuss the benefits of the low glycemic index (GI) diet and supplements that can help to accelerate weight loss.

Keywords: glycemic index; green tea; Coleus forskohlii; Citrus aurantium; chromium; Glucosol; 5-hydroxytryptophan; Phaseolamin

## INTRODUCTION

Preserving muscle mass and losing weight predominantly as body fat is the key to improve metabolic control. Muscle mass dictates metabolism. Very overweight and obese individuals have extremely high body fat relative to muscle mass, and this can effectively slow their metabolism as well as promote insulin resistance. A total program is one that incorporates diet and exercise with supplements that will help improve some of the metabolic control.

Crash dieting and fad dieting that induces "quick" weight loss generally promotes muscle and water loss and less fat loss. This keeps patients in the "yo-yo" syndrome since when they gain the weight back they gain it as fat, not muscle. Studies have shown that during low caloric intakes energy expenditure can be decreased by 10%. When normal food intake is resumed, it can further decrease by as much as 15%. Our bodies don't know we are cutting calories just to lose weight: they are programmed to reduce our metabolism to adjust for food shortages that occurred during our hunter-gatherer existence. Crash dieting leads to further slowing of metabolism since most of the weight is lost as muscle and water and later gained back as body fat.

## THE LOW GLYCEMIC INDEX DIET

In reviewing the scientific data, it is clear that a low glycemic index (GI) diet appears to promote weight loss more effectively than other types of diets. Those following this type of diet feel full faster, are more satisfied with what they have eaten, and have better glucose tolerance. Their weight loss is predominantly as fat. That is because low GI diets prevent the metabolic switch that increases fat storage rather than fat burning from being thrown. Simply restricting carbohydrates and treating them all the same still allows dieters to consume high GI carbohydrates, which will throw the metabolic switch to store more body fat.

A low GI diet allows carbohydrates that do not elicit a high GI response such as fiber, beans, lentils, oats, yams, and sweet potatoes, as well as a host of other foods. Even most fruits such as apples, oranges and grapefruit which are all high in pectin, elicit a low to moderate GI, which would make them also permissible on a diet plan.

Simply restricting calories has not resulted in the preferential change in body composition of losing body fat rather than muscle mass. Also, significantly cutting calories in an attempt to lose weight can decrease energy expenditure by 10% and during re-feeding by as much as 15%. Simply restricting calories and/or carbohydrates does not insure that high GI foods will not be consumed. High GI foods can cause a metabolic switch that preferentially stores protein, fat, and carbohydrate rather than promoting oxidation of these nutrients.

Low GI diets also improve insulin resistance and other risk factors for coronary artery disease such as elevated blood lipids. High protein, high fat diets promote insulin resistance, lower levels of protective HDL cholesterol and raise C-Reactive Protein levels, a risk factor for coronary artery disease.

Unlike other diets, a low GI plan can be followed indefinitely. The best plan to follow is one that targets the change in body composition and preferentially enhances the lost of body fat rather than muscle mass. It is also important to incorporate exercise into the program to significantly improve body composition. Walking, dancing, cycling, and stepper machines are all examples of aerobic exercise. Some extremely overweight and obese people may have pain even when walking so water aerobics may be a better place to start for these people. Everyone should start slowly if they are out of shape and start with 5-10 minutes three times each week building up slowly to 30-45 minutes 3-5 times each week. Strength training can be added later to further preserve body composition. Remember that muscle dictates your metabolism and high body fat slows metabolism. Preserving or even building a little more muscle can have dramatic effects on metabolism.

## SUPPLEMENTS THAT ACCELERATE WEIGHT LOSS

There are many dietary supplements that can help enhance weight loss when a low GI diet and exercise plan is followed. Also, these supplements can help improve blood sugar control, metabolism and body composition. They may also help prevent long periods of plateau that can be quite frustrating and can cause people to "fall off the wagon". It is also possible that these supplements may help to prevent weight gain with occasional cheats, and that means occasional!

### Green Tea

The thermogenic effect of green tea (*Camellia sinensis*) was originally attributed to its caffeine content. However, green tea stimulates brown fat thermogenesis at a far greater level than a comparable amount of pure caffeine. It appears that the catechin-polyphenols, in particular epigallocatechin gallate (EGCG), and caffeine that naturally occur in green tea work synergistically to stimulate thermogenesis and augment and prolong sympathetic stimulation of thermogenesis. It has been shown to increase 24-hour energy expenditure and fat oxidation (caffeine only increases metabolism during the time you take it). Drinking several cups of green tea each day has well documented anti-cancer effects particularly with respect to the prostate, breast, uterus and ovary.

Green tea is generally taken as a standardized extract in capsule or tablet form to provide 50 mg of caffeine and 90 mg of epigallocatechin gallate to be taken three times daily before meals. Although green tea contains a small amount of caffeine, it is generally not enough to create any adverse side effects. Drinking several glasses of green tea each day may yield a similar thermogenic effect to the supplement although this has not been studied thus far.

### *Coleus Forskohlii*

Coleus has a long history of use in Ayurvedic medicine. Forskolin, one of its active compounds, has been studied as a weight loss aid. Animal studies have shown that forskolin has anti-inflammatory and anticancer effects. Human studies have shown that forskolin may be effective for glaucoma (as eye drops) and may have other therapeutic effects. Numerous animal studies have shown that forskolin can raise cyclic AMP (3'5' adenosine monophosphate), a naturally occurring compound in our bodies that releases fatty acids from adipose tissue storage, which may result in enhanced thermogenesis, and loss of body fat, and may increase lean body mass. Coleus appears to be thermogenic and may also decrease body fat and preserve muscle mass.

Standardized extracts of Coleus generally provide 10% of forskolin. Thus, 500 mg of standardized Coleus will provide 50 mg of the active compound forskolin. Forslean® has published the research on this herb.

### *Citrus Aurantium*

Citrus aurantium is also known by its Chinese name Zhi Shi. It is an herb that has a long history in Traditional Chinese Medicine. It is commonly known as bitter orange. A standardized extract provides 6% amines and the most studied extract is known as Synephrine.

Synephrine has thermogenic properties. The amines are similar in action to ephedrine (found in Ma Huang/Ephedra) in terms of thermogenesis, but they do not cause the stimulant side effects associated with ephedrine or large amounts of caffeine, such as nervousness, fast heart beat, high blood pressure, dry mouth, insomnia, or even more serious side effects recently reported. This is because these active amines work through a different pathway than either caffeine or ephedrine.

An effective dose of Citrus aurantium would be 975-1000 mg and would be standardized to provide 6% of the active amines.

### *Chromium*

Chromium is an essential mineral for glucose tolerance. It improves glucose tolerance and insulin resistance, and lowers elevated blood sugar levels. It may also improve blood levels of cholesterol, triglycerides, and HDL cholesterol.

The majority of chromium is removed from processed foods, and if you eat a lot of refined carbohydrates and/or sugar it is virtually impossible to get enough of this mineral just through food. There are many forms of chromium readily available, including: polynicotinate (Chromate®), dinicotinate, and GTF. Each of these forms is effective in improving glucose tolerance and insulin resistance. Human studies using 400-1000 mcg of chromium have yielded better blood sugar lowering results than when lower doses are used.

Chromium does not stimulate metabolism nor is it thermogenic. It is important because it can blunt the rise in blood sugar when a high GI carbohydrate is consumed, thus helping to prevent the metabolic switch into fat storage mode. That does not mean that by simply taking chromium you can continue to routinely eat high GI carbohydrates and achieve weight loss. But it can help if cheats are occasional as evidenced in studies with diabetic patients who did not modify their diet had improvements in glucose control. What also makes chromium interesting is that is shifts weight loss to favor body fat and preserve muscle mass, the very thing we want to achieve with a total program.

### *Glucosol*

Glucosol is an herbal extract from the herb *Lagerstroemia speciosa*. Its active ingredient, corosolic acid, is responsible for its blood sugar lowering and normalizing effect. Numerous animal and human studies have shown that Glucosol improves glucose tolerance, lowers serum blood sugar levels, and improves insulin resistance very much like chromium.

What is most remarkable about Glucosol is that it can blunt the rise in blood sugar rise associated with high glycemic index foods. In some of the studies, a modest weight reduction occurred without the use of a restricted diet. Since Glucosol significantly blunts the blood sugar rise associated with high GI foods, insulin levels are also blunted. This would prevent the metabolic switching to the storage of body fat associated with elevated glucose and insulin levels. It appears that both Glucosol and chromium may help dieters to better tolerate carbohydrates and help control blood sugar and insulin levels.

### *5-Hydroxytryptophan*

Several studies have shown that L-tryptophan (which is currently not available as a dietary supplement) can blunt carbohydrate cravings by increasing brain serotonin levels. Brain serotonin levels have an inhibitory effect on eating behavior and helps curb appetite. Since L-tryptophan has been removed from the market place, 5-hydroxytryptophan (5-HTP) has been made available and appears to have the same benefits. This form of tryptophan is the intermediate metabolite of L-tryptophan in the serotonin pathway.

Low serotonin levels in obese patients have been associated with carbohydrate cravings and binge eating behavior. Studies have shown that carbohydrate intake may decrease by as much as 50% when 5-HTP is given without dietary restriction and it also has an appetite suppressant effect in very overweight, obese and diabetic patients. Other benefits of 5-HTP administration may include significant improvement in depression, insomnia, fibromyalgia and chronic headaches when taken as 50-300 mg three times daily.

Some researchers (including myself) have expressed concern that the level of 5-HTP used in the studies (300 mg three times daily) was very high and may over time cause a neurotransmitter imbalance by increasing serotonin levels well beyond normal. In the published studies those taking 5-HTP were not eating a low GI diet. Therefore it is possible that lower levels such as 50-100 mg given one to three times daily may have a similar effect if combined with a low GI diet and exercise program.

### *Phaseolamin*

Phaseolamin is also known as Phase 2®. It is a non-stimulant, all-natural nutritional ingredient that is derived from the white kidney bean. Preliminary research has demonstrated that it neutralizes the enzyme alpha amylase before it can digest starch into glucose. Thus, allowing some of the starch in foods such as potatoes, breads, pasta, rice, corn and crackers to pass safely through your system without being digested or absorbed. Therefore it can reduce the absorption of some starch calories. This appears to be an exciting new ingredient that can be an excellent adjunct to a low GI diet and exercise program.

## CONCLUSION

A review of the scientific literature reveals that the best diet to follow for life is a low GI diet. It can be followed indefinitely and helps correct many of the metabolic alterations that overweight and obese people must over come. Furthermore, it appears that given the mechanism of action of dietary supplements such as green tea, Coleus forskohlii, Citrus aurantium, chromium, Glucosol, 5-HTP, and Phaseolamin they may assist achieving weight loss goals along with a low GI diet and exercise plan. The other benefits of 5-HTP administration at lower doses than used in the weight loss studies include significant improvement in depression, insomnia, fibromyalgia, and chronic headaches: many of the conditions associated with overweight and obesity that make it difficult for individuals to stick to a program for life.


## REFERENCES

Agus MS, Swain JF, Larson CL, Eckert EA, Ludwig DS. Dietary composition and physiologic adaptations to energy restriction. *Am J Clin Nutr.* 2000;71:901-907.

Bahadori B, Wallner S, Schneider H, Wascher TC, Toplak H. Effect of chromium yeast and chromium picolinate on body composition of obese, non-diabetic patients during and after a formula diet. *Acta Medica Austriaca* 1997;24:185-187.

Bell SJ, Goodrick GK. A functional food product for the management of weight. *Crit Rev Food Sci Nutr.* 2002;42:163-178.

Cangiano C, Ceci F, Cairella M, Cascino A, Del Ben M, Laviano A, Muscaritoli M, Rossi-Fanelli F. Effect of 5-hydroxytryptophan on eating behavior and adherence to dietary prescriptions in obese adult subjects. *Adv Exp Med Biol.* 1991;294:591-593.

Cangiano C, Ceci F, Cascino A, Del Ben M, Laviano A, Muscaritoli M, Antonucci F, Rossi-Fanelli F. Eating behavior and adherence to dietary prescriptions in obese adult subjects treated with 5-hydroxytryptophan. *Am J Clin Nutr.* 1992;56:863-867.

Ceci F, Cangiano C, Cairella M, Cascino A, Del Ben M, Muscaritoli M, Sibilia L, Rossi Fanelli F. The effects of oral 5-hydroxytryptophan administration on feeding behavior in obese adult female subjects. *J Neural Transm.* 1989;76:109-119.

Chantre P, Lairon D. Recent findings of green tea extract AR25 (Exolise) and its activity for the treatment of obesity. *Phytomedicine* 2002;9:3-8.

Dulloo AG, Duret C, Rohrer D, Girardier L, Mensi N, Fathi M, Chantre P, Vandermander J. Efficacy of a green tea extract rich in catechin polyphenols and caffeine in increasing 24 hour energy expenditure and fat oxidation in humans. *Am J Clin Nutr.* 1999;70:1040-1045.

Dulloo AG, Giradier L. Adaptive changes in energy expenditure during refeeding following low-calorie intake: evidence for a specific metabolic component favoring fat storage. *Am J Clin Nutr.* 1990;52:415-420.

Kao YH, Hiipakka RA, Liao S. Modulation of endocrine systems and food intake by green tea epigallocatechin gallate. *Endocrinology* 2000;141:980-987.

Kaats GR, Blum K, Fisher JA. Effects of chromium picolinate supplementation on body composition: a randomized, double-masked, placebo-controlled study. *Curr Ther Res.* 1996;57:747-756.

Lieberman S, Bruning N. *Dare To Lose: 4 Simple Steps to a Better Body.* New York: Avery/Penguin Putnam;2003.

Ludwig DS. Dietary glycemic index and obesity. *J Nutr.* 2000;130:280S-283S.

Preuss HG, Grojec PL, Lieberman S, Anderson RA. Effects of different chromium compounds on blood pressure and lipid peroxidation of spontaneously hypertensive rate. *Clin Nephrol.* 1998;47:325-330.

Samaha FF, Iqbal N, Seshadri P, Chicano KL, Daily DA, McGrory J, Williams T, Williams M, Gracely EJ, Stern L. A low-carbohydrate as compared with a low-fat diet in severe obesity. *N Engl J Med.* 2003;348:2074-2081.

5-Hydroxytryptophan Monograph. *Altern Med Rev.* 1998;3:224-226.

## USEFUL RESOURCES
Phaseolamin: www.phase2info.com

## ABOUT THE AUTHOR

Dr. Lieberman holds her Ph.D. in Clinical Nutrition and Exercise Physiology. She is a Certified Nutrition Specialist (C.N.S.); a Fellow of the American College of Nutrition (FACN); a member of the New York Academy of Science; a member of the American Academy of Anti-Aging Medicine (A4M); a former officer and present board member of the Certification Board for Nutrition Specialists; and President of the American Association for Health Freedom. She is the recipient of the National Nutritional Foods Association 2003 Clinician of the Year Award and a member of the Nutrition Team for the New York City Marathon.

Dr. Lieberman's best-selling book *The Real Vitamin & Mineral Book* is now in its third edition (Avery/Penguin Putnam 2003). She is the author of *Dare To Lose: 4 Simple Steps to a Better Body* (Avery/Penguin Putnam 2002) and *Get Off the Menopause Roller Coaster* (Avery/Penguin Putnam 2002).

Dr. Lieberman is a faculty member of the University of Bridgeport, School of Human Nutrition graduate program; a published scientific researcher, and a presenter at numerous scientific conferences. Dr. Lieberman is a frequent guest on television and radio and her name is often seen in magazines as an authority on nutrition. She has been in private practice as a clinical nutritionist for more than 20 years. She can be contacted through her website at www.drshari.net.

Chapter 24

# Cutting-Edge Technology in the Prevention and Treatment of Cardiovascular Disease: A Picture Tells a Thousand Words: The Case for IMT Heart™ Scan

*Jacques D Barth, M.D., Ph.D.*
*Associate Professor, Keck School of Medicine, University of Southern California,*
*Director of Research, SPARC*
*Medical Director, Prevention Concepts, Inc.*

## ABSTRACT

IMTHeartScan™ is an accepted surrogate endpoint in atherosclerosis studies. Atherosclerosis may be viewed as an aging of the arteries. Reversal of this process is possible with dietary intervention and by treatment with specific antioxidants and growth hormone (GH). By sequentially giving patients IMTHeartScan™ the physician can follow the benefits of intervention on an individual basis. Furthermore, IMTHeartScan™ provides the physician with the facility to provide patients with an image of their artery that shows disease and the effect of the aging process itself, thus motivating the individual to adhere to the intervention regimen prescribed.

**Keywords:** atherosclerosis; carotid artery; non-invasive artery imaging; ultrasound diagnostic technology

## INTRODUCTION

The aim of this paper is to discuss how to use carotid artery intima media thickness (IMT) as a marker for surrogate cardiovascular disease. What are the current applications, and why should you have it in your office.

Most health professionals agree on how atherosclerosis develops. A normal, healthy endothelium is exposed to a variety of damaging factors. Eventually, the healthy tissue is injured and endothelial dysfunction occurs. If the damage persists, raised lesions in the vessel wall and atherosclerotic plaque occur. Plaque vulnerability and likelihood of rupture ensue. A cardiac event lies at the end of the scenario. Researchers are currently examining various points in the atherosclerotic process to determine surrogate endpoints for prevention and treatment of cardiac events.

A surrogate endpoint is a biomarker established for the purpose of creating interim determinations in a clinical trial. In the past, surrogate markers had inherent limitations. For example, response may not translate into clinical benefit or survival benefit, and may not be intervention dependent. Waiting for the clinical endpoint determination in the pre-clinical phase can take a decade. However, the development of surrogate markers allows us to establish prevention measurements during this timeframe, hopefully providing us with a safe, non-invasive, reproducible method to assess the progression of the disease. Additional advantages of surrogate endpoints are customization of a patient's intervention/management and increasing adherence to healthcare professional recommendations. What is the leading surrogate endpoint available in cardiovascular disease? We believe it is the IMTHeartScan™.

## THE IMTHeartScan™

Atherosclerosis doesn't start in the center of the artery, the lumen; it starts in the wall. Thus, it would make sense to develop a technique that would identify the initial faces of atherosclerosis, using non-invasive techniques. So, I started working with ultrasound and found that the carotid artery is a great surrogate endpoint to assess the thickness of atherosclerosis in the beginning, and the changes of atherosclerosis. It correlates well with coronaries; it correlates well with other symptoms. So we are talking about the intima, the media, and the adventitia. Those are the inner layers of every blood vessel. Most people don't even realize they have atherosclerosis until they have a complication, possibly a fatal one. We want to prevent that from happening. As we all know, prevention is basically a form of anti-aging.

Why the carotid artery? The carotid artery is fairly accessible. Blood flow is better in the common carotid area, and correlates very well with the flow in the coronary arteries. Basically, the carotid artery is a very good area to do a study.

The result of my research is the IMTHeartScan™. IMTHeartScan™ is the quantitative cardiovascular risk measurement of the far wall of the common carotid artery using ARTIS® automatic tracking and analysis system and the interactive database. IMTHeartScan™ is suitable for all stages of atherosclerosis and can be used to diagnose and track the disease. The carotid IMT has predictive value for likelihood of cerebrovascular and cardiovascular events in men and women.

A comparison between IMTHeartScan™ computer software program and caliper IMT revealed that the computer program was four times as accurate as the caliper IMT. Repeated caliper measurements were, in fact, within the normal variation of the technique, resulting in a significantly less accurate method to track IMT than the ARTIS® computerized edge contour measurement technique.

IMTHeartScan™ is a safe, standardized and validated method that uses ultrasound images. With IMTHeartScan™ is portable, has a large reference database, and is relatively inexpensive. It has a proven track record and improves patient compliance and adherence to a prescribed regimen. Data shows that IMTHeartScan™ correlates with cardiac and cerebrovascular outcome (cardiac outcome is even more accurate than stroke). It also provides the physician with an indicated risk (absolute and relative) for the individual patient and enables the physician to track the change of risk during management. It can be used on all populations, including children.

The first indication of atherosclerosis is a thickening of the intima-medial area. If you have a computerized ultrasound system, you can calculate the likelihood of that person, given the fact that we know the mean of this area, having a stroke or heart attack within the next 6 years. What other test can do that? An IMTHeartScan™ report looks like a school report card; the patient is given a grade of A, B, C, D, or E. A is normal. B is above normal. C is above the $95^{th}$ percentile, D is twice the relative risk, and E is basically bad news.

A study done by a group from the University of California at Irvine compared different non-invasive imaging techniques for detecting atherosclerosis, including automatic carotid IMT analysis, ankle-brachial index, EBT (electron beam tomography), ultrafast CT (computed tomography), and MRI (magnetic resonance imaging). The automatic carotid IMT analysis was shown to have a very high specificity, and very high sensitivity, at a relatively low cost.

### *Clinical Applications*

What are the clinical applications of the IMTHeartScan™? We are clinicians. We are interested in what it brings to us. Well, for the clinical manifestations of atherosclerosis, there is coronary heart disease, cerebrovascular disease, and arterial disease: intima-medial thickness is relevant in all three. One study that showed the capabilities of the IMTHeartScan™ was the Cholesterol Lowering Atherosclerosis

Study (CLAS), a placebo-controlled, angiographic trial designed to test the hypothesis that lowering of LDL cholesterol with concomitant increase in HDL cholesterol will reverse or retard atherosclerosis in coronary artery bypass patients. CLAS was conducted in the days before the introduction of cholesterol-lowering statin drugs, and was designed to determine whether combined therapy with colestipol, a bile acid sequestrant, and niacin (Vitamin B3) would produce clinically significant changes in coronary, carotid, and femoral artery atherosclerosis and coronary bypass graft lesions. The participants were given a sequential coronary angiogram every second year, and an IMT every six months. With the IMT results it was possible to predict 10 years ahead of time, those who would suffer a stroke or a myocardial infarction, if no further intervention was prescribed.

What are the other clinical applications of IMTHeartScan™? IMTHeartScan™ is very useful for monitoring the effects of intervention. What are the interventions that have been tested using IMTHeartScan™? The effect of specific diets on an individual has been well tested. There are many antioxidants on the market. Several studies have been done with antioxidants, and one of them that stands out is lycopene, which is found in tomatoes. Lycopene prevents progression of disease. IMT is certainly reactive to the antioxidant effect of lycopene. If you look at other vitamins in chronic disease prevention, benefit have been shown in specific populations with folate, Vitamin B6, Vitamin B12, and Vitamin A. The jury is still out on vitamin E. Some people benefit tremendously from it. Others do not. Most people appear to benefit from fish oils. On hormones, if we are talking testosterone or growth hormone, it varies. Some people think that more is better. That is not always the case. The effect of exercise on IMT has also been tested. What is the impact of exercise on IMT? Tests show that a thickened IMT can be reversed by exercise, which is amazing; to get reversal just by doing exercise. The effect of psychological stress and stress reduction has also been investigated. A study looking at the effect of psychological stress in the workplace on IMT was conducted by *Kamarck* et al. More and more pressure was put on people in order to see if their IMT thickened, which it did. When the psychological pressure was removed, the IMT went thin again. Thus, the results of that study provided further proof that psychological stress plays an important role in development of coronary artery disease.

One of the focuses of my current research is obesity. If you look at the percentage of people who are obese in the US in 1918 it was 15%, in 1999 that figure had nearly doubled to 27%. If you look at children and young adults, it has jumped from 3% to 13%. Of every child that was born in the US in 2003, one in three will develop diabetes. More than 50% will be obese. I participate in a program called KidShape®, which is sponsored by the school educational board of LA County. KidShape® impacts three aspects on obese kids: nutrition, psychological health, and physical exercise. It doesn't last that long, only 16 weeks; but the impact is tremendous. Some of the children have adult-onset or Type II diabetes. Right now, I am screening children as young as 3 up to the age of 12. At the start of the program, the average insulin level of the 12-year-old participants was 81. By the end, 16-weeks later, it had dropped significantly to 37. What did we do? We just taught them about a healthy diet. We gave them an hour of exercise a day. These simple measures also had an impact on IMT, triglyceride levels, and blood pressure.

IMTHeartScan™ is particularly good at detecting asymptomatic cardiovascular disease, and disease that is not detectable by other methods. We did a screening of more than 7000 people in a large power company. Results showed that approximately 4% of the workforce had significant abnormalities that were not detectable in any other fashion. They were asymptomatic. The IMT analysis will give you the average value, the standard deviation, the standard error minimum, the standard error maximum. We also have for every age, and every ethnic group, a specific normal range. Thus, as well as detecting disease, the IMTHeartScan™ can determine a patient's relative risk.

The State of California was interested to find out whether or not heart disease occurs among high school children. So we carried out IMT tests on pupils from three different high schools: a Latino school, a Caucasian school, and a Seventh Day Adventists school. The Latinos, and certainly in Southern California, are the largest minority group, about 30% of the population is Latino. If we look at serum LDL cholesterol, 37% of Latino pupils had elevated levels, compared with 90% of Caucasians. Low HDL cholesterol was 18% in the Latino population versus 10% in the Caucasian. 8% of the Latino population already had diabetes. We are talking about 13 to 17 year olds. Seven of the diabetics also had advanced plaques.

Another interesting case that highlights the potential of IMTHeartScan™ is that of a man who came to be tested. He was very happy when he arrived, and very depressed when he left. Why was that? He just had undergone a whole body scan and been told he was perfectly healthy and there were no problems whatsoever, especially his coronaries were excellent. No problem. I did an IMT on him. He had a lot of soft plaque and a very thick IMT on both sides. Whole body scans, or ultrafast CT pick up calcification, but do not pick up soft plaque. Soft plaque is a problem. So, I had to prescribe him several medications, in addition to changing his lifestyle, which he didn't like because he thought, I'm healthy and now I have to do all these things.

Thus, the IMTHeartScan™ is good at detecting asymptomatic cardiovascular disease. The type of plaque we want to detect and treat as soon as possible are vulnerable plaques, because those are the ones that tend to rupture: IMTHeartScan™ can differentiate between stable and vulnerable plaques.

*Improving Compliance*

We did a study in patients who had some kind of cardiovascular risk factors. What is one of the problems that people with cardiovascular risk factors or chronic diseases have? They have to take medication. They listen to you and how many people really follow your orders? We did a test where we had a microchip in the cap of a bottle and I told the patients that they had to take this pill once a day. After 30 days, I did a pill count. Results showed that compliance in general was 40%. They opened the bottle once a day. They closed the bottle once a day. Another 40% opened the bottle only once during the 30 days, and that one day was the day prior to the doctor's visit. 20% were totally erratic. When we provided the patient with an image of their artery along with the risk calculation of their likelihood of having a stroke and a heart attack, we found that compliance increased significantly from 40% to 76%. So, providing patients with an image of their artery that shows disease and the effect of the aging process itself along with a printout of their risk calculation appears to significantly improve their resolve to change their diet and lifestyle for the better.

## INTRODUCING IMTHeartScan™ TO YOUR PRACTICE

What is needed to introduce IMTHeartScan™ into your practice? You need to have a technician with some sonographic experiencel; in some states, an RVT is required; a registered vascular technician. You need to have an ultrasound machine with a linear array 7.5-10 MHz probe, which costs between 10 and 15 thousand dollars. It needs to have a mode equipment component and it needs to be able to download either to a VCR or digital format, and it has to be sent to a validated certified core imaging lab for certification.

## CONCLUDING REMARKS

In conclusion, IMTHeartScan™ assesses the extent of cerebrovascular health and disease and aging. It can be used to assess the impact of any intervention for progression or reversal of disease. It increases compliance and can be given also to people who are pre-aging. Right now we have a database of over 40,000 people with an average follow-up of 6 years, so we can calculate on an individual basis for that person, if that person will get a stroke or a heart attack within the next six years.

## REFERENCES

Blankenhorn DH, Johnson RL, Nessim SA, Azen SP, Sanmarco ME, Selzer RH. The Cholesterol Lowering Atherosclerosis Study (CLAS): design, methods, and baseline results. Control Clin Trials. 1987;8:356-387.

Kamarck TW, Everson SA, Kaplan GA, Manuck SB, Jennings JR, Salonen R, Salonen JT. Exaggerated blood pressure responses during mental stress are associated with enhanced carotid atherosclerosis in middle-aged Finnish men: findings from the Kuopio Ischemic Heart Disease Study. *Circulation* 1997;96:3842-3848.

## ABOUT THE AUTHOR

Dr. Barth received his medical degree in 1968 from Maimonides Lyceum, Amsterdam, The Netherlands. He continued his medical training with a Residence in Internal Medicine at Erasmus University in Rotterdam, a Fellowship in Cardiology with Erasmus University, and a PhD with California Institute of Technology. Dr. Barth has a distinguished record of academic appointments, having served as Assistant Professor of Cardiology with Erasmus University, Director of Cardiovascular Disease Prevention, University of British Columbia School of Medicine, and currently as Associate Professor, Keck School of Medicine, University of Southern California, Los Angeles, CA. Dr. Barth has been involved in a number of research projects and currently serves as Director of Research with SPARC (Southern California Atherosclerosis Prevention Center). Dr. Barth is a published author and serves as a reviewer for the University of California on TRDPD studies concerning different ethnic groups, and for the journal *Atheroclerosis* and the *American Journal of Epidemiology*.

Chapter 25

# Event-Related Potential (P300) Prolonged Latency Is Differentially Negatively Correlated with Sex Hormones and Insulin Growth Factors as a Function of Gender: A Preliminary Study of Hormones in Neurocognition

*Eric R. Braverman MD, Thomas JH.Chen PhD, Arpana Rayannavar, Neeta Makhija, John Schoolfield MSc, Matthew S. Stanford PhD, and Kenneth Blum PhD.*

## ABSTRACT

In this large clinically based study we found a number very important findings. Specifically; in males, both IGF-1 and IGFBP-3 significantly associated negatively with prolonged P300 at different age periods; in males the spearman correlation between P300 latency and Free Testosterone was significant at different age periods; in males aged 50-69 there was a significant negative correlation between P300 latency and DHEA levels; in females only IGFBP-3 not IGF-1 significantly associated negatively with prolonged P300 latency; in females there was no significant correlations between estrogen and progesterone and P300 latency; in females there were significant negative correlations between DHEA levels and P300 latency at different age periods. Moreover there were no statistically significant correlations between any hormone and WMS (Weschler Memory Scale)-111. However, there was a significant negative correlation between estrogen levels and the number of ADD complaints. If these results could be confirmed, it may have important value in the diagnosis, prevention and treatment of cognitive function.

**Keywords:** IGF-1, IGFBP-3, free testosterone, DHEA, P300 latency, estrogen, Attention Deficit Disorder; cognitive decline

## INTRODUCTION

A review of the literature reveals that sex hormones have often been associated with changes in behavioral and mental abilities.[1] Generally, estrogen, the female sex hormone, seems to have a positive effect in preventing, but not treating Alzheimer's disease. Moreover, estrogen use may improve mood amongst women with postnatal or perimenstrual depression[2]: however, it may contribute to increasing depressive symptoms in women with premenstrual dysphoria.[3] The behavioral effects of the male sex hormone testosterone and dehydroepiandrosterone (DHEA) remain unclear but preliminary reports suggest that their use is associated with improved mood. At present, there is not enough hard data to support the use of sex hormones and DHEA, the adrenal androgen, for the treatment of depression or cognitive decline or memory deficits. Additionally, the GH/insulin-like growth factor -1 (GH/IGF-1) axis is known to be involved in aging of physiological functions including low levels associating with cognitive decline[4] as a function of age. In fact, deficiency of growth hormone (GH), an important regulator of IGF-1, is associated with reduced wellbeing. Furthermore, because plasma IGF-1 levels are reported to be enhanced by DHEA administration, it has been suggested that IGF-1 may be implicated in some of the reported associations between low DHEA sulfate levels and impaired health measures in elderly subjects.[5]

With regard to estrogens there is a plethora of scientific literature that has provided biological plausibility for the hypothesis that estrogen replacement therapy (ERT) would protect against cognitive aging in healthy women. The weight of the evidence from randomized controlled trials of estrogen and cognition in women shows that this hormone preferentially protects verbal memory in postmenopausal women,[6] whereas findings from observational studies are less consistent and show a more diffuse effect of estrogen on a range of brain functions including: protection against cognitive decline, [7-8] reduction of Alzheimer's disease risk,[9] treatment of schizophrenia,[10] modulation of brain aging in females,[11] protection against beta-amyloid, presenelin and apolipoprotien-E-4 deposits,[12] regulation of the function of the immune-brain barrier,[12] decreased risk of dementia during menopause,[13] antioxidant "chemical shield" for neurons,[14] protection against degeneration of cholinergic innervation reducing memory decay,[15] reduction of risk of Parkinson's disease,[16] enhancement of tests of learning and memory,[17] and improvement of cerebral blood flow.[18]

Studies demonstrate a decline in androgens with age and this results in the andropause in males. High endogenous testosterone levels predicted better performance on visual spatial tests in several studies, but not in all studies.[19] Likewise, testosterone replacement in hypogonadic patients improved cognitive functions in some but not in all studies.[19] Testosterone has also been shown to improve cognitive function in eugonadal men and several studies have shown that decline in DHEA may contribute to Alzheimer's disease.[20]

A recent Medline search revealed that IGF-1 can improve well-being in GH-deficient adults,[21] and improve cognitive function.[22] Low levels of IGF-1 may be involved in the progression of dementia[22] and cognitive decline,[23] and have been associated with a decline in verbal memory.[24] Whereas higher IGF-1 levels have been associated with better cognitive performance by increasing mental processing speed.[25] IGF-1 may also play a role in determining the speed of information processing and intelligence.[22,26] IGF-1 levels were directly correlated with Mini-Mental State Examination scores (MMSE), in that they were lower in patients with more advanced cognitive deterioration and neuronal function.[27]

After insulin-like growth factor binding protein-3 (IGFBP-3) was identified in serum as the carrier protein for most circulating IGF's, its variations were shown to be regulated by GH secretion,[28] and like IGF-1 levels are age-dependent. However, recent work now suggests that IGFBP-3 in humans is regulated directly by IGF-1 and is GH-independent.[29] A recent Medline search could not find even one study that associated IGFBP-3 with cognitive function.

In looking at the statistics of the aging population in the US we are reminded of the dramatic increase in the prevalence of dementia. Three to 11% of persons older than 65 years of age and 25% to 47% of those older than 85 years of age have dementia. In fact, in 1997, the number of people in the US diagnosed with Alzheimer's disease was estimated to be 2.3 million: more than 90% of whom were 60 years of age and older. Besides the suffering dementia causes for society, for patients, and for their families, the annual societal cost of dementia has sky rocketed.[30]

Event-Related Potential P300 is frontally generated and travels temporally, parietally and occipitally across the entire brain as a global wave measurement of brain health. P300 reflects cognitive events of information processing. Reduced P300 amplitude and prolonged P300 latency occurs with age, while dementia often exhibits P300 latency in excess of 400ms (oddball auditory task). This may be contrasted with decreased amplitude that is frequently observed in the earliest stages of psychopathological conditions.[31-32]

P300 is documented to be a nonspecific, but sensitive marker of brain (mind-body) dysfunction for neurological, psychiatric, medical, and developmental problems. In neurology association of P300 variables include: epilepsies (childhood epilepsy, partial seizure), migraine and post-traumatic headache, Parkinson's disease, multiple-system atrophy, progressive supranuclear palsy, multiple sclerosis, hypertension, orthostatic hypotension, stroke, ischemia, cerebral hypoxia, obstructive sleep apnea, spinal cord injury, brain stem injury, diffuse brain damage, coma, Alzheimer's disease and memory disorders, tumor/amnesia, attention deficit hyperactivity disorders, narcolepsy, organic solvent and toxic metal exposures, various forms of closed head injury, visual and acoustic disorders, myotonic dystrophy, and metabolic encephalopathies. In psychiatry: schizophrenia, alcoholism, substance use disorder, nicotine dependence, criminals and psychopaths, affective disorders, anxiety, panic and obsessive compulsive disorders, bipolar depression, suicidal and various personality disorders (Borderline, Schizoid, Avoidant), social adjustment disorder, and posttraumatic stress disorders. In medicine it can be useful for: diabetes and endocrine disorders, anemia, fatigue, menopause and pre-menstrual syndrome, status post oophorectomy, bypass surgery, dialysis, HIV, chronic pulmonary disease, cirrhosis and other liver diseases, impaired neurocognitive performance and abnormal development of structures such as: amygdala, hippocampus, left temporal, and the cerebellar vermis.[31-32] Another important measure of cognition is the Weschler Memory Assessment (WMS-111). Thus, WMS-111 is a standardized measure used to assess learning and memory abilities especially in the elderly.

To determine the possible associations of various sex hormones and growth hormone on their ability to effect cognition, we utilized brain function measures as evaluated by both P300 latency and WMS-111.

## METHODS
### Subjects

A total of 905 patients were evaluated in this study. Gender and age were recorded for these patients. Average age for females was 51.6 and 50 for males. These patients were selected for study from an outpatient private medical clinical practice (Medical and Neuropsychiatric) and research foundation in New York City.

All subjects signed an approved IRB consent form based on an approval from the PATH Medical IRB committee (registration # IRB00002334) and ethics board approval from the PATH Foundation. Criteria for study inclusion were that the patients had to be tested on the WMS-111 and have had at least one P300 test. Trained EEG medical and psychometric technicians conducted the tests. All test interpreters were blinded to other patient results. All subjects were part of a catchment study involving brain electrical activity mapping and aging research.

### Analysis of Hormones

Venipuncture was carried out on non-fasting subjects between 8:30 AM and 7:30 PM at baseline examination of the PATH Medical Clinic Program. Blood samples were collected in 5-ml tubes containing a 0.5ml sodium citrate solution. All tubes were stored on ice before and after blood sampling. Platelet-free plasma was obtained by 2-stage centrifugation (10 minutes at 1600g at 4°C and 30 minutes at 7000g at 4°C). Platelet-free samples were immediately frozen in liquid nitrogen and stored at -80°C. Assays were performed blinded to information on the subject. Plasma levels of estradiol and sex hormone-binding globulin (SHBG) were estimated with double anti-body radioimmunoassays (Bioreference Lab, New York, NY). Measures of the levels of bioavailable and free estradiol, testosterone, DHEA, and nonprotein-bound estradiol, respectively, were calculated in the basis of hormone and binding protein levels.[33-34] For the analysis of GH and IGF-1 and IGF-3 binding proteins the laboratory performed standardized procedures. [29, 35]

*P300 latency*

All patients in this study were analyzed by the BEAM. A 24-channel EEG recorder was used. The standard International 10/20 System of electrode placement was used. In addition, there were two electrodes placed on earlobes, two EKG electrodes connected to the cervical spine and electrocap, and two supraorbital electrodes were also used. Digital EEG was recorded in a monopolar (LR linked ears left over right) and bipolar (LR 3,4 linked ears left over right) montage.

Impedances were measured for 3K ohms and data were collected at a sampling rate of 128 Hz. P300 tests were conducted: 15 minutes by standard auditory oddball paradigm eliciting burst tones of 1 Khz (frequent/common) and 2Khz (rare/oddball), at a .75-1.5 sec interval stimulus and 85 dB SPL-Sound Pressure Level. Rare tones were intermittently distributed amongst common tones, and the test was discontinued when a total of 20 rare tones were delivered. The frequency of common tones varied with each test and was pre-set by the computer. Data was collected during eyes closed with a pre-stimulus baseline. The tones were presented through headphones. The subjects were instructed to lift their finger each time a rare tone was heard, indicating that the sounds were audible and that task performance was equitable across subject groups and ages. LFF (low frequency filter) was set at 1hz, and HFF (high frequency filter) was set at 300hz, with a sensitivity of 200 microvolts.

The computer averaged evoked potentials. The system mathematically adjusted the baseline to the average value of stimulus signal per channel. P300 results were read at the maximum voltage (dV differential voltage; amplitude is relative to the mean voltage of the entire waveform) electrode (i.e. usually at PZ). Neuropsychiatric patients frequently have peaks that occur at FZ, CZ, OZ, P3, P4, O1, and O2. Review by a neurologist showed our computerized QEEG-P300 test to be 100% inter- and intra-reliable.

### Memory Assessment: WMS-111

WMS-111 is a standardized measure we used to assess learning and memory abilities of 631 patients between 40 and 89 years. Results are organized unto summary index scores, reflecting Verbal, Visual, Immediate and Working Memory, and interpreted accordingly. Scores of 130 and above demonstrates very superior abilities, 120-129 is considered superior , 110-119 demonstrates high average abilities, 90-109 indicates abilities, 80-89 is considered low average , 70-79 indicates borderline abilities, and 69 and below demonstrates impairment.

## RESULTS
### Hormone Correlates
#### P300 Latency

This analysis was performed separately for males and females aged 30 to 90. The hormone data was standardized by assigning a percentile ranking of 1 to 20 to each hormone measure, with 1 representing values ranging from the minimum to the 5th percentile and 20 representing values ranging from the 95th percentile to the maximum. Partial correlations were performed to check for associations between hormone rankings and P300 latency controlling for age.

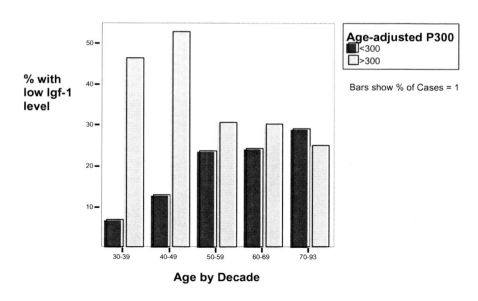

*Table 1. Percentage of Men with Low IGF-1 Levels Correlated with P300 Latency*

## Males

In males, rankings of IGF-1, IGF-3, free testosterone, and DHEA were correlated with P300 latency. There were 213 males with IGF-1 values, 211 males with IGF-3 values, 191 males with free testosterone values, and 176 males with DHEA values. All partial correlations were small, with r-squares less than 0.02, so hormone levels explained less than 2% of the age-adjusted variance of P300 latency in males. However, among the 188 males having both IGF-1 and IGF-3 values, the rankings for the IGF hormones were significantly correlated ($r = 0.521$, $p<0.001$) after age adjustment.

For age 30-39 (46.2% vs. 6.7%) and 40-49 (52.6% vs. 12.8%), males with elevated P300 had a higher percentage of IGF-1 in the lowest quartile (IGF-1 <170 for 30-39 and IGF-1 <140 for 40-49) compared with males with normal P300. For the 28 males aged 30-39 with IGF-1 data, this percentage difference was statistically significant ($c2=5.791$, $p<0.025$), and the Spearman correlation between P300 Latency and IGF-1 was marginally significant (rho = -0.356, p=0.063). For the 58 males aged 40-49 with IGF-1 data, this percentage difference was statistically significant ($c2=10.561$, $p<0.005$), and the Spearman correlation between P300 Latency and IGF-1 was statistically significant (rho = -0.401, $p<0.005$). For the 86 males aged 30-49 with IGF-1 data, the percentage difference for elevated vs. normal P300 (50.0% vs. 11.1%) was statistically significant ($c2=15.962$, $p<0.001$), and the Spearman correlation between age-adjusted P300 Latency and IGF-1 was statistically significant (rho = -0.357, $p<0.005$), and the Spearman correlation between P300 Latency and IGF-1 was also statistically significant (rho = -0.374, $p<0.001$).

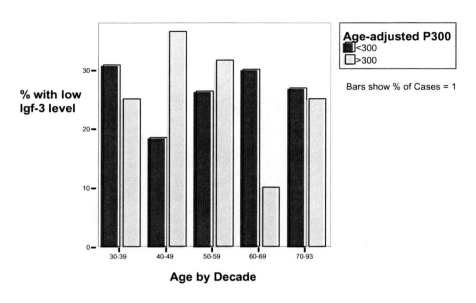

*Table 2. Percentage of Men with Low IGF-3 Levels Correlated with P300 Latency*

For age 40-49 (36.4% vs. 18.4%), males with elevated P300 had a higher percentage of IGF-3 in the lowest quartile (IGF-3 <2.7) compared with males with normal P300. For the 60 males aged 40-49 with IGF-3 data, this percentage difference was not statistically significant (c2=2.392, p>0.10), but the Spearman correlation between P300 Latency and IGF-3 was significant (rho = -0.267, p<0.040).

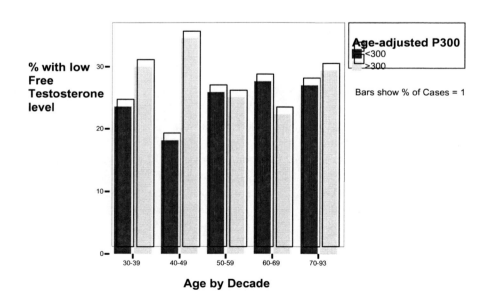

*Table 3. Percentage of Men with Low Free Testosterone Levels Correlated with P300 Latency*

For age 40-49 (34.6% vs. 18.2%), males with elevated P300 had a higher percentage of free testosterone in the lowest quartile (free testosterone <10) compared with males with normal P300. For the 59 males aged 40-49 with free testosterone data, this percentage difference was not statistically significant (c2=2.071, p>0.10), but the Spearman correlation between P300 Latency and free testosterone was significant (rho = -0.296, p<0.025). For the 86 males aged 30-49 with free testosterone data, the percentage difference for elevated vs. normal P300 (33.3% vs. 20.0%) was not significant (c2=1.955, p>0.15), but the Spearman correlation between age-adjusted P300 Latency and free testosterone was statistically significant (rho = -0.281, p<0.010), while the Spearman correlation between P300 Latency and Free Testosterone was statistically significant (rho = -0.305, p<0.005).

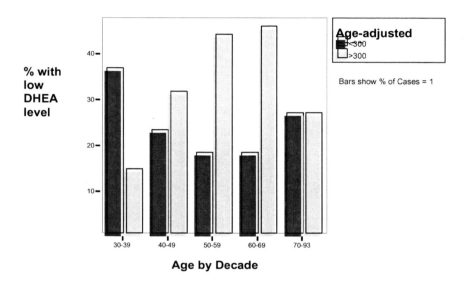

*Table 4. Percentage of Men with Low DHEA Levels Correlated with P300 Latency*

For age 30-39 (14.3% vs. 36.4%), males with elevated P300 had a lower percentage of DHEA in the lowest quartile (DHEA <200) compared with males with normal P300. For the 18 males aged 30-39 with DHEA data, this percentage difference was not statistically significant (c2=1.039, p>0.30), and the Spearman correlation between P300 Latency and DHEA was not significant (rho = 0.051, p>0.80). For age 50-59 (43.8% vs. 17.9%) and 60-69 (45.5% vs. 17.9%), males with elevated P300 had a higher percentage of DHEA in the lowest quartile (DHEA <130 for 50-59 and DHEA <80 for 60-69) compared with males with normal P300. For the 44 males aged 50-59 with DHEA data, this percentage difference was marginally significant (c2=3.442, p=0.064), but the Spearman correlation between P300 Latency and DHEA was not significant (rho = -0.125, p>0.40). For the 39 males aged 60-69 with DHEA data, this percentage difference was marginally significant (c2=3.155, p=0.076), and the Spearman correlation between P300 Latency and DHEA was significant (rho = -0.326, p<0.045). For the 83 males aged 50-69 with DHEA data, the percentage difference for elevated versus normal P300 (44.4% vs. 17.9%) was statistically significant (c2=6.610, p<0.010), but the Spearman correlation between age-adjusted P300 Latency and DHEA was not significant (rho = -0.174, p>0.10), however the Spearman correlation between P300 Latency and DHEA was significant (rho = -0.228, p<0.040).

*Females*

When the procedure was repeated for females, rankings of IGF-1, IGF-3, estrogen, progesterone, and DHEA were correlated with P300 latency. There were 261 females with IGF-1 values, 247 females with IGF-3 values, 287 females with estrogen values, 258 females with progesterone values, and 207 females with DHEA values. All partial correlations were small, with r-squares less than 0.03, so hormone levels explained less than 3% of the age-adjusted variance of P300 latency in females. 220 females had both IGF-1 and IGF-3, which had rankings that were significantly correlated ($r = 0.343$, $p<0.001$) controlling for age. 239 females had both estrogen and progesterone, which had rankings that were significantly correlated ($r = 0.302$, $p<0.001$) controlling for age. 181 females had both IGF-1 and progesterone, which had rankings that were significantly correlated ($r = 0.156$, $p<0.035$) controlling for age. 149 females had both DHEA and progesterone, which had rankings that were significantly correlated ($r = 0.254$, $p<0.005$) after age adjustment.

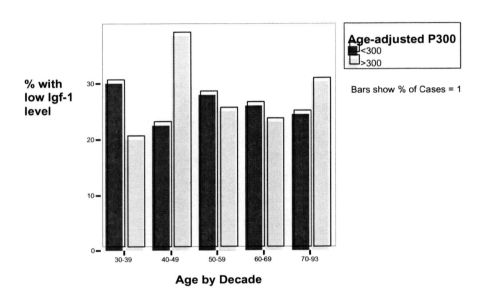

*Table 5. Percentage of Women with Low IGF-1 Levels Correlated with P300 Latency*

For age 40-49 (38.5% vs. 22.5%), females with elevated P300 had a higher percentage of Igf-1 in the lowest quartile (IGF-1 <135) compared with females with normal P300. For the 53 females aged 40-49 with IGF-1 data, this percentage difference was not statistically significant ($c2=1.286$, $p>0.25$), and the Spearman correlation between P300 Latency and IGF-1 was not significant (rho = -0.061, $p>0.60$).

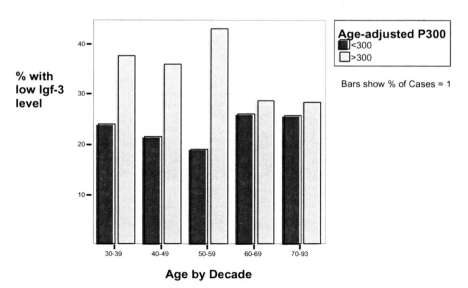

*Table 6. Percentage of Women with Low IGF-3 Levels Correlated with P300 Latency*

For age 30-39 (37.5% vs. 23.8%), 40-49 (35.7% vs. 21.4%), and 50-59 (42.9% vs. 18.9%), females with elevated P300 had a higher percentage of IGF-3 in the lowest quartile (IGF-3 <3.1 for 30-39, IGF-3 <3.0 for 40-49, and IGF-3 <2.7 for 50-59) compared with females with normal P300. For the 29 females aged 30-39 with IGF-3 data, the percentage difference was not statistically significant ($c2=0.544$, $p>0.45$), and the Spearman correlation between P300 latency and IGF-3 was not significant (rho = -0.153, $p>0.40$). For the 56 females aged 40-49 with IGF-3 data, the percentage difference was not statistically significant ($c2=1.143$, $p>0.25$), and the Spearman correlation between P300 latency and IGF-3 was not significant (rho = -0.147, $p>0.25$). For the 74 females aged 50-59 with IGF-3 data, the percentage difference was statistically significant ($c2=4.536$, $p<0.035$), and the Spearman correlation between P300 latency and IGF-3 was significant (rho = -0.247, $p<0.035$). For the 159 females aged 30-59 with IGF-3 data, the percentage difference for elevated vs. normal P300 (39.5% vs. 20.7%) was statistically significant ($c2=5.822$, $p<0.020$), and the Spearman correlation between age-adjusted P300 Latency and IGF-3 was statistically significant (rho = -0.186, $p<0.020$), while the Spearman correlation between P300 Latency and IGF-3 was also significant (rho = -0.222, $p<0.005$).

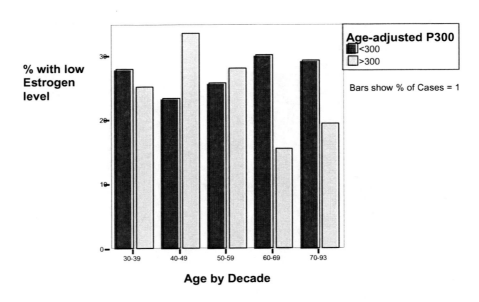

*Table 7. Percentage of Women with Low Estrogen Levels Correlated with P300 Latency*

For age 40-49 (33.3% vs. 23.2%), females with elevated P300 had a higher percentage of estrogen in the lowest quartile (estrogen <37) compared with females with normal P300. For the 71 females aged 40-49 with estrogen data, the percentage difference was not statistically significant ($c2=0.640$, $p>0.40$), and the Spearman correlation between P300 latency and estrogen was not significant ($rho= -0.117$, $p>0.30$). For age 60-69 (15.4% vs. 30.0%) and 70-93 (19.2% vs. 29.1%), females with elevated P300 had a lower percentage of estrogen in the lowest quartile (estrogen <17 for 60-69 and estrogen <20 for 70-93) compared with females with normal P300. For the 43 females aged 60-69 with estrogen data, the percentage difference was not statistically significant ($c2=1.018$, $p>0.30$), and the Spearman correlation between P300 latency and estrogen was not significant ($rho= -0.094$, $p>0.50$). For the 81 females aged 70-93 with estrogen data, the percentage difference was not statistically significant ($c2=0.894$, $p>0.30$), and the Spearman correlation between P300 latency and estrogen was not significant ($rho= 0.080$, $p>0.45$).

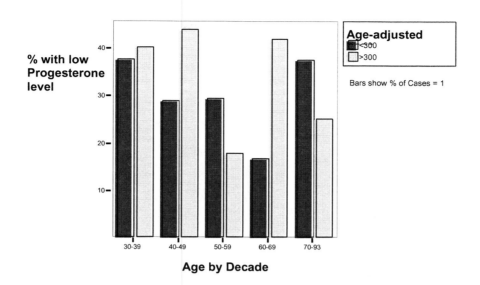

*Table 8. Percentage of Women with Low Progesterone Levels Correlated with P300 Latency*

For age 40-49 (43.8% vs. 28.8%) and 60-69 (41.7% vs. 16.7%), females with elevated P300 had a higher percentage of progesterone in the lowest quartile (progesterone <0.70 for 40-49 and progesterone <0.20 for 60-69) compared with females with normal P300. For the 68 females aged 40-49 with progesterone data, the percentage difference was not statistically significant ($c2=1.242$, $p>0.25$), and the Spearman correlation between P300 latency and progesterone was not significant (rho= -0.170, $p>0.15$). For the 36 females aged 60-69 with progesterone data, the percentage difference was not statistically significant ($c2=2.667$, $p>0.10$), and the Spearman correlation between P300 latency and progesterone was not significant (rho= -0.073, $p>0.60$).

For age 40-49 (55.6% vs. 18.8%), 50-59 (35.3% vs. 21.3%), and 60-69 (33.3% vs. 21.1%), females with elevated P300 had a higher percentage of DHEA in the lowest quartile (DHEA <105 for 40-49, DHEA <65 for 50-59, and DHEA <54 for 60-69) compared with females with normal P300. For the 41 females aged 40-49 with DHEA data, the percentage difference was statistically significant ($c2=4.847$, $p<0.030$), but the Spearman correlation between P300 latency and DHEA was not significant (rho= -0.122, $p>0.40$). For the 64 females aged 50-59 with DHEA data, the percentage difference was not statistically significant ($c2=1.308$, $p>0.25$), and the Spearman correlation between P300 latency and DHEA was not significant (rho= -0.071, $p>0.50$). For the 31 females aged 60-69 with DHEA data, the percentage difference was not statistically significant ($c2=0.579$, $p>0.40$), and the Spearman correlation between P300 latency and DHEA was not significant (rho= -0.204, $p>0.25$). For the 136 females aged 40-69 with DHEA data, the percentage difference for elevated vs. normal P300 (39.5% vs. 20.4%) was statistically significant ($c2=5.208$, $p<0.025$), but the Spearman correlation between age-adjusted P300 Latency and DHEA was not significant (rho = -0.125, $p>0.100$), while the Spearman correlation between P300 Latency and DHEA was significant (rho = -0.170, $p<0.050$).

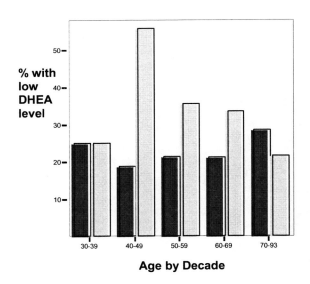

Table 9. Percentage of Women with Low DHEA Levels Correlated with P300 Latency

## Weschler Memory Scores

This analysis was performed separately for males and females aged 30 to 90. Using the standardized values described above for hormone levels, partial correlations were performed with Wechsler Memory controlling for age.

### Males

Among 311 males with Wechsler Memory scores, 142 had IGF-1, 138 had IGF-3, 126 had free testosterone, and 123 had DHEA. No partial correlations were observed that were significantly different from 0 (p>0.06).

### Females

Among 326 females with Wechsler Memory scores, 150 had IGF-1, 141 had IGF-3, 163 had estrogen, 143 had progesterone, and 138 had DHEA. No partial correlations were observed that were significantly different from 0 (p>0.07).

## Number of ADD Complaints

From the DSM IV Attention Deficit Disorder Statistical Checklists that the patients at PATH Medical fill out, 72.8% of the patients who filled them out had more than one attention complaint out of sixteen. 41.5% had more than five complaints out of the sixteen.

This analysis was performed separately for males and females aged 40 to 90. Partial correlations between the number of ADD complaints and rankings of hormone levels controlling for age were performed.

### Males

Among the 128 males with the number of ADD complaints recorded, 56 had IGF-1, 52 had IGF-2, 47 had free testosterone, and 42 had DHEA. None of the partial correlations were statistically significant, with all r-squares less than 0.01 (p>0.70).

*Females*

Among the 152 females with the number of ADD complaints recorded, 70 had IGF-1, 71 had IGF-3, 68 had estrogen, 63 had progesterone, and 46 had DHEA. The partial correlation for ADD and estrogen ranking was statistically significant ($r = 0.309$, $p<0.010$). No other partial correlations were statistically significant, with r-squares less than 0.02 ($p< 0.35$).

## COMMENTS

In this large clinically based study we found a number very important findings. Specifically: in males, both IGF-1 and IGFBP-3 significantly associated negatively with prolonged P300 at different age periods; in males the Spearman correlation between P300 latency and free testosterone was significant at different age periods; in males aged 50-69 there was a significant negative correlation between P300 latency and DHEA levels; in females, only IGFBP-3 and not IGF-1 was significantly associated negatively with prolonged P300 latency; in females there was no significant correlations between estrogen and progesterone and P300 latency; in females there were significant negative correlations between DHEA levels and P300 latency. Moreover there were no statistically significant correlations between any hormone and WMS-111. However, there was a significant negative correlation between estrogen levels and the number of ADD complaints.

In terms of the findings related to the female sex hormone estrogen and either the p300 latency or the WMS-111 results, the literature has not consistently shown that estrogens prevent cognitive decline or Alzheimer's disease. In fact, while there is consistent support for the hypothesis that estrogens prevent dementia in animals,[7-8] observational studies in humans on endogenous levels of estrogen in relation to cognitive function have been inconclusive. Some reported negative effects of higher endogenous estrogen levels on delayed visual reproduction,[13] and attention tasks in women,[36] Mini-Mental State Examination memory tasks,[13] and special performance in men.[37] Recent randomized trials with ERT in patients with Alzheimer's disease showed no beneficial effect of exogenous estrogen on cognitive decline.[38] In fact, one study showed a small negative effect of higher estradiol levels in memory performance in both females and males.[1] Thus our negative findings of the relation between estrogen and WMS-111 are in agreement with similar negative findings from other laboratories. With regard to our negative findings with both testosterone and DHEA there are no supportive data to date in the scientific literature that offer support for an improvement of either memory or cognitive function following testosterone or DHEA treatment.[1]

In terms of the present study it is noteworthy, that binding sites for GH and IGF-1 contribute to the function of various brain areas.[39] Their distribution suggests that GH and IGF-1 contribute to the function of the hippocampus, a brain structure important for the maintenance of cognitive functions such as learning and memory. Evidence for cognitive deficits in GH-deficient individuals has been found in various studies, some of which have shown that these deficits can be reversed by GH substitution therapy. Based on available data, one might hypothesize that relative GH or IGF-1 deficiency could contribute to the deterioration of cognitive function observed in the elderly. However, we can not as yet provide an explanation for the differential gender findings with regard to IGFBP-3 significantly associating with P300 latency in females, but not IGF-1, whereas both growth hormones significantly associated with P300 prolonged latency in males. Evidently it appears that both DHEA and free testosterone levels negatively correlate with prolonged P300 latency especially in older individuals. Similar findings were obtained for DHEA levels and older women and prolonged P300. These finding could have very significant importance in targeting both prevention and treatment of cognitive dysfunction in both males and females.

The present study also addressed attentional complaints and the potential relation to hormone levels. Attention problems have a multimodal dimension. ADHD, including attentional complaints, are related to memory, electrophysiology, genetic, and psychiatric factors. The least biological factor that affects attention failure in adults is of course the environment that the specific individual is exposed to. Various unpredictable occurrences such as a sudden death in the family or an act of terrorism can cause an individual to have a certain degree of attention failure. Although an individual can certainly protect himself or herself from his or her environment; the environment does affect an individual's ability to focus and concentrate on various things.

Attention complaints also have Advanced Psychiatric Disease Performance Test (Axis I) sources, such as anxiety disorders, depression, schizophrenia, delusions, etc. It turns out that attention deficits and impaired memory are common to patients with depression.[40] Another study also suggests that an apathy syndrome is associated with poor executive function in older adults with major depression. The operational definition of apathy in this study involves four items from the Hamilton Psychiatric Rating Scale for Depression and it included characteristics such as diminished work/ interest, and psychomotor retardation, etc.[41]

The only hormone we found in the present study to significantly associate with ADD complaints was estrogen. While there is evidence to support both the negative and the potential positive role of estrogen in both visual memory[42] and cognitive decline,[43] more research is warranted to decipher the exact nature of this association. Moreover, the present study does not reject the possibility that exogenous estrogens, testosterone, DHEA, and growth hormones may be beneficial in protecting against cognitive decline and Alzheimer's disease, and may act as a protectant against cell loss and an antioxidant, amongst other positive hormonal effects on brain function.

## CONCLUDING REMARKS

To our knowledge this is the first report showing a significant negative association of IGF-1, IGFBP-3, free testosterone, and DHEA, and prolonged P300 latency (a predictor of memory impairment and cognitive decline,[31-32]) in males, and a significant negative association of only IGFBP-3 and DHEA and prolonged P300 latency in females. In addition, it is also the first study to report a significant negative association of endogenous levels of estrogen and the number of ADD complaints in a clinical setting. If these results could be confirmed, it may have important value in the diagnosis, prevention and treatment of cognitive function.

## REFERENCES

1. Morley JE. Hormones and the Aging Process. *J Amer Ger Soc.* 2003;51:5333-5337.
2. Almeida OP, Barclay L. Sex hormones and their impact on dementia and depression: a clinical perspective. *Expert Opinion on Pharmacotherapy.* 2001:2:527-535.
3. Cauley JA, Gutal JP, Kuller LH, LeDonne D, Powell JG. The epidemiology of serum sex hormones on postmenopausal women. *Am J Epidemiol.* 1989:129:1120-1131.
4. Kalmijn S, Janssen JA, Pols, HA, Lamberts SW, Breteler MM. A prospective study on circulating insulin-like growth factor-1 (IGF-1), IGF-binding proteins, and cognitive function in the elderly. *J Clin Endocrin Metab* 2000;85:4551-4555.
5. Raynaud-Simon A, Lafont S, Berr C, Dartigues JF, Baulieu EE, Le Bouc Y. Plasma IGF-1 levels in the elderly: relation to plasma dehydroepiandeosterone sulfate levels, nutritional status, health and mortality. *Gerontology* 2000;47:198-206
6. Sherwin BB. Estrogen and cognitive functioning in women. *Endocrine Reviews* 2003;24:133-151.
7. Kawas C, Resnick S, Morrison A, Brookmeyer R, Corrada M, Zonderman A, Bacal C, Lingle DD, Metter E. A prospective study of estrogen replacement therapy and the risk of developing Alzheimer's disease: the Baltimore Longitudinal Study of Aging. *Neurology.* 1997;48:1517-1521. Erratum in: *Neurology* 1998;51:654.

8. Tang MX, Jacobs D, Stern Y, Marder K, Schofield P, Gurland B, Andrews H, Mayeux R. Effect of oestrogen during menopause on risk and age at onset of Alzheimer's disease. *Lancet.* 1996;348:429-432.
9. Mulnard RA, Cotman CW, Kawas C, van Dyck CH, Sano M, Doody R, Koss E, Pfeiffer E, Jin S, Gamst A, et al. Estrogen replacement therapy for treatment of mild to moderate Alzheimer disease: a randomized controlled trial. Alzheimer's Disease Cooperative Study. *JAMA.* 2000;283:1007-1015. Erratum in: *JAMA* 2000;284:2597.
10. Kolsch H, Rao ML. Neuroprotective effects of estradiol-17beta: implications for psychiatric disorders. *Archives of women's Mental Health.* 2000;5:105-110.
11. Compton J, Van Amelsvoort T, Murphy D. HRT and its effect on normal ageing of the brain and dementia. *Brit J Clin Pharmacol.* 2001;52:647-653.
12. Behl C, Skutella T., Lezoualc'h F. et. al. Neuroprotection against oxidative stress by estrogens: structure -activity relationship. Mol. Pharmacol. 1997. 51: 535-541.
13. Barrett-Conner E, Goodman-Gruen D. Cognitive function and endogenous sex hormones in older women. *J Am Geriatr Soc.* 1999;47:1289-1293.
14. Behl C, Manthey D. Neuroprotective activities of estrogen: an update. *J Neurocytol.* 2000;29:351-358. Review.
15. Sano M. Understanding the role of estrogen on cognition and dementia. *J Neural Transm Suppl.* 2000;59:223-229. Review.
16. Cyr M, Calon F, Morissette M, Grandbois M, Di Paolo T, Callier S. Drugs with estrogen-like potency and brain activity: potential therapeutic application for the CNS. *Current Phamaceutical Design.* 2000:6:1287-1312.
17. Cholerton B, Gleason CE, Baker LD, Asthana S. Estrogen and Alzheimer's Disease: The story so far. *Drugs and Aging.* 2002;19:405-427.
18. Wang PN, Liao SQ, Liu RS, Liu CY, Chao HT, Lu SR, Yu HY, Wang SJ, Liu HC. Effects of estrogen on cognition, mood, and cerebral blood flow in AD: a controlled study. *Neurology.* 2000;54:2061-2066.
19. Tan RS, Pu SJ. The andropause and memory loss: is there a link between androgen decline and dementia in the aging male? *Asian J Andrology* 2001:3:169-174.
20. Huppert FA, Van Niekerk JK, Herbert J. DHEA supplementation for cognition and wellbeing. Cochrane Database of Systemic Reviews.2000;2:CD000304.
21. Pavel ME, Lohmann T, Hahn EG, Hoffman M. Impact of growth hormone on central nervous activity, vigilance, and tiredness after short-term therapy in growth hormone in deficient adults. *Hormone & Metabolic Research.* 2003;35:114-119.
22. Aleman A, Verhaar HJ, De Haan EH, De Vries WR, Samson MM, Drent ML, Van der Veen EA, Koppeschaar HP. Insulin-like growth factor-I and cognitive function in healthy older men. *J Clin Endocrinol Metab.* 1999;84:471-475.
23. Arai Y, Hirose N, Yamamura K, Shimizu K, Takayama M, Ebihara Y, Osono Y. Serum insulin-like growth factor-1 in centenarians: implications of IGF-1 as a rapid turnover protein. *J Gerontol A Biol Sci Med Sci.* 2001;56:M79-82.
24. Asthana S, Craft S, Baker LD, Raskind MA, Birnbaum RS, Lofgreen CP, Veith RC, Plymate SR. Cognitive and neuroendocrine response to transdermal estrogen in postmenopausal women with Alzheimer's disease: results of a placebo-controlled, double-blind, pilot study. *Psychoneuroendocrinology.* 1999;24:657-677.
25. Aleman A, de Vries WR, de Haan EH, Verhaar HJ, Samson MM, Koppeschaar HP. Age-sensitive cognitive function, growth hormone and insulin-like growth factor 1 plasma levels in healthy older men. *Neuropsychobiology.* 2000;41:73-78.
26. Baum HB, Katznelson L, Sherman JC, Biller BM, Hayden DL, Schoenfeld DA, Cannistraro KE, Klibanski A. Effects of physiological growth hormone (GH) therapy on cognition and quality of life in patients with adult-onset GH deficiency. *J Clin Endocrinol Metab.* 1998;83:3184-3189.
27. Rollero A, Murialdo G, Fonzi S, Garrone S, Gianelli MV, Gazzero E, Barreca A, Polleri A. Relationship between cognitive function, growth hormone and insulin-like growth factor I plasma levels in aged subjects. *Neuropsychobiology.* 1998;38:73-79.
28. Binoux M.GH, IGF's, IGF-Binding protein-3 and acid-labile subunit: What is the pecking order? European J Endocrin. 1999;137:805-809.

29. Baxter RC, Martin JL. Radioimmunoassay of growth hormone-dependent insulin-like growth factor binding protein in human plasma. *J Clin Investigation*. 1986;78:1504-1512.
30. Brookmeyer R, Gary S, Kawas, C. Projections of Alzheimer's disease in the United States and the public health impact of delaying disease onset. *Am J Pub Health*. 1998;88:1337-1342.
31. Braverman ER, Blum K. P300 (Latency) event-related potential: an accurate predictor of memory impairment. *Clin EEG*. 2003;34:124-139.
32. Braverman ER, Blum, K. Substance use disorder exacerbates brain electrophysiological abnormalities in a psychiatrically-111 Population. *Clin EEG*. 1996;27:1-21.
33. Sodergard R, Backstrom T, Shanbhag V, Carstensen H. Calculation of free and bound fractions of testosterone and estradiol-17 beta to human plasma proteins at body temperature. *J Steroid Biochem*. 1982;16:801-810.
34. Van den Beid AW, de Jong FH, Grobbee DE, Pois HAP, Lamberts SW. Measures of bioavailable serum testosterone and estradiol and their relationships with muscle strength, bone density, and body composition in elderly men. *J Clin Endocrinol Metab*. 2000;85:3276-3282.
35. Brondu NE, Drake BL, Moser DR, Lin M, Boses M, Bar RS. Regulation of endothelial IGFBP-3 synthesis and secretion by IGF-1 and TGF-beta. *Growth Regulation* 1996;6:1-9.
36. Yaffle K, Grady D, Pressman A, Cummings S. Serum estrogen levels, cognitive performance, and risk of cognitive decline in older community women. *J Am Geriatr Soc*. 1998;46:816-821.
37. Durante R., Lachman M, Mohr B. Longcope C, Mckinlay JB. Is there a relation between hormones and cognition in older men? *Am J Epidemiol*. 1997;145: (suppl) S2.
38. Henderson VW, Paganini-Hill A, Miller BL, Elble RJ, Reyes PF, Shoupe D, McCleary CA, Klein RA, Hake AM, Farlow MR. Estrogen for Alzheimer's disease in women: randomized, double-blind, placebo-controlled trial. *Neurology*. 2000;54:295-301.
39. Lobie PE, Zhu T, Graichen R, Goh EL. Growth hormone, insulin-like growth factor I and the CNS: localization, function and mechanism of action. *Growth Horm IGF Res*. 2000;10 Suppl B:S51-6. Review.
40. Ellwart T, Rinck M, Becker ES. Selective memory and memory deficits in depressed inpatients. *Depression and Anxiety*. 2003;17:197-206.
41. Feil D, Razani J, Boone K, Lesser I. Apathy and cognitive performance in older adults with depression. *Int J Geriatr Psychiatry*. 2003;18:479-485.
42. den Heijer T, Geerlings MI, Hofman A, de Jong FH, Launer LJ, Pols HA, Breteler MM. Higher estrogen levels are not associated with larger hippocampi and better memory performance. *Arch Neurol*. 2003;60:213-220.
43. LeBlance E, Janowsky J, Chan BKS, Nelson HD. Hormone replacement therapy and cognition: systematic review and meta-analysis. *JAMA*. 2001;285:1489-1499.

## ABOUT THE PRIMARY AUTHORS
*Eric Braverman, M.D.*

Dr. Eric Braverman is the Director of The Place for Achieving Total Health (PATH Medical), with locations in New York, NY, Penndel, PA (Metro-Philadelphia), and a national network of affiliated medical professionals. Dr. Braverman received his BA Summa Cum Laude from Brandeis University and his MD with honors from New York University Medical School, after which he performed postgraduate work in internal medicine with a Yale Medical School affiliate in Greenwich, CT. Dr. Braverman is a recipient of the American Medical Association's Physician Recognition Award.

Dr. Braverman has published and presented more than 90 research papers to the medical community. His lectures include topics on "Melatonin, Tryptophan, and Amino Acids" given at Los Alamos National Laboratories, and The Core Neurotransmitters and Hormones and "How They Affect the Aging Process" given at Brookhaven National Laboratories. One of his most recent lectures was on "P300 Evoked Response as a Predictor of Alzheimer's Disease" at Oxford University in England.

He is the author of five medical books, including the *PATH Wellness Manual,* which is a user's guide to alternative treatment. He has appeared on CNN (Larry King Live), PBS, AHN, MSNBC, FOX News Channel and local TV stations. Dr. Braverman has been quoted in the *New York Post, New York Times*, and the *Wall Street Journal*. Dr. Braverman's 26 years of medical education, training, and clinical practice have focused on the brain's overall health.

*Kenneth Blum, Ph.D*

Dr. Blum graduated with a doctorate in pharmacology in 1968 from New York Medical College. He completed post-doctorate research in psychopharmacology at Southwest Foundation for Research and Education, and pharmacogenetics at the University of Colorado. Dr. Blum has held several academic appointments in his career, most notably Professor, Department of Pharmacology and Chief of the Division of Addictive Disease with the University of Texas Health Science Center at San Antonio, TX. He currently serves as Adjunct Professor with the University of Northern Texas. Dr. Blum has been involved with pharmaceutical research for more than 25 years. In 1990 together with Ernest Noble of UCLA and his colleagues at the University of Texas, Dr Blum found the first specific molecular link to alcoholism, the D2 receptor gene. He is the author of *"Alcohol and the Addictive Brain."*

Chapter 26

# Developing an Anti-Aging Clinical Operation: The European Model

*Heather Bird, MBA*
*Founder & President of HB Health*
*Director, World Academy of Anti-Aging Medicine*

## ABSTRACT

The focus of this article is on how anti-aging professionals can expand their practices and provide enhanced opportunities for growing numbers of people to experience optimal health and a youthful appearance well into their later years. Specifically, we will examine how our industry can expand beyond the borders of the United States and function successfully in European countries.

**Keywords:** Europe, anti-aging, clinical operation, health, life expectancy, health spending.

## INTRODUCTION

Although this article is primarily dedicated to advancing and expanding our knowledge of the science and practice of anti-aging, we will focus on how anti-aging professionals can expand their practices and provide enhanced opportunities for growing numbers of people to experience optimal health and a youthful appearance well into their later years. Specifically, we will examine how our industry can expand beyond the borders of the United States and function successfully in European countries.

## DEMOGRAPHIC PROFILE OF THE UNITED STATES

Census Bureau figures tell us that 12.5% of Americans are 65 or older today and it is projected that this number will grow to 25% in less than 25 years: this increase is being driven by the aging baby boomer population (those born between 1946 and 1964). Close to 80 million Americans inhabit this demographic, which accounts for approximately 30% of the population. More significantly, in light of the anti-aging industry, is the large portion of disposable income they control. This number stands at 55%, of which 12% is spent on drugs and cosmetics.

### A Growing Market

According to figures compiled by the United States General Accounting Office, $30 billion was spent on anti-aging products in 2002. Half of that was for cosmeceuticals. Spending on skincare products alone has increased by more than 30% in just 3 years and, at $1 billion a year, sales of anti-aging supplements are expected to experience similar growth.

As impressive as the above numbers are, when the demographic information on the baby boomers is added to it we have reason to be very optimistic about the growth prospects in our industry for many years to come. For practitioners of anti-aging science in the United States the timing is, indeed, ideal.

*Why Grow Beyond the United States?*

Having established the extraordinary strength of our market in the United States, is it possible to improve on the picture? Consider these questions: First, what if the population was even older and living longer? And second, what if you were one of the first into the market, arriving even earlier than you already have? Is that a situation you could take advantage of? Well, that is precisely the opportunity that is available to each of us by expanding into European markets today.

Once a successful business model has been established here in the United States it is usually a straightforward process to duplicate it in other locations around the country, so long as the demand exists. A more challenging task, however, arises when foreign markets are considered. How do you determine where to expand, and, when you do, should you keep the same business model, or restructure?

## EVALUATING EXPANSION ABROAD

Prior to opening up a facility in a new country, it is vital to invest the necessary resources in conducting advance research. It will cost time and money, but the knowledge gained will outweigh the costs by a wide margin. Below is a discussion of the general areas to consider.

*Market Research*

What is the current level of demand in a potential location? What could it be with the right promotion? Do consumers have the financial capacity to buy your goods and services? What kind of government regulations will you encounter? These are important questions that must be answered as accurately as possible. There are plenty of firms that specialize in market research that may be hired for this task, or, given all the information that is available online and in academic and public libraries, you can do it yourself.

*Demographics*

As with market research, reports can be purchased online, while general demographic information can be found at no charge. Even a simple search using the name of your target country and terms like "demographics" or "consulate" will yield plenty of initial data.

*Business Structure*

Evaluate your current business model and structure to get an idea of the pros and cons that come with operating in another country. For example, whether your current business is a sole proprietorship, corporation, partnership, etc. how will this translate to a new environment given factors such as international legal structures and financial requirements?

Will you initiate a start-up business abroad without partners, where you make all the decisions, provide financing, and carry the risk alone, while having the potential for sole enjoyment of the rewards? Or will you work jointly with others, so that they can help shoulder the risk and contribute their expertise, which means you will keep a smaller piece of the pie?

Other alternatives exist, too. Maybe franchising is available, where you can take on a working business model and a proven brand. Another possibility is licensing. In this case you purchase the right to a particular brand or the right to sell a product or group of products.

*Management From Afar*

A new challenge for those who move into international markets is managing from a distance. Are the medications, or suitable equivalents, that clients purchase in your home location available abroad? When they need specialist diagnostics, are there competent people to refer them to? Most important of all, how is continuity of care to be assured from a distance?

Management from afar will bring on a variety of new challenges. Be sure you have identified them and answered the right questions before proceeding any further.

## A BOOMING MARKET, FOR THE RIGHT APPROACH

MTV learned a hard lesson when they thought they could just present American music and culture anywhere and succeed. Instead, they found themselves resented by the locals in foreign countries, which translated into poor ratings. Then they "got the picture." MTV began supporting and featuring local artists and hiring from the communities they served. One indicator of their success is that fact that today MTV Asia is bigger than MTV in the United States.

A more recent error can be seen in the embarrassment suffered by General Motors when they promoted the Buick LaCrosse in Canada, only to discover that LaCrosse is a sexual slang term in Quebec. Though this is an extreme example, it does represent something that happens often: companies run into problems because they have not taken the time to get to know the foreign markets into which they are expanding.

Here in America there is cultural continuity in the sense that advertising and marketing techniques are similar across the country. For example, the same techniques will generate similar responses within different major cities, but they may not abroad. In the anti-aging industry we have a strong incentive to be culturally sensitive because the opportunities for expansion into Europe have the potential to be very lucrative. Our sector of the economy is only starting to boom there and the market is far from saturated. There is not only room for new competition, but also simply a need to fill a growing demand for what we provide.

### *Fitting America's Business Culture to New Environments*

When heading overseas do not expect that you can do things the same way in Europe as you do in the United States. Remember: different cultures have different expectations. Are there elements of America's business culture that cross borders successfully? You bet! Good old-fashioned American determination and our work ethic translate into most other cultures very well; but you still have to apply them correctly in the context of that new culture. An example of a trait that often does not translate well is the American tendency to be aggressive in business. This can be problematic, especially in more socialistic countries where nepotism sometimes thrives and Americans come into conflict with it when they expect results according to merit.

Here is an example of the kind of thing you might face: I hired an American doctor to work for my practice, early on, in the United Kingdom. This doctor was very upfront and open-minded; things we might expect here in the United States. But in the United Kingdom these same traits often turned patients off. In an area like hormone therapy, where Americans tend to be open, the British were more reserved, which proved to be a barrier to the success of this therapy.

From another angle, imagine the frustration of the American doctor who wanted to prescribe hormones such as DHEA and melatonin, which are over the counter supplements in the United States, but require a prescription in the United Kingdom. Compounding this were the challenges of not having all the same prescriptions available, not being able to find equivalents, and having to order certain hormones from the United States. These and other differences, such as work permits and pay, added up to it not working out for this particular doctor. Armed with foreknowledge of such challenges, however, they can be overcome.

## OVERVIEW OF POTENTIAL LOCATIONS

The obvious goal is to land in a market that highly values our products and services, has plenty of money to spend, and wants to spend that money on what you have to offer. So how do you pick the right country, or the right locale within it? As we mentioned earlier, of course, the answer is specific market research. Because there are so many possible choices, we will look at an overview of the European market.

### National Rankings of Spending per Person

If you have a busy clinic here in the United States, can you expect the same kind of demand in Europe? It is important to understand from the beginning that there is nowhere else in the world where healthcare spending per person equals the United States. Here it averages over $4,200 for every individual. There are some countries where the government provides healthcare where the spending is close, such as Switzerland, Norway, and Denmark, but the markets we will spend the most time looking at lag a little further behind, but not by enough to discourage us. For example, among the more robust world economies Germany and France are in the top 10 of spending per person on health, and the United Kingdom comes in at 18th. What this means is that these countries, among others in Europe, show promise for business expansion even though the spending level does not equal America's. In addition, because these are relatively stable economies the outlook for continued healthcare spending is favorable.

### European Life Spans

Beyond just healthcare spending per capita it is important to consider the age distributions of different nations. Despite all the money the United States spends on healthcare, it comes in surprisingly low on rankings of life expectancy in industrialized countries and the percentage of citizens who will not live past the age of 60. In fact, the United States is the 26th worst country for living beyond 60, where a whopping 12.8% of the population will not reach the age of 61. In comparison, France loses 1% less, and Germany and the United Kingdom 2% and 3% less respectively.

In France more than 90% of the female population reaches the age of 65. Germany and the United Kingdom stand at approximately 89%. In the United States less than 86% of women reach the age of 65. On a global list of life expectancy Italy, Spain, and France have the best in Europe: each around 79. Germany and the United Kingdom come in just below 78. The United States is #42 on the list with an average life expectancy of a bit over 77.

In France and Germany approximately 17% of the population is age 65 or over. In Italy the number is close to 19%. In the United Kingdom it is just under 16%. And the United States? Less than 13% of the population is 65 or older.

What these numbers tell us is that a larger percentage of the overall European market is suited to the anti-aging industry. So, although they spend less per capita on healthcare, our goods and services have the potential to appeal to a greater proportion of the population. Now let us take a look on spending trends, not just in healthcare, but on anti-aging products.

### European Spending Patterns

One good indicator is spending on facial skincare. In Europe last year volume sales were up both in sales to new customers and sales to current customers. Considering its generally older population, is it any surprise that France spends the most on facial skincare: nearly 2 billion Euros a year just on facial skincare? This speaks to a healthy future for our industry in Europe as the population continues to age and people in general live longer.

If we look at Germany we find that spending per person on facial skincare is less. However, here we have an example of how a little persistence in our research can paint some interesting pictures of where to set up shop in Europe. For instance, Germany has been suffering an economic slump for the last few years, a factor that would make a nation cut back on anti-aging spending, which is considered a luxury in comparison to weekly groceries. It is important to remember, though, that Germany's economy is a relatively stable one and economic improvement is very likely to follow a slump, which improves the prospects for the anti-aging industry. In Germany we are already starting to see this with our sample indicator of facial skincare sales: it has recently increased to 500 million euros per year.

Economic consistency is why I am focusing most on the European countries of Germany, France, and the United Kingdom. In choosing a location for expansion it is very important to locate in markets that are both substantial and stable, and these countries meet the criteria. In Germany increasing stability could prove to be very encouraging. West and East Germany were only reunited a little over a decade ago and money has been pouring into East Germany to "bring it up to speed." If economic strength in the East begins to approach what the West already has, we have a sound location for an anti-aging practice.

## *Lessons from London*

Now that we have an array of raw numbers for the European market and have outlined a general approach for evaluating it, we will narrow the focus to some specific examples based on personal experiences in London that can be applied to much of the rest of Europe.

### *Location*

Location is not just about setting up shop where there is a large older population with money. In Europe the trick is to be near a highly respected hospital or in proximity to the medical community. Not only does this bring the potential for more business, but it also makes it more convenient for clients to get screenings, blood work, or any other medical services you may recommend but do not offer on site. Keeping things easy is a good way to promote repeat business.

### *Products and Presentation*

Once the right location has been chosen, we must choose the most appropriate products, services, and marketing techniques for the European community we are operating in. Let me begin this section with a question: What would happen if McDonald's simply picked up its American business and duplicated it all over the globe? In many cases, they have done this successfully. But how do you think their famous all-beef patty would be received in India, home of the sacred cow? In India, McDonald's is extremely sensitive to this issue and provides a substantial vegetarian menu. If you visit McDonald's India web site you will see how carefully they spell things out: all of the vegetarian food is cooked separately from anything containing meat. In fact, you can identify the workers who are cooking only vegetarian food by their green aprons.

Let's consider another worldwide icon, Coca-Cola, one of the most consumed beverages in the world. If, however, Coca-Cola decided to only push its cola into every market it would miss out on a lot of dollars. In Japan, for example, the world's $3^{rd}$ largest economy, Coca-Cola does not sell mainly cola. Its biggest seller there is a canned coffee beverage. Right here in the United States bottled water has surpassed soda in sales and is now the number three drink in the nation, behind non-bottled water and coffee. If Coca-Cola ignored what the market wanted it would lose market share and be headed into a dead end. But Coca-Cola would never fall into that. What is their relatively new label that we see everywhere? Dasani bottled water, which competes with Pepsi's Aquafina.

How does this relate to you if you are considering an expansion of your practice into Europe? Here is an example: Here in the states, internal and external anti-aging products and services can readily join forces. In some European countries, the public sees these as separate entities and selling them together would be seen as unprofessional. So, if you marched into certain parts of Europe and starting marketing your external anti-aging wares beside internal medicines, you might find yourself not being taken seriously, no matter how common that is here in the States. Knowing this in advance allows you to separate the two or plan a strategic approach.

*Adapting For Success*

To take the idea of separating services a step further, you may find that making such accommodations can bring you numerous advantages. Say your operation, as others have, sets up an external clinic apart from the internal clinic. This allows for cross selling between the two and the opportunity to lure patients in with "quick fix" aesthetic products and services such as massage, microdermabrasion, mesotherapy, and many others. Once there, they can be educated about the benefits of optimizing the aging process from the inside out. In other words, a certain kind of clientele can be brought in: those who think they are only interested in external treatments and, perhaps, are not aware of all the internal work that is available. The external services act as a "cushioned bridge" that gives us a chance to earn their trust and slowly introduce them to, and educate them about, internal options at the other clinic, like diagnostics, hormonal balancing and lifestyle. This is a simple and valuable approach you can use to meet the market's expectations and reach customers that might otherwise be too timid to step into a unified clinic.

## MARKETING TOOLS FOR SUCCESS

The education and level-of-awareness-raising spoken of above is generally a useful marketing tool. On the other hand, blatant forms of advertising in our industry are restrictive and a poor use of marketing funds. They are seen as too self-serving and neither educate or build trust. What you are really after is positive word of mouth exposure, whether by media or directly from clients. Of course, we all know word of mouth is the ideal in any market. After all, it's free. But how do you get that word of mouth going?

We have found extraordinary success with one simple technique: invite the press in to experience what is on offer. Granted, if you invite the press you had better give them a spectacular experience! If not, you won't succeed in any market, and that's just common sense.

Most of the above refers to getting people in the door, but what about getting people back in the door; what about return patients? In the United States it has been said that the average grocery store spends more than $100 in advertising for each new customer. You can bet that once they have someone inside they don't want that money going to waste. They have got to provide the best possible experience so that new customer becomes a regular customer.

You may have heard of the Rule of Five, that it takes five impressions of your business before a customer will walk in the door. This can mean seeing you in ads, reading about you in articles or newsletters, or hearing about you by word of mouth. Five impressions can mean a big investment. How many reporters did you have to woo? How much did you spend to produce and ship newsletters? Surely you do not want to waste that time and money by causing first-time patients to walk out the door, never to return, or, worse yet, to share bad word of mouth!

*The Tipping Point*

When it comes to keeping patients much insight can be gained from a book called The Tipping Point, by Malcolm Gladwell. He theorizes that that there are three primary ways for a business to reach a tipping point, then suddenly surge ahead in the marketplace. These are, "The Law of the Few," the "Stickiness Factor," and the "Power of Context."

He uses the Law of the Few to point out that it does not take a lot of people to create a tipping effect; it just takes the right people. In the case of a new clinic, the right people can easily be those members of the media who have the power to "spread the word" to many thousands of people with a single article. This part of the equation has to do with getting people in the door. The next two address how to keep people coming back.

The Stickiness Factor, in our industry, has to do with the experience of an actual treatment. Do the treatment and its results create such a positive impression that it sticks forever?

Does a patient feel so rejuvenated that she can't wait to have that sensation again? In order to create this effect it is important not only have to have the best treatments and products available, but also the best practitioners.

The third component of the tipping point, the Power of Context, means, according to Gladwell, that the environment where something takes place has a greater impact on people than we generally realize. This is nothing new. Fast food restaurants have used bright, flashy colors for years to get customers to eat more quickly.

For our purposes, the idea of context concerns the entire experience of an office visit. This means something much more than the results of the product or service you are offering. The more you can create a total experience for someone where they are taken away from the world that is aging them, where they are brought to a place that whisks away their stresses the moment they enter, the closer you are coming to that tipping point where your practice will surge to the head of its class.

Think of how the city of Las Vegas does this. It is not just a place to go gambling; that can be done in many places across the United States. So why not go to a less expensive, closer spot? Because Las Vegas is not about an activity, it is about an experience. It makes people feel like kings and queens. By walking down the street you can visit Venice, Paris, then ancient Rome. There is no end of activity and entertainment, 24 hours a day. Who, besides kings and queens, ever used to get that kind of experience?

As one more example, there is a restaurant called "The Rainforest Café" that people talk about just because it's a blast of sensory intake. Just walking by it you see rain falling along the outside of the restaurant, creating walls of water rather than walls of plaster. You enter and a crocodile roars at you; a monkey swings past. When you sit down to eat you experience tropical rainstorms, complete with lightning and thunder; aquariums and robotic animals that further enhance the spectacular experience surround you. You do not go there just to eat; you go for the smells, sights, and sounds, too.

## *Providing the Perfect Experience*

With demand rising we know that the anti-aging industry is going to become more and more competitive. You have the option of being the "complete experience" clinic or the average clinic. The average clinic won't necessarily run out of customers, especially if it benefits from a good location, but being average means failing to ever experience a real boom in your business.

Whether we are talking about a practice in the States or an expanded practice in Europe, what are the first things that clients hear, see, smell, or feel as they walk through the door? Are they met with appealing music or the clinical sound of nothing, maybe punctuated from time to time by somebody turning a magazine page or the ring of a telephone? Are they overwhelmed by the receptionist's perfume or too much incense, or soothed with the delicate smell of fresh flowers? Are colors vivid or calming; are lines sharp or curved? How is the temperature, do people hesitate to take off their jackets? What are the chairs like, rigid and hard, or soft and forgiving? These are simple questions that need to be addressed right away.

Then there are the more subtle issues, which are also important to creating the perfect experience. For example: Does the staff know the clients by name, or do they have to sign in as they would in any other clinical setting? Are people welcomed with a smile, maybe even by someone who will take their coats and hang them up for them? Are there healthy snacks out for those arriving early who have to wait? Do you have a newsletter in the office that educates customers about everything you can offer them? Will they be made more comfortable by understanding how different products and procedures work and knowing the staff they will see during the visit? Is it possible for you to do even more, like offer free foot massages to people who are waiting? Do you want their experience to be average, or extraordinary?

None of the questions and comments above are about how you should run your clinic. They are simply meant to inspire some productive thought. You should always be asking yourself, where are the strengths; where are the weaknesses; what can be done to create such a wonderful experience from beginning to end so that patients cannot wait to return?

### *Atmosphere and Staffing*

The goal in our practices is to do away with the feel of a traditional medical center because the philosophy is one of "be healthy and stay healthy." The patient should not be made to feel as if they are sick and in the doctor's office. This can be achieved with cushioned chairs and sofas to give a home-like atmosphere. Doctors can forgo wearing white coats. Patients are on a first-name basis with administrative staff and greeted by name when they arrive. This approach lends itself to a team effort where the goal is to stay healthy rather than coming in to be fixed. After all, who wants to feel like they're broken?

In addition to employing people in general who show a sincere interest in your clients and treat them wonderfully, the quality of the clinical staff is vital. Not only do they have to be familiar with the latest technologies and research, they have to be the kind of people who will stay up-to-date. As part of this you must be willing to invest in them so they can stay up-to-date.

## CONCLUDING REMARKS

A great deal of what has been said in this article can be applied immediately to anti-aging practices in the United States, particularly the emphasis on providing the best possible overall experience for every patient. The anti-aging industry in Europe is growing and is rife with untapped market opportunities for practitioners to expand their businesses along with it. If you act on this potential you will be on the unique footing of an industry pioneer, positioned to capture substantial profits and bring health and vitality to a population in need.

## REFERENCES

Gladwell M. The Tipping Point: *How Little Things Can Make a Big Difference.* New York, NY: Little Brown & Company; 2000.

United States Census Bureau. 2002 Data Profiles. Available at: http://www.census.gov/acs/www/Products/Profiles/Single/2002/ACS/index.htm

US General Accounting Office (GAO). Health Products for Seniors: "Anti-Aging" Products Pose Potential for Physical and Economic Harm. Washington, DC: US General Accounting Office; 2001. Publication GAO-01-1129. Available at: http://www.gao.gov/new.items/d011129.pdf.

World Bank. 2002. World Development Indicators 2002. Health Spending per Person. NationMaster.com. Available at: http://www.nationmaster.com/graph-T/hea_spe_per_per.

World Health Organization, Reducing Risks, Promoting Healthy Life. In: World Health Report 2002. Chapter 7, page 9. Available at: http://www.who.int/whr/2002/chapter7/en/index8.html.

## ABOUT THE AUTHOR

Ms Bird received her Master's degree in 1999 from Stern Business School NYI, New York University of Southern Europe. After completing her Masters of Business Administration, she began to learn about anti-aging medicine from doctors in the field and established her own clinics. Heather Bird is the Founder and President of HB Health, with two clinics: HB Health of Harley Street and HB Health of Beauchamp Place in London, United Kingdom. She travels extensively searching for the latest breakthroughs in medical science. Ms Bird was a co-sponsor and co-organizer of the 3rd Annual Monte Carlo Anti-Aging Conference in September of 2002. She has been recently appointed a Director of the World Anti-Aging Academy of Medicine.

Chapter 27

# Melatonin: More Than Just a Brake for Jet-Lag

*Dr. Jan-Dirk Fauteck, Proverum GmbH*
*Münster, Germany*

## ABSTRACT

Melatonin, the hormone of the pineal gland, is under discussion as a multi-potent hormone for different indications. However, more clinical studies are needed to evaluate all these indications. Research as well as first-hand clinical experience, suggests that the use of melatonin to treat sleep disorders caused by a deficit of melatonin might be appropriate.

**Keywords:** sleep disorders; hormone replacement therapy; chronotherapy

## INTRODUCTION

Melatonin, or 5-Methoxy-N-acetyl-tryptamine, is a hormone produced by the pineal gland. This synthesis and subsequent secretion occurs only during night, which is why melatonin is sometimes called the "hormone of darkness". Due to its special secretion pattern, it is one of the most important regulators for circadian rhythms in all species studied so far, including humans. Light acts on hypothalamic nuclei, which are linked by a polysynaptic inhibitory pathway with the ganglius suprachiasmaticus. From here, post-synaptic nerves reach the pineal gland. Therefore, during the night, the pineal gland secretes high amounts of melatonin, but during the day, or when the hypothalamic nuclei are exposed to light, secretion is blocked and melatonin serum levels drop to extremely low levels.[6]

During the last 50 years, a number of studies have been conducted concerning the therapeutic use of melatonin in physiological or pharmaceutical doses. There are data for different medical indications, including fertility control, anti-cancer therapy, and treatment of age-related sleep disorders, psychiatric diseases, and jet lag. Unfortunately these studies often reported controversial results that are not reproducible. One of the reasons for this might by the non-existence of a well-defined pharmaceutical product for melatonin. Most of these studies were performed with so called food supplements, which are often lacking for standardized concentrations and/or purity. Nevertheless, the clinical use of melatonin might by justifiable if we take into account the basic research, and our knowledge of receptor distribution, mechanism of action, and the circadian rhythm of secretion of this hormone.

## RECEPTOR DISTRIBUTION AND MECHANISM OF ACTION

The literature describes two different mechanisms of action: receptor-mediated and nonreceptor-mediated: in the non-receptor mediated mechanism of action melatonin acts as an unspecific free radical scavenger. The interaction between melatonin and its cell-specific binding site is the best described mechanism and probably the most important one. Different receptor types,[4-5] which act by different intra-cellular mechanisms, have been described, however the most important findings are the differences concerning the species-specific distribution of these receptors. In all species the highest density of receptors is found within the central nervous system. In all animals studied so far, receptors have been found on structures involved with the reproductive system, such as the nucleii suprachiasmaticea (SCN), and the nucleii paraventricularea (PVN). The greatest number of receptors is typically found on the pars tuberalis (PT). Cortical structures and the cerebellum are often completely lacking melatonin receptors.[8]

## Human SCN                               ## Human cerebellum

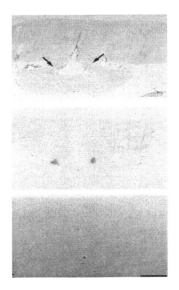 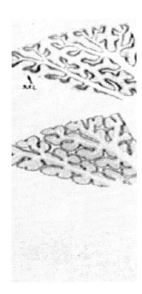

*Figure 1. Human Melatonin receptors within the SCN and cerebellum*

The central nervous system is also the primary target of melatonin in humans. However, in contrast to animals, the highest density of specific receptors is found on the cerebellum, followed by the SCN, where the internal clock is located, and neocortical structures that involved in sleep regulation (Fig 1). Structures involved in reproduction do not express any significant functional binding sites.[2-3]

Based on these histological differences, it is possible to explain the different effects of Melatonin. Given the fact, that the SCN of all species expresses melatonin receptors, and that this nucleus is considered the internal clock, exogenous melatonin is able to re-set the biological clock. Therefore, persons suffering from jet lag or shift workers might benefit from treatment with melatonin if used appropriately. Additionally, in animals, which express the highest density of melatonin receptors on the PT, melatonin is able to regulate the hypothalamic-hypophyseal-gonadal axis. By a still unknown mechanism, melatonin is able to regulate the reproduction capacity of long-day and short-day breeders. In humans, who do not express these receptors on the PT, but on neocortical structures, no direct effect on reproduction is observed if Melatonin is consumed.

These morphological differences between animals and humans might represent a kind of evolution. Where in animals, the melatonin signal is important to regulate the reproduction of the species, for humans the regeneration of the central nervous system during the night might be the principle role of melatonin. Therefore, an intact melatonin signal, in terms of physiological concentration during the whole, might be the basis of a healthy sleep pattern and alteration of this signal will be expressed in different sleep disorders.

Independently from these receptor-mediated effects, melatonin is also discussed as a free radical scavenger. This mechanism of action suggests that melatonin might act as an anti-cancer and anti-aging agent; however, these indications are not yet proven.

## CIRCADIAN SECRETION RHYTHM OF MELATONIN AND THE IMPORTANCE FOR TREATMENT

One of the central characteristics of melatonin is its 24-hour secretion rhythm. This pattern is identical for all species studied so far. Under physiological conditions, the pineal gland begins to secrete large amounts of melatonin immediately after light is removed. Normally, these concentrations will be kept for the whole night, before dropping down to the lowest daytime levels just before dawn. At present, no standard values for daytime and nighttime concentrations are available, because of intra- individual changes. Additionally, the nighttime concentration decreases with age. Thus, elderly patients often have serum levels 10-times lower than those measured in young persons.

Generally the secretion pattern respects the following minimal characteristics: night levels are 6-8 times those measured during day, and these night concentrations will be detectable for at least 6-7 hours.[6] Different diseases that are directly linked to different pathologies may lead to variations of this normal secretion pattern. The most common changes of this pattern are represented by secretion deficits in terms of partial or complete deficit, followed by secretion patterns with normal melatonin amount secreted out of the normal time. Extremely rare cases of melatonin overproduction are reported. In all of these occasions a pineal tumor was found.

If a partial deficit is diagnosed, the clinical outcome depends on the deficit. Low melatonin concentrations during the first part of night will cause difficulties in falling asleep. Patients suffering from early awakenings often do not secrete melatonin for 6-7 hours, and daytime concentrations will be found within the second part of night. A third type of partial deficit might be diagnosed in patients who are suffering by frequent awakenings during night. Their melatonin pattern is frequently interrupted and different peaks of melatonin might be detected within one night. The pathological agents that are responsible for these deficits are still unknown, but several factors have been implicated. Often, light exposure during the night, stress, and certain medications are considered as the principle causes.

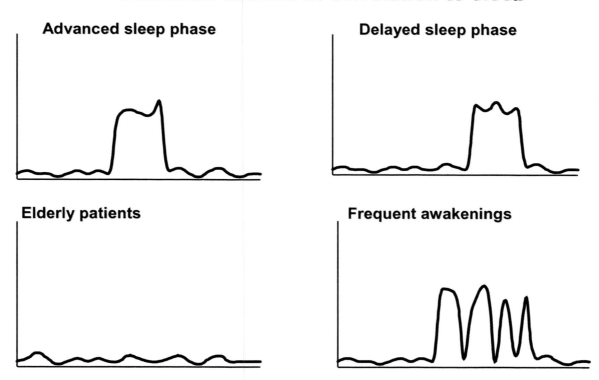

Figure 2 Specific Melatonin deficits in correlation to sleep disorders

A total lack of a melatonin pattern will be discovered in elderly patients. With age, the pineal gland becomes unable to synthesis melatonin and these patients suffer from complex sleep problems classified as endogenous sleep disorder (Fig 2).

Melatonin secretion out of phase might be responsible for so-called desynchronising disorders. One of the best known disorders in this context is jet-lag. Patients travelling over several time zones or shift workers do not secrete melatonin at the time that their body normally considers to be bedtime.

Nevertheless, within 5-7 days the new day-night rhythm will reorganise the function of the pineal gland and the patient will be synchronised again. The situation is different if the patient is blind. Because no light could be seen, no external trigger is given to the pineal gland. Without this external trigger the pineal gland secretes melatonin about every 25 hours instead of 24 hours. Therefore, these patients are sometimes synchronised with the normal day-night circle and sometimes desynchronised. Those patients are classified as free-running patients and they are suffer from sleep problems that occur periodically.

## RATIONALITY OF THE CLINICAL USE OF MELATONIN

Taken into account the results of the basic research concerning melatonin secretion and the distribution of melatonin-specific receptors, two therapeutic approaches are possible. The first one is classical hormone replacement therapy (HRT). Melatonin is well known as a sleep inducer, however short-acting preparations are able to promote sleep but are unable to maintain it. If a complete deficit has to be treated, long-acting formulations are needed. Additionally, the delivery patterns of these formulations have to mimic the physiological pattern: immediate release to promote sleep followed by constant release for at least 4-5 hours to guarantee a total sleep period of 6-7 hours.

Melatonin may also be used as a "Zeitgeber". This therapeutic approach is called "chronotherapy" and melatonin is the first choice. If given at the right time it is possible to shift all circadian rhythms in both directions. Once the patient is synchronised with the day-night pattern a dose of melatonin given just before bedtime will help to maintain this rhythm.

## CONCLUDING REMARKS

In conclusion, melatonin is useful for treating a number of sleep disorders, as well as jet lag. Some researchers believe that the hormone may also prove useful in the treatment of cancer and epilepsy, and as an anti-aging agent, however more clinical studies are needed.

## REFERENCES

1. Fauteck JD, Bockmann J, Böckers TM, Wittkowski W, Köhling R, Lücke A, Straub H, Speckmann E-J, Tuxhorn I, et al. Melatonin reduces low $Mg^{2+}$ epileptiform activity in human temporal slices. *Exp Brain Res*. 1995;107:321-325.
2. Fauteck JD, Lerchl A, Bergmann M, Möller M, Fraschini F, Wittkowski W, Stankov B. The adult human cerebellum is a target of the neuroendocrine system involved in the circadian timing. *Neurosci Lett*. 1994;179:60-64.
3. Mazzucchelli C, Pannacci M, Nonno R, Lucini V, Fraschini F, Stankov BM. The melatonin receptor in the human brain: cloning experiments and distribution studies. *Brain Res Mol Brain Res*. 1996;39:117-126.
4. Morgan PJ, Barrett P, Howell HE, Helliwell R. Melatonin receptors: localization, molecular pharmacology and physiological significance. *Neurochem Int*. 1994;24:101-146.
5. Reiter RJ. Normal patterns of melatonin levels in the pineal gland and body fluids of humans and experimental animals. *J Neural Transm*. 1986;21:35-54.
6. Stankov B, Capsoni S, Lucini V, Fauteck J-D, Gatti S, Gridelli B, Biella G, Cozzi B, Fraschini F. Autoradiographic localization of putative melatonin receptors in the brain of two old world primates: Cercopithecus aethiops and Papio ursinus. *Neuroscience*. 1992;52:459-468.

## ABOUT THE AUTHOR

Dr Fauteck received his medical degree in 1992 from the University of Milan, Italy (Summa cum laude). He continued his education qualifying as a specialist in human anatomy, histology and embryology in 1997 after Post Doctorate Fellowship at the Institute of Anatomy, University of Munster, Germany. Dr Fauteck has made more than 60 presentations before national and international professional meetings and has had over 20 original peer-reviewd publications. Dr Fauteck is currently emplyed by the German comany PROVERUM GmgH as General Manager and Head of Medical Affairs. He has focused his most recent research on melatonin and new drug delivery forms.

Contact Dr. Jan-Dirk Fauteck, Proverum GmbH, at: postal: Münsterstrasse 111, 48155 Münster, Germany. Tel.:+49 2596 864217; Fax: +49 2506 864222; E-mail: fauteck@proverum.de.

Chapter 28

# Clinical Study in Patients with Sleep Disorders Treated with a New Chronobiotic Melatonin Formulation Compared to Normal-Release and Delayed-Release Formulations: Effects on Sleep Parameters

*Dr. M. Gervasoni and Dr. B.M. Stankov*
*University of Milan, Milan, Italy*
*AMBROS Pharma, s.r.l., Milan, Italy*

## ABSTRACT

The effects of three different formulations of melatonin on a series of sleep parameters were analyzed in patients with sleep disorders. The three different formulations of melatonin used in the study were a normal (fast) release, a delayed-release, and a new chronobiologically-correct release formulation (Melachron®), developed by AMBROS Pharma. This new chronobiotic has been demonstrated to be able to reproduce plasma melatonin patterns similar to the physiological one.

Melachron® produced a significant increment in the sleep time, reduced the sleep latency, and enhanced the stability of sleep, as evaluated by wake after sleep onset (WASO), the number of awakenings (NA), and a calculated parameter sleep efficiency-1 (SE1%), much better than the retard formulation. It also enhanced the quality of sleep evaluated by subjective parameters as the score (S), as well as by objective parameters sleep efficiency-2 (SE2%), in a manner significantly superior to both comparators. While the effects of the standard melatonin were concerted on the sleep latency and those of the retard formulation on wake after sleep onset, Melachron® acted on all sleep parameters.

**Keywords:** melatonin replacement; sleep disorders; chronotherapy

## INTRODUCTION

Melatonin levels drastically decrease with age, and this has particularly negative consequences on the sleep-wake cycle. An accurate melatonin-replacement therapy has to be oriented in the reproduction of the physiological kinetic biphasic pattern of the secretion of this substance during the nighttimes. The two phases consist of a rapid increase in the beginning of the sleep period over a threshold level, essential for the sleep initiation, and a maintenance phase of the peripheral blood concentrations for a period of time no longer than 5-6 hours, followed by a rapid decrease coincident with awakening.

The currently available formulations do not reproduce the physiological pattern of melatonin release. The results obtained with the approach utilized up to now, consisting in administration of high doses of either standard or slow-release melatonin formulations, do not satisfy the circadian body requirements, because melatonin has a very short half-life (ß1/2 approx. 30-40 min in the human), and the hormone has to be bioavailable continuously for 5-7 hours, from the beginning to the end of the scotophase.

In an attempt to achieve this goal of an appropriate melatonin treatment, especially in sleep disorders, a new, chronobiologically-correct formulation has been developed. The dissolution characteristics of this product result in a plasma melatonin pattern with peripheral blood levels that closely mimic the physiological release, and with concentrations above a threshold level that would influence sleep parameters. Variation in pH conditions does not influence the dissolution in the gastrointestinal tract.

The aim of the study was to evaluate the effects of this new product in patients with sleep disorders in comparison with melatonin formulations currently available, declared as standard-release or delayed-release. All the formulations are actually available as "dietary supplements".

## MATERIALS AND METHODS

Analysis has been performed through in-depth statistical evaluation on the modifications in the following parameters: Total Sleep Time (TST), Sleep Latency (SL), Wake After Sleep Onset (WASO), Number of Awakenings (NA), and a Score (S - ranged between 1 to 10), the latter attributed by the patient to the quality of sleep induced by treatment with Melachron® (MEL I) compared with placebo (Basal - Bas) and with two formulations of melatonin, a standard normal-release formulation (Standard Melatonin - MEL S) and a delayed-release "Retard" product (Melatonin Retard - MEL R).

In the study, 15 subjects (7 females and 8 males) with sleep disorders, aged between 45 and 65 years were enlisted.

For each treatment, all the parameters of the study were evaluated every day for a period of a one treatment-week. In the basal estimation for each subject the mean values of the weekly raw data was calculated. In the case of treatment with the three melatonin formulations (MEL S, MEL R, MEL I) the value of the first day was not used in mean evaluation to avoid the possibility of bias induced by the adaptation of the subject to the pharmacological treatment, notwithstanding the three days placebo-washout between treatments.

The mean data of the week relating to TST, SL and WASO are expressed in minutes, NA and S are expressed as absolute values. For all parameters the mean weekly values are in the form of real numbers, used up to the first decimal.

Two additional parameters [(Sleep Efficiency, SE1(%) and SE2(%)] were calculated from the data related to the sleep time for every individual subject, for every study point, in accordance with the following formula:

$$SE\ 1\% = \frac{TST-WASO}{TST} \times 100$$

$$SE\ 2\% = \frac{TST}{TB} \times 100$$

SE1(%) is therefore an index of the sleep stability, while SE2(%) is a measure of the overall quality of sleep. The mean week evaluation for these values belongs as well to the real numbers and they were used up to the first decimal.

No side effects were noted, and there were no patient dropouts because of problems related to compliance in all groups.

## STATISTICAL ANALYSIS

The experimental design therefore permits the evaluation of the effects of the pharmacological treatment in the normalization of the sleep measured as TST, SL and WASO, and sleep efficiency in term of stability [(NA, SE 1(%)] and quality [(S and SE2 (%)].

For all the parameters in the study if the single value is assumed to be in the form of discrete quantity, the computation of the mean for the treatment-week can transform the data to be submitted to analysis to ones belonging to real numbers and this allows the application of classic statistical system, as One-way ANOVA. Besides, the discreet number of samples assures a suitable analytical strength. For the post hoc analysis, a multiple comparison test was applied (Tukey's test) to investigate the differences among all couples of treatment.

The data was evaluated with the program PRISM, version 3.0 of the GraphPad Software Inc.

## RESULTS

Table 1 is a summary of the complete analysis of the parameters: TST, SL, WASO, NA, S, SE1(%) and SE2(%) divided by treatment, with the one-way ANOVA test, and Tukey's multiple comparison test.

|  | BASELINE | MEL S | MEL R | MEL I |
|---|---|---|---|---|
| **TST** | 268.4 ± 25.2 | 289.8 ± 19.1 $_A$ | 305.0 ± 21.3 $_A$ | 367.3 ± 42.9 $_{A,B,C}$ |
| **SL** | 51.8 ± 8.5 | 31.1 ± 8.8 $_A$ | 53.6 ± 10.9 $_B$ | 27.9 ± 7.8 $_{A,C}$ |
| **WASO** | 42.7 ± 16.5 | 43.5 ± 10.4 | 22.8 ± 7.1 $_{A,B}$ | 18.8 ± 5.5 $_{A,B,C}$ |
| **NA** | 6.1 ± 1.7 | 5.8 ± 1.6 | 3.3 ± 0.5 $_{A,B}$ | 3.0 ± 0.6 $_{A,B}$ |
| **SCORE** | 2.9 ± 0.5 | 4.3 ± 0.5 $_A$ | 4.6 ± 0.5 $_A$ | 6.3 ± 0.5 $_{A,B,C}$ |
| **SE1%** | 73.9 ± 4.0 | 84.6 ± 4.1 $_A$ | 92.3 ± 2.4 $_{A,B}$ | 94.6 ± 1.9 $_{A,B}$ |
| **SE2%** | 74.0 ± 3.9 | 79.6 ± 2.7 $_A$ | 80.0 ± 3.3 $_A$ | 88.6 ± 2.8 $_{A,B,C}$ |

A = significantly different from baseline
B = significantly different from MEL S
C = significantly different from MEL R

*Table 1: Tabular Summary of the One-way ANOVA results*

In figures 1 and 2 we present a graphical summary of all the parameters evaluated in confront to a "normal-sleep" situation for literature.

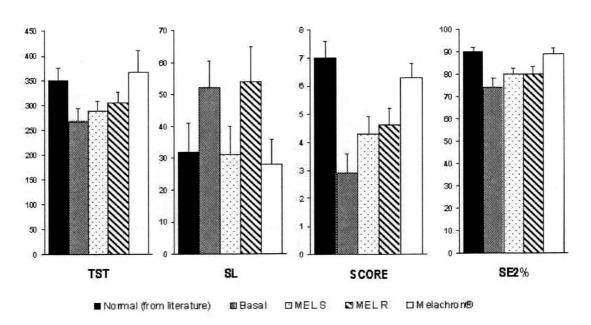

Fig. 1. Influence of different melatonin treatments on sleep quality.

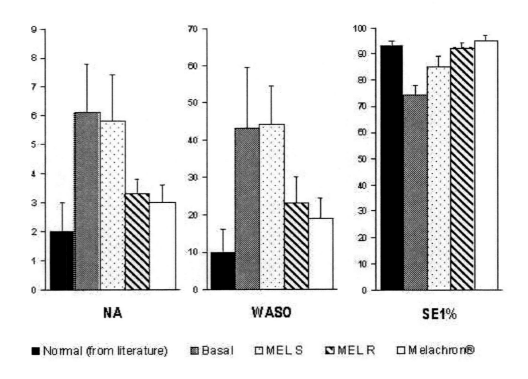

Fig. 2. Influence of different melatonin treatments on sleep stability.

In the case of TST, the overall p value is highly significant (p<0.0001) and the most part of the variance may be explained by the treatment (between columns). The results of the post hoc tests identify the most significant difference (p<0.001) between the MEL I group and all the other treatments. The comparison of all the treatment groups (MEL S, MEL R, MEL I) with basal set (BAS) is significant (BAS vs MEL S p<0.05; BAS versus MEL R or MEL I p<0.001).

In the case of SL, the result of the one-way ANOVA was already highly significant (p<0.0001). The results of Tukey's test indicate that there were no differences (p>0.05) between the basal and the MEL R group and between MEL S versus MEL I. The differences between BAS or MEL R versus MEL S or MEL I (p<0.001) can explain the result obtained in one-way ANOVA.

A highly significant outcome (p<0.0001) was obtained also in one-way ANOVA for the WASO parameter. Significant differences (p<0.001) were found between BAS and MEL R or BAS versus MEL I only. Similar results were obtained between MEL S versus MEL R or MEL I treatment (p<0.001). No differences (p>0.05) were found in the BAS versus MEL S or MEL R versus MEL I comparison.

In the NA parameter we may identify the same pattern obtained for WASO in the one-way ANOVA (p<0.0001) and Tukey's multiple comparison test: BAS was not different from MEL S (p>0.05) as MEL R versus MEL I (p>0.05). All the variance may be explained by the difference between BAS versus MEL R or MEL I (p<0.001), and by the difference between MEL S versus MEL R or MEL I (p<0.001).

In the analysis of the results for S we can identify a highly significant difference between BAS versus all the treatments (p<0.001) and between MEL I versus MEL S or MEL R (p<0.001). No difference could be identified between MEL S versus MEL R (p>0.05).

For SE1 (%) all the comparisons performed among the groups in the analysis were different. Probability will result lesser than 0.001 for all contrasts with the exception of MEL R versus MEL I were p<0.05 values were obtained.

In SE2 (%), however, the results obtained from the Tukey's test will identify three levels of difference: the first between BAS group and all the treatments groups (p<0.001), the second level include MEL S and MEL R that comes not different in-between (p>0.05), and the third level is represented by MEL I that is significantly different from all the other groups (p<0.001).

## CONCLUDING REMARKS

It is well established that melatonin replacement therapy in sleep disorders is necessary because of the deterioration of the circadian system with the age. The existing methods consist of administering various doses (3-5 mg) of either standard or slow-release melatonin, but this approach does not satisfy the circadian body requirements, because melatonin has a very short half-life, but has to be bioavailable from the beginning of the scotophase. None of the existing formulations are able to reproduce the physiological pattern that, in normal subjects, participates in the control of the sleep-wake cycle. Many fast-release formulations produce transient serum melatonin elevations with and a successive rapid decline, while with retard formulations melatonin levels grow slowly, reaching the threshold late in the scotophase. The consequence of this incorrect kinetics is sleep instability and/or difficulty to fall asleep.

We carried out a statistical evaluation by means of one-way ANOVA on the induced modification in the Total Sleep Time (TST), Sleep Latency (SL), Wake After Sleep Onset (WASO), Number of Awakening (NA), Score (S) and two calculated parameters for Sleep Efficiency [SE1 (%) and SE2 (%)] following treatment with Melachron® (MEL I) as compared to placebo (BAS) and two reference treatments Standard Melatonin (MEL S) and Melatonin Retard (MEL R) in a group of 8 males and 7 females for each treatment (for a total of 15 subjects in 4 groups-treatments at a stable crossover design conditions).

From the comparisons described above is possible to deduce that: All products are able to produce some variations in the TST, however the most significant increment was produced by Melachron® in comparison with the two other products (Standard Melatonin and Melatonin Retard). This increase is about 100 minutes greater as compared to the Basal state. With regards to SL, the retard formulation did not exhibit any significant modification with respect to the basal values. On the contrary, the results with Standard Melatonin and Melachron® demonstrated the capacity of both formulations to reduce the latency of the sleep (influence positively the sleep initiation). The effects on the normalization of the stability of the sleep may be deduced from a series of parameters [WASO, NA and SE1 (%)]. In this case Melachron® normalized the sleep period by decreasing both NA and WASO, with an expansion of the total sleep period. In the estimation of SE1 (%) the effect of Melachron® is much more marked than that of the retard comparator.

The overall evaluation of the quality of sleep induced by the three melatonin formulations may be figured out from the Score attributed by the patient and by the objective SE2 (%) parameter (Calculated from TST, SL and WASO). From the statistical evaluation of the score attributed it is possible to infer that all the patients on Melachron® have had an improvement in the quality of the sleep that was significantly higher than that obtained with any of the two comparators. Also, by objective evaluation through analysis of the SE2 (%) parameter it is possible to conclude that the sleep induced by Melachron® is without bias of better quality than that induced by either the standard or the retard formulations.

## REFERENCES

Alvarez B, Dahlitz MJ, Vignau J, Parkes JD. The delayed sleep phase syndrome: clinical and investigative findings in 14 subjects. *J Neurol Neurosurg Psychiatry*. 1992;55:665-670.

Arendt J. Use of melatonin in circadian rhythm disturbances. *Biogenic Amines*. 1993;9:469-471.

Armstrong SM, Redman JR. Melatonin: a chronobiotic with anti-aging properties? *Medical Hypotheses*. 1991;34:300-309.

Attenburrow ME, Cowen PJ, Sharpley AL. Low dose melatonin improves sleep in healthy middle-aged subjects. *Psychopharmacology* (Berl). 1996;126:179-181.

Cagnacci A, Elliott JA, Yen SS. Melatonin: a major regulator of the circadian rhythm of core temperature in humans. *J Clin Endocrinol Metab*. 1992;75:447-452.

Dahlitz M, Alvarez B, Vignau J, English J, Arendt J, Parkes JD. Delayed sleep phase syndrome response to melatonin. *Lancet*. 1991;337:1121-1124.

Dawson D, Encel N. Melatonin and sleep in humans. *J Pineal Res*. 1993;15:1-12.

Deacon S, Arendt J. Melatonin-induced temperature suppression and its acute phase-shifting effects correlate in a dose-dependent manner in humans. *Brain Res*. 1995;688:77-85.

Dollins AB, Zhdanova IV, Wurtman RJ, Lynch HJ, Deng MH. Effect of inducing nocturnal serum melatonin concentrations in daytime on sleep, mood, body temperature, and performance. *Proc Natl Acad Sci USA*. 1994;91:1824-1828.

Dollins AB, Lynch HJ, Wurtman RJ, Deng MH, Kischka KU, Gleason RE, Lieberman HR. Effect of pharmacological daytime doses of melatonin on human mood and performance. *Psychopharmacology* (Berl). 1993;112:490-496.

Ferini-Strambi L, Zucconi M, Biella G, Stankov B, Fraschini F, Oldani A, Smirne S. Effect of melatonin on sleep microstructure: preliminary results in healthy subjects. *Sleep*. 1993;16:744-747.

Folkard S, Arendt J, Clark M. Can melatonin improve shift workers' tolerance of the night shift? Some preliminary findings. *Chronobiol Int*. 1993;10:315-320.

Haimov I, Lavie P. Potential of melatonin replacement therapy in older patients with sleep disorders. *Drugs Aging*. 1995;7:75-78.

Haimov I, Laudon M, Zisapel N, Souroujon M, Nof D, Shlitner A, Herer P, Tzischinsky O, Lavie P. Sleep disorders and melatonin rhythms in elderly people. *BMJ*. 1994;309:167.

Hoffmann H, Dittgen M, Hoffmann A, Bartsch C, Breitbarth H, Timpe C, Farker K, Schmidt U, Mellinger U, Zimmermann H, *et al*. Evaluation of an oral pulsatile delivery system for melatonin in humans. *Pharmazie*. 1998;53:462-466.

Iguichi H, Kato KI, Ibayashi H. Age-dependent reduction in serum melatonin concentrations in healthy human subjects. *J Clin Endocrinol Metab*. 1982;55:27-29.

Kabuto M, Namura I, Saitoh Y. Nocturnal enhancement of plasma melatonin could be suppressed by benzodiazepines in humans. *Endocrinol Jpn*. 1986;33:405-414.

Lewy AL. Melatonin shifts human circadian rhythms according to a phase-response curve. *Chronobiol Int*. 1992;9:380-392.

Lewy AL, *et al*. The influence of melatonin on the human circadian clock. In: Fraschini F, Reiter RJ, Stankov B, eds. *The Pineal Gland and Its Hormones: Fundamentals and Clinical Perspectives*. New York, NY: Plenum Press; 1995:173-182.

Dollins AB, Lynch HJ, Wurtman RJ, Deng MH, Kischka KU, Gleason RE, Lieberman HR. Effect of pharmacological daytime doses of melatonin on human mood and performance. *Psychopharmacology* (Berl). 1993;112:490-496.

Matsumoto M, Sack RL, Blood ML, Lewy AJ. The amplitude of endogenous melatonin production is not affected by melatonin treatment in humans. *J Pineal Res*. 1997;22:42-44.

McIntyre IM, Norman TR, Burrows GD, Armstrong SM. Alterations to plasma melatonin and cortisol after evening alprazolam administration in humans. *Chronobiol Int*. 1993;10:205-213.

Moline ML, Pollak CP, Monk TH, Lester LS, Wagner DR, Zendell SM, Graeber RC, Salter CA, Hirsch E. Age-related differences in recovery from simulated jet lag. *Sleep*. 1992;15:28-40.

Oldani A, Ferini-Strambi L, Zucconi M, Stankov B, Fraschini F, Smirne S. Melatonin and delayed sleep phase syndrome: ambulatory polygraphic evaluation. *Neuroreport*. 1994;6:132-134.

Palm L, Blennow G, Wetterberg L. Correction of non-24-hour sleep/wake cycle by melatonin in a blind retarded boy. *Ann Neurol*. 1991;29:336-339.

Petrie K, Conaglen JV, Thompson L, Chamberlain K. Effect of melatonin on jet lag after long haul flights. *BMJ*. 1989;298:705-707.

Petrie K, Dawson AG, Thompson L, Brook R. A double-blind trial of melatonin as a treatment for jet lag in international cabin crew. Biol Psychiatry. 1993;33:526-530.

Reiter RJ. Pineal melatonin: cell biology of its synthesis and of its physiological interactions. *Endocrine Reviews*. 1991;12:151-179.

Reiter RJ, Robinson J. Drugs that deplete melatonin. In: Reiter RJ, Robinson J. *Melatonin*. New York, NY; Bantan Books; 1995:181-191.

Sack RL, Lewy AJ. Human circadian rhythms: lessons from the blind. *Ann Med*. 1993;25:303-305.

Sack RL, Lewy AJ, Erb DL, Vollmer WM, Singer CM. Human melatonin production decreases with age. *J Pineal Res*. 1986;3:379-388.

Sack RL, Blood ML, Lewy AJ. Melatonin rhythms in night shift workers. *Sleep*. 1992;15:434-441.

Stankov BM, Gervasoni M. Dissolution tests with eight melatonin formulations. 2004 (in press).

Stankov B, Biella G, Panara C, Lucini V, Capsoni S, Fauteck J, Cozzi B, Fraschini F. Melatonin signal transduction and mechanism of action in the central nervous system: using the rabbit cortex as a model. *Endocrinology*. 1992;130:2152-2159.

Stankov B, *et al*. The melatonin receptor: distribution, biochemistry, and pharmacology. In: Yu Hs, Reiter RJ, eds. *Melatonin Biosynthesis, Physiological Effects, and Clinical Applications*. Boca Raton, FL: CRC Press; 1993:155-186.

Tzischinsky O, Lavie P. Melatonin possesses time-dependent hypnotic effects. *Sleep*. 1994;17:638-645.

Wehr TA. The durations of human melatonin secretion and sleep respond to changes in daylength (photoperiod). *J Clin Endocrinol Metab*. 1991;73:1276-1280.

## RESOURCES
Melachron®): AMBROS Pharma, Milan, Italy
GraphPad Software Inc.: San Diego, CA 92121, USA.

## ABOUT THE PRIMARY AUTHOR
Dr. Stankov is a 1976 graduate of the University of Sofia with a degree in Biochemistry. He received specialized training from Cornell University, NY and Institute of Biology and Immunology in Sofia, Bulgaria, in Radiobiology. He has also expanded his education by obtaining two doctorate degrees, one in Biology from the Bulgarian Academy of Sciences and the other in Pharmacology at the University of Milan, Italy. Dr. Stankov is a member of the New York Academy of Sciences, the Endocrine Society, and the World Federation of Scientists. He is currently a Professor in the Department of Pharmacology at the University of Milan, Milan, Italy.

# Chapter 29
# Nutritional Factors Including Antioxidants in Dementia and Anti-Aging

*Luis Vitetta, B.Sc. (Hons), Ph.D.*
*Deputy of Research, Graduate School of Integrative Medicine,*
*Swinburne University, Melbourne, Australia*

## ABSTRACT

Both normal cognitive aging and diseases that cause dementia, such as Alzheimer's disease (AD) and vascular dementia, can impair vital cognition in old age. Although the cognitive impairments associated with normal aging have been defined and may impair quality of life, cognitive decline with aging is believed not to be inevitable. Recent research has resulted in data identifying clinical risk factors for cognitive aging that are potentially modifiable. These new data support an emerging basis for primary and secondary prevention efforts that could achieve and maintain a vital cognitive brain in late life. Strategies that would promote this vitality in cognition with aging include lifelong learning, social engagement, and occupational complexity. Within this framework, lifestyle modifications that include nutritional factors and antioxidant supplementation with a mind-body medicine approach to health could significantly prevent and possibly stop further cognitive decline in adults.

**Keywords:** Alzheimer's Disease; vascular dementia; essential fatty acids; antioxidants; B-vitamins; folate; vitamin C; dietary macronutrients; mind-body connection

## INTRODUCTION

The longevity revolution has increased the focus on many aspects of health in aging. The older population is growing rapidly, and individuals are typically living longer with more active lives. Nevertheless, many older individuals still face late life with cognitive function changes that affect quality of life and increase mortality. Both normal cognitive aging and diseases that cause dementia, such as Alzheimer's disease (AD) and vascular dementia, can impair vital cognition in old age. Although the cognitive impairments associated with normal aging have been defined and may impair quality of life, cognitive decline with aging is believed not to be inevitable. However, many older adults, including some centenarians, appear to avoid cognitive decline even into the eleventh decade of life.

Recent research has resulted in data identifying clinical risk factors for cognitive aging that are potentially modifiable. These new data support an emerging basis for primary and secondary prevention efforts that could achieve and maintain a vital cognitive brain in late life. Strategies that would promote this vitality in cognition with aging include lifelong learning, social engagement, and occupational complexity. Within this framework, lifestyle modifications that include nutritional factors and antioxidant supplementation with a mind-body medicine approach to health could significantly prevent and possibly stop further cognitive decline in adults.

In this paper we shall discuss the aging brain and examine trends in cognitive decline, in particular, the increasing incidence of cognitively impaired people, most notably the aged. We will also consider the link between nutrition, brain function and cognitive performance, and discuss whether nutrition may play a role in the causation of cognitive decline in the elderly.

## DEMENTIA AND THE BRAIN

Cognitive function is a chronic disease. We all recognize that dementia in its most chronic form, AD, is associated with multiple domains on different chromosomes, as well as the amyloid precursor protein (APP). We can actually see changes in the general level anatomy of the brain, and these are exemplified by cellular disruption mechanisms. What is particularly interesting for us, in terms of the study and the epidemiology evidence that we have, is the oxidative stress that is actually a primer of the disease.

If you think about lifestyle factors that may influence the risk of an illness like AD, you may consider high blood pressure that remains undetected, or high cholesterol that remains unmanaged. Other things that need to be considered are the increase in body mass index that persists throughout the adult life, high blood sugar, and also the most important: sedentary lifestyle. Sedentary lifestyle is an overall factor that is basically associated with mind/body medicine attitudes within the community.

Cognitive impairment is a major component of dementia syndromes, and this is what we understand is influencing the ability to function in a community. As the population ages, cognitive impairment is actually expected to increase, and when you establish an early diagnosis the benefit of that is that you have additional treatment options for that particular patient.

Clinical definitions are important because we need to identify those in the community that are suffering from a true frank dementia, from those that actually have a dementia that is associated with an increasing aging process. When cognitive impairment is greater than that found in normal aging a person will be diagnosed as having dementia, whereas normal age-associated cognitive impairment is classed as mild cognitive impairment (MCI), which is actually the most widely used term in psychiatry and in neurology. In terms of the common causes of dementia, the two overwhelming reported conditions are AD, which accounts for about 70% of cases, and vascular dementia, which comprises around 30% of the cases.

Recent data shows that the risk of dementia increases with age, and projected figures from the United States National Institutes on Health (NIH) and from a recent publication in the *Journal of Neurology* suggest that within two decades the baby boomers will be the predominant group in our community, and that within the next four or five decades the number of people with AD will be into the tens of millions. If these estimates prove to be true we will have a significant clinical and community problem.

Now if you look at depression and dementia, depression is significantly associated with dementia. Depression is a risk for dementia, and dementia is a mind/body medicine factor: a very important factor in terms of the lives of individuals that are in the community. Depression may be a prodrome of dementia. There is a question mark on this at the moment, however, depression could play a causal role in dementia, and dementia has numerous attenuants associated with chronic disease. The link between depression and dementia is thought to be via a glucocorticoid cascade type mechanism that affects the hippocampus.

The adult brain weighs about 3 pounds. It looks like a medium cauliflower in terms of size. The brain contains billions of neurons and trillions connections, and consumes more oxygen than any other organ in the body. It has a high concentration of easily oxidizable lipids, and a relative deficiency of antioxidant enzymes when you compare it with other tissues. It also consists of 50% of essential fatty acids. Iron and copper have been getting a lot of publicity in the last few years, and rightly so. It is though that the two minerals could play an important role in free radical generation, and free radicals have been found in high concentration in the brains of those suffering from AD.

In a study of centenarians, Thomas Perls and his study group at Boston University found that healthy cognitive function is actually a better predictor of independent functioning than physical health. This is an extremely important clue as to the fact that it is independent function at late age that may show us the factors that are required to prevent dementia. In a follow-up study on the centenarians, Perls found that a third did not have dementia, and that those with no dementia were cognitively intact. Furthermore, neuropathologic examination of the participants brains after death revealed that the brains of those with no dementia looked like the brains of 60 year olds. Further evidence tends to show that some people are able to escape age associated disease such as AD and cerebrovascular disease by virtue of the lifestyle that they lead. Lifestyle choices associated with a reduced risk of dementia include: good nutrition, maintaining an active life, and proper anti-oxidant supplementation. There is also evidence to suggest that the brain may possess a cognitive reserve that offers people who keep their brains' active some sort of protection from cognitive decline. Perls et al also found that dementia-free centenarians tended to weigh less, and therefore have a lower body mass index. This suggests that fat metabolism may have an important role to play as a marker for achieving a long-life without any form of dementia.

## THE EFFECT OF NUTRITION AND MACRONUTRIENTS ON DEMENTIA AND COGNITIVE DECLINE
*Fats*

In an Italian study by Solfrizzi *et al*, it was suggested that diet plays a significant role in age-related cognitive decline. This study was concerned with a Mediterranean diet, which is associated with a high consumption of fresh produce, olive oil, and essential fatty acids. Results showed that a high consumption of monounsaturated fatty acids was associated with a significant reduction in cognitive decline.

Other studies of macronutrients suggest that a high consumption of monounsaturated fats, a low saturated fat intake, and a high plant food intake, are all beneficial. Meanwhile, results of a study by Kalminj *et al* linked high linoleic acid intake with increased risk for cognitive impairment, and high fish consumption with reduced risk of cognitive impairment. Both linoleic acid and fish are rich sources of polyunsaturated fatty acids, however linoleic acid contains high levels of n-6 poyunsaturated acids, while fish oils are a rich source of n-3 polyunsaturated acids. Additional nutritional epidemiological data from longitudinal studies actually clouds the issue with respect to which type of essential fatty acid or which type of fat is actually protective and minimizes the risk of cognitive impairment and which type increases the risk. There are studies that have found that consuming high levels of saturated fat improves cognitive function. However, However, in those particular studies, participants were also being given supplementary antioxidants, vitamins, and minerals, so the evidence then becomes somewhat controversial.

There is a mechanistic hypothesis going around that looks at polyunsaturated fatty acids and maintains that their consumption is associated with maintaining the structural integrity of neuronal membranes, which then leads to a fluidity of synaptic membranes between neurons as well as regulation of neuronal transmission. Some neurologists doing research in this particular area think that essential fatty acids may actually be initiating neuronal transmission.

In terms of unsaturated fat consumption, that unsaturated fat consumption is probably a marker for other dietary factors, for example polyphenols. So if it really is the high consumption of olive oils that is the preventative nutrient with respect to reducing the risk of age-related cognitive decline and AD, it is probably something to do with the polyphenols present in the olive oil, and the oil itself if just a marker for that.

Epidemiological investigations actually show that there is a significant correlation between the consumption of n-3 polyunsaturated fatty acid, which are obtained from eating fish, and the development of dementia problems like AD. The Japanese are renowned for living long, healthy lives. These people meditate every day and consume fish twice a day, and many of the oldest people in the World live in Japan.

Studies of the link between AD and n-3 consumption have shown that regular fish eaters are significantly less likely to develop AD: people who ate fish just once a week were found to have a 60% lower risk of AD in a study by Morris *et al;* people with AD tend to have significantly lower plasma n-3 fatty acids levels than age-matched people who do not have AD or any other type of dementia. So, the evidence suggests that essential fatty acids of the type found in fish are primarily important in preventing some sort of cognitive deficit in later life.

As the all the evidence suggests that fish is good for the brain, doctors often recommend that their patients should eat fish regularly. However, it is important to remember that many types of fish are contaminated with mercury to such a degree that it may be deleterious to health. Therefore, with respect to consumption of fish, it may be prudent to advise patients that the essential fatty acids in fish can also be obtained from other sources, such as oil in salad dressings and nuts. If fish is not an option with respect to the mercury content, as it is in the North American content, it may also be worthwhile to advise patients that they need to be taking essential fatty acids in capsule form if there is any clinical sign that they are in a minor cognitive impairment state with no dementia.

### Antioxidants, Vitamins, and Minerals

Antioxidant supplementation often improves memory performance in aged individuals. In terms of the epidemiology, it has been shown that low serum levels of a number of B vitamins and vitamin C and folate are correlated with cognitive decline in older people. Decreasing levels of serum vitamin A have also shown the same trend.

Poor cognition has actually joined the list of adverse outcomes that are associated with hyperhomocysteinemia. With respect to this, the homocysteine/folate relationship as shown in Seshadri *et al's* study of participants from the Framingham Heart Study, is actually the proof of the evidence. Results of this study showed that over the follow-up period of eight years, 10% of participants developed dementia, and 75% of these participants were diagnosed with AD. Increased plasma homocysteine levels were found to be strongly linked to dementia risk, and individuals who were found to have a plasma homocysteine level greater than 14 micromol per liter were nearly twice as likely to develop AD than those with normal levels. With today's evidence, it appears that increased homocysteine levels are a strong independent risk factor for the development of AD or some form of minor dementia. .

Some very interesting results have been obtained from studies on blueberry supplementation in rodents. Joseph *et al* found that blueberry supplementation led to a reversal of the effects of aging on motor behavior and neuronal signaling in senescent rodents. This is a very interesting result as blueberries are loaded with phytochemicals, and we still do not fully understand what it is that they do. Joseph found that blueberry fed mice models of AD showed no deficits in Y-maze performance and had no alterations in amyloid-beta burden. They concluded that these protective benefits appear to be derived from blueberry-induced enhancement of memory-associated neuronal signaling and alterations in neutral sphingomyelin-specific phospholipase C activity. Thus, suggesting that it may be possible to overcome genetic predispositions to Alzheimer disease through diet.

### The Importance of a Healthy Diet and Other Factors

Pharmaceutical medicine has a place in treating any form of dementia but the physician needs to be involved in an overall integrative approach for management that can enhance the medical care of that patient with dementia. Thus, it is important to discuss micronutrients, macronutrients, herbal therapies, the use of ginkgo biloba, the use of DHEA and other hormonal treatments, and more, with patients.

Encourage them to eat healthily, that is try to make sure that they eat plenty of complex carbohydrates, fibers, cereals, red wine, fresh fruit and vegetables, and try to keep animal fat consumption as low as possible, as this is the type of diet that is thought to offer protection against age-related cognitive decline. This kind of a diet is also independently aging stopping, as shown by the epidemiological data of those people that actually live a long life; and by the way, only one person in two billion lives to 114, and only a handful actually die from old age. Most people actually die from a chronic disease or the complications thereof. The diet should also include a high intake of monounsaturated fatty acids from olive oil, and vitamin supplementation to correct minor deficiencies that could have an effect upon cognitive impairment. Foods containing large amounts of aluminum-containing additives should be avoided, as should aluminum from drinking water, and anything else that might add a risk to an aberrant process. So, a healthy diet, antioxidant supplements, and the prevention of nutritional deficiencies, could be considered the first line of defense against the development and progression of any form of dementia.

## OXIDATIVE STRESS AND DEMENTIA

If the number of reactive oxygen species (ROS) present in a cell exceeds the antioxidant capacity of the cell, it is in a deleterious state of condition known as oxidative stress. The evidence tends to suggest that oxidative stress in the brain is a source of neuronal damage. In terms of oxidative damage and oxidative reactions, what is actually going on is that the ROS are actually damaging the cellular membrane in terms of reacting with that cell membrane through lipid peroxides.

Mitochondria have been touted as being at the center of aging, and at the center of chronic diseases like dementia and AD. Just 1% of the mitochondrial electron flow leads to free radical formation, and this 1% produces the superoxide radical, or $O_2^-$, as a result of the process of converting oxygen to energy. If you interfere with that electron process, you skyrocket the amount of free radicals that are actually being produced.

Cells actually possess quite a few mechanisms that actually balance this reaction out and the superoxide radical is actually converted to hydrogen peroxide. However, hydrogen peroxide can actually give rise to the hydroxyl radical, which is a much more potent free radical, and it can cause havoc for DNA, RNA, proteins, and carbohydrates, as well as lipid membranes. If you look at free radical formation with respect to the risk of producing an abnormal cell, you are looking at DNA damage, and there are the biological antioxidants that we recognize, such as glutathione, and the vitamins and carotenoids, that can actually limit the harm caused by oxidative damage. There are a number of different systems that are associated with free radicals and oxidative stress. The body itself has numerous mechanisms to mop up the free radical activity that is actually being produced. What is significant though is that if you are under an excessive amount of physical stress, you could actually exceed the capacity of these antioxidants to balance the free radicals and be in a synthetic state of oxidative stress. An unchecked excess of ROS species can actually lead to the destruction of cellular components, and this can then lead to cell death and necrosis.

*In vitro* studies implicate the ROS in neuronal death; however, we do not really have any clear *in vivo* evidence, although, markers for oxidative stress have been found in neurofibrillary tangles (NFTs) and senile plaques present in the brains of AD sufferers. Furthermore, significantly increased levels of 8-hydroxyguanine (8-OHG), the most prominent marker of DNA oxidation, have been found in the cerebrospinal fluid (CSF) of patients with AD.

Changes in the cellular balance of certain transition metals, in particular iron and copper, have also been implicated in the etiology of AD and other neurodegenerative diseases. Researchers are currently studying clioquinol, an old antibiotic that actually sequesters iron and copper from the brain as an alternative treatment for patients with AD.

So the questions that we ask in terms of our research domain, are: Can antioxidants actually prevent wear and tear on human cells? And if so, can this affect aging of the brain? Furthermore, are we able to actually show that we are displaying an age-related deficit if we don't have the adequate amounts of antioxidants, and is this actually manifested as a cognitive and minor performance aberration in those patients that have got an underlying disease?

## MIND-BODY MEDICINE

You cannot improve dementia, and you cannot improve chronic disease until you talk about the mind-body medicine approach. The mind-body medicine approach is associated with the stresses in life, and there are very few, if any, people out there who can honestly say that they have not got any stress. The major stressors in life are associated with doing your job, changing jobs, moving house, breaking up a relationship, and the death of a loved one: all of these are major stress factors. In terms of mind-body medicine this is really interesting because it is not just about what you eat; and with respect to actually eating all the right food, there is always somebody out there that is going to stress you, that is going to cause to actually get something. So, when you look at mind-body medicine, what is the definitive point? It is the brain. The brain is at the center of health. It is the conductor of the body orchestra. If the brain is happy, the rest of the body is happy as well. There are enormous amounts of data to show that stress and certain forms of minor cognitive impairment associated dementia are associated with a bidirectional flow of information between the brain, the nervous system, the hormonal system, and the immune system.

When we look at the cause of disease, it is a balance between stress and pleasure. Obviously, there are other factors associated with it: whether you smoke or you don't smoke; whether you are overweigh or not; whether you have got the genetic background; and so on. So, there are multiple factors. The critical one to associate in terms of a mind-body medicine approach is that balance between the stressors in life and the pleasures in life. A good example is cancer. A number of studies have shown that there is an increased cancer incidence in those that are depressed and those that have multiple life stressors on a continuous basis. Osteoporosis is something else that is associated with that, as is platelet function. Platelet function is associated with stress as well as numerous other factors, but stress is up at the top. In terms of heart disease, the epidemiological data says that if you are a stressful person, you are at increased risk of heart attack. Stress is also a predetermining significant factor for AD. It alters brain structures. It affects dendrites. It atrophies the areas in the hippocampus. There is some evidence to suggest that stress can actually kill neurons.

So what can be done to solve this problem? With regards to heart disease or a minor cognitive impairment there is a sort of reversal program that patients can actually partake in. This includes going to stress management classes, taking up meditation and yoga, taking regular exercise, and eating a low-stress diet: that is a diet that is low in saturated fats, low in animal fats, and high in vegetables and fish.

## CONCLUDING REMARKS

Mind-body medicine is at the center of health. It is what determines what we do with the hand. The hamburger that we pick up and put to the mouth is not an automatic action. This is a conditioned action. The cigarette that you put in your mouth is a conditioned action. As a matter of fact, some great research in the US showed that if you give depressed patients an antidepressant, they actually stop smoking quicker. So the mind is hugely important.

Get some sunlight in your life. That does not mean go out and burn your skin, just get some sunlight. It improves serotonin levels. Exercise and walk rather than go up the escalator. Go up the stairs. Drink red wine with meals, red wine contains potent phytochemicals. Eat non-mercury-polluted fish daily. Eat dark chocolate: it's an antidepressant. Last year a group from Australia published an article, a leading article in the *American Journal of Psychiatry* where they showed that actually dark chocolate was more effective at treating depression than Zoloft®. This probably has something to do with the antioxidant effect of the cocoa and extra phytochemicals. Take supplementary folic acid, as well as other antioxidants. Folic acid is a potent genetic corrective agent, and is hugely important in health and maintaining health in order to prevent disease rather than actually cure it. None of these things are cures. These are all preventative approaches that can help to thwart the adverse outcome.

If you want to talk anti-aging, and you want to talk about stunting dementia indefinitely, one needs to be thinking out of the box, not within it.

## REFERENCES

Conquer JA, Tierney MC, Zecevic J, Bettger WJ, Fisher RH. Fatty acid analysis of blood plasma of patients with Alzheimer's disease, other types of dementia, and cognitive impairment. *Lipids*. 2000;35:1305-1312.

Joseph JA, Denisova NA, Arendash G, Gordon M, Diamond D, Shukitt-Hale B, Morgan D. Blueberry supplementation enhances signaling and prevents behavioral deficits in an Alzheimer disease model. *Nutr Neurosci*. 2003;6:153-162.

Kalmijn S, Feskens EJ, Launer LJ, Kromhout D. Polyunsaturated fatty acids, antioxidants, and cognitive function in very old men. *Am J Epidemiol*. 1997;145:33-41.

Morris MC, Evans DA, Bienias JL, Tangney CC, Bennett DA, Wilson RS, Aggarwal N, Schneider J. Consumption of fish and n-3 fatty acids and risk of incident Alzheimer disease. *Arch Neurol*. 2003;60:940-946.

Solfrizzi V, Panza F, Torres F, Mastroianni F, Del Parigi A, Venezia A, Capurso A. High monounsaturated fatty acids intake protects against age-related cognitive decline. *Neurology*. 1999;52:1563-1569.

## ABOUT THE AUTHOR

Dr. Luis Vitetta is the Director of Research for the Swinburne University Graduate School of Integrative Medicine. Dr. Vitetta is an Honors Graduate from Monash University (1981) in the Department of Biochemistry/Faculty of Medicine, and a PhD Graduate from the University of Melbourne (1985) and the Faculty of Medicine's Department of Surgery (Austin & Repatriation Medical Centre) where he studied the epidemiological and etiological factors of biliary disease. He was a Senior Research Associate with the University of Melbourne's Faculty of Medicine/Centre for Palliative Care at Caritas Christi Hospital and St Vincent's Hospital. Prior to that, he was a University of Melbourne Research Fellow with the Faculty of Medicine and the Department of Surgery at the Austin & Repatriation Medical Centre. His interests are predominantly in clinical epidemiology. He has collaborated extensively in numerous epidemiological projects related to chronic diseases, such as large bowel cancer, breast cancer, and skin cancer. His interests include nutrition, immune system function, and mind/body medicine.

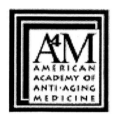

# Application for NEW INDIVIDUAL MEMBERSHIP

Name: _____ _____ _____  Title: _____
            FIRST      MI      LAST

Degree(s)   [ ]MD   [ ]DO   [ ]MBBS   [ ]DC   [ ]DDS   [ ]ND
             [ ]DPM  [ ]PhD [ ]DVM   [ ]RPh [ ]RN   [ ]NP
             [ ]PA   [ ]other (specify):_____

Practice/Company: _____
Mailing Address: (STREET OR POSTAL DELIVERY):_____
                  (STREET:)_____
                  (CITY):_____(STATE/PROVINCE):_____( ZIP CODE):_____
                  (COUNTRY):_____
                  (PHONE):_____ (FAX):_____ (E-MAIL):_____

| Membership Category | 1-year | Save! 2-year | Save More! 5-year |
|---|---|---|---|
| [ ] Physician Member (MD, DO, MBBS) | [ ] US$ 150 | [ ] US$ 250 | [ ] US$ 500 |
| [ ] Scientific/Healthcare (DC, DDS, ND, DPM, RPh, PhD, RN, NP, PA) | [ ] US$ 95 | [ ] US$ 150 | NA |
| [ ] Preferred General Public | [ ] US$ 89.95 | NA | NA |

I wish to be accepted as a member of the American Academy of Anti-Aging Medicine and agree to abide by its By Laws and Code of Ethics: Signed: _____

Please Select a Voluntary Contribution Level (optional): [ ] US$50  [ ] US$100  [ ] US$150  [ ] _____
                                                                                                                            (other)

Payment in the amount of US$_____ is enclosed (membership dues + contribution)
    [ ] Check Enclosed
    [ ] I authorize A4M to process payment to the following credit card:
        [ ] VISA   [ ] MASTERCARD   [ ] AMEX
        Card Number: _____  Expiration Date: _____
        Name (as appears on card): _____
        Signature: _____  Today's Date: _____

---

REMIT COMPLETED FORM TO:
**American Academy of Anti-Aging Medicine**
1510 West Montana Street
Chicago, IL 60614 USA
Phone: 773-528-1000
Fax: 773-528-5390
Attn: Membership Coordinator

ccspat

www.worldhealth.net

- An Organizational Membership affords you extended benefits. Conttact the A4M Membership Department for details.
- Allow 6-8 weeks for processing your new membership application and receipt of your Welcoming Kit and Member Certificate.
- Applicants wishing to return their A4M membership are required to comply to A4M's Membership Return Policy. Instructions are available on the "Membership" page at www.worldhealth.net and from the A4M Membership department.
- For inquiries, contact Membership Coordinator at 773-528-1000 or e-mail info@worldhealth.net

# AMERICAN ACADEMY OF ANTI-AGING MEDICINE
## Publications & Multimedia Products
*State-of-the-Science Anti-Aging Clinical Educational Materials*

[ ] _____
$24.95
$18.95 [A4M member]
**BEST SELLER**

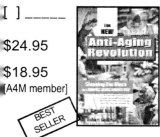

***The NEW Anti-Aging Revolution***
[softcover; 627 pp; 2003]
Synthesizes the latest cutting-edge research findings and clinical observations on anti-aging medicine, the newest and most important healthcare model in this millennium.

[ ] _____
$14.95
$12.00 [A4M member]

***Brain Fitness***
[softcover; 347 pp; 1999]
How to strengthen the mind as we age.

[ ] _____
$14.95
$12.00 [A4M member]

***Death in the Locker Room II***
[softcover; 386 pp; 1992]
Covering the epidemic of steroid drug abuse in sports.

[ ] _____
$24.95
$12.00 [A4M member]

***The E Factor***
[hardcover; 575 pp; 1988]
Based on ergogenics, read secrets of new tech training and fitness for the winning edge.

[ ] _____
$14.00
$13.00 [A4M member]
**BEST SELLER**

***Grow Young with HGH***
[softcover; 372 pp; 1997]
The best-selling book that started the anti-aging medical movement.

[ ] _____
$24.95
$17.50 [A4M member]

***Infection Protection***
[hardcover; 448 pp; 2002]
Explores the connection between infectious diseases and the onset and/or progression of the chronic degenerative diseases of aging.

**MORE PRODUCTS LISTED ON OTHER SIDE ...**

[ ] _____
$150.00
$ 65.00 [A4M member]

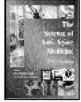

***The Science of Anti-Aging Medicine -- 2003 Update*** [softcover; 268 pp; 2003]
Covering theories of aging, innovative anti-aging therapies, and the future of anti-aging medicine at its decade anniversary.

[ ] _____
$22.95
$15.00 [A4M member]

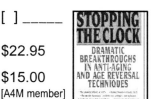

***Stopping the Clock***
[hardcover; 369 pp; 1996]
Covering nutritional supplementation, hormone replacement, diet, lifestyle changes, and other approaches that may reverse aging.

[ ] _____
$15.95
$10.00 [A4M member]

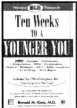

***Ten Weeks to a Younger You***
[softcover; 336 pp; 1999]
Definitive age reversal text outlines real life measures that you can implement to optimize mental and physical well being.

[ ] _____
$229.00
$199.00 [A4M member]

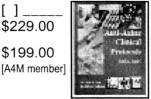

***Anti-Aging Clinical Protocols, 2004-2005*** [softcover; 280 pp; 2004]
The first "how to" and "hands on" publication covering the latest diagnostic and therapeutic procedures involved in preventing, treating and reversing metabolic dysfunctions that are implicated in the aging process.

Subscription Update Service (2 updates in 2004-2005):
[ ] _____ $99.00
[ ] _____ $79.00 [A4M member]

**NEW in 2004**

[ ] _____
$16.95
$10.00 [A4M member]

***Yearbook 2003 (Anti-Aging Physicians Directory & Resource Guide)***
[112 pp; 2003 Edition]
The annual showcase of physicians, practitioners, clinics, and suppliers involved in the anti-aging field. The Anti-Aging Desk Reference in this Yearbook reviews 135+ anti-aging interventions.

---

ORDERED BY:
Name: _____ (first) _____ (last)
Shipping Address: _____ (street)
_____ _____ (city/state)
_____ _____ (zipcode/country)
Telephone: _____ Fax: _____
Email: _____
**PAYMENT METHOD:**  [ ] Cash   [ ] Check
[ ] Credit Card: [ ] Visa [ ] MasterCard [ ] AmericanExpress
Number: _____ Exp Date: _____

# AMERICAN ACADEMY OF ANTI-AGING MEDICINE
## Publications & Multimedia Products
*Continued from front side*

[ ] _____
$175.00
$125.00
[A4M member]
*BEST SELLER*

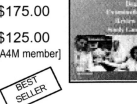

**Board Examination Review & Study Guide**
[softcover; 750 pp; 2002 Edn]
A must-have clinical anti-aging reference, this review text facilitates preparation for physicians and practitioners pursuing anti-aging board certification.

[ ] _____
$399.00
$199.00
[A4M member]

**Official ABAAM Board Exam Video Series** [DVD]

[ ] _____
$595.00
[ABAAM kit]
*HIGHLY RECOMMENDED*

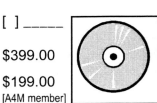

**Board Examination Review Kit**
Combination of the Study Guide, Official Video Series (DVD), and selected books. An ideal way to start or expand your anti-aging professional reference library.

[ ] _____
$250.00
$149.00
[A4M member]

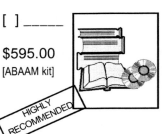

**Master Series on Anti-Aging Endocrinology** [DVD]
Learn from this collection of lectures on anti-aging endocrinology by some of A4M's best speakers.

[ ] _____
$250.00
$149.00
[A4M member]

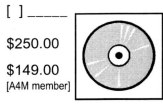

**Master Series on Antioxidant Therapy** [DVD]
Learn from this collection of lectures on antioxidant therapy by some of A4M's best speakers.

[ ] _____
$169.00

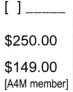 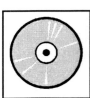

**35-mm Presentation Slides, volume 1** [39-slide set]
Essential for physicians and practitioners who regularly give public seminars on health promotion.

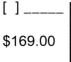 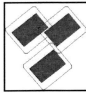

[ ] _____
$65.00
$50.00
[A4M member]

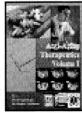

**Anti-Aging Medical Therapeutics, vol. 1**
[softcover; 218 pp; 1996 conference yr]
Proceedings of the Fourth International Congress on Anti-Aging Medicine and Biomedical Technologies.

[ ] _____
$65.00
$50.00
[A4M member]

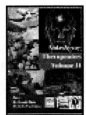

**Anti-Aging Medical Therapeutics, vol. 2**
[softcover; 213 pp; 1997 conference year]
Proceedings of the Fifth International Congress on Anti-Aging Medicine and Biomedical Technologies.

[ ] _____
$129.00
$99.00
[A4M member]

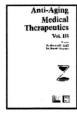

**Anti-Aging Medical Therapeutics, vol. 3**
[hardcover; 381 pp; 1998 conference year]
Proceedings of the Sixth International Congress on Anti-Aging Medicine & Biomedical Technologies and Summer Seminar for Office-Based Health Professional.

[ ] _____
$129.00
$99.00
[A4M member]

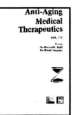

**Anti-Aging Medical Therapeutics, vol. 4**
[hardcover; 355 pp; 1999 conference year]
Proceedings of the Seventh International Congress on Anti-Aging Medicine & Biomedical Technologies and Summer Seminar for Office-Based Health Professional.

[ ] _____
$259.00
[softcover]
[ ] _____
$199.00
[on CD]
A4M member:
[ ] _____
$149.00
[softcover]
[ ] _____
$99.00
[on CD]

**Anti-Aging Medical Therapeutics, vol. 5**
[softcover; 540 pgs; 2000-2001-2002 conference years (spans 3 years)]
Proceedings of the Eighth, Ninth, and Tenth International Congresses on Anti-Aging Medicine & Biomedical Technologies and Summer Seminars for Office-Based Health Professional.

[ ] _____
$179.00
[softcover]
[ ] _____
$139.00
[on CD]

**Anti-Aging Medical Therapeutics, vol. 6**
[softcover; 250 pp; 2003 conference year]
Proceedings of the Eleventh International Congress on Anti-Aging Medicine & Biomedical Technologies, Summer Seminars for Office-Based Health Professional, and the Second Asia-Pacific Anti-Aging Conference (Singapore).

*NEW in 2004*

All prices quoted in US $ Dollars. Shipping and handling charges to be calculated and applied at time of order processing. Allow 4-6 weeks for processing of your order. Active A4M membership required for "A4M Member" pricing and will be confirmed at time A4M receives your order form.

**... CONTINUED FROM OTHER SIDE**

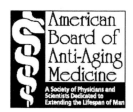

# Anti-Aging Board Certification
# Physician's Program

The **American Board of Anti-Aging Medicine (ABAAM)** was founded in 1997 as a professional certification and review board for individuals with M.D. (Doctor of Medicine), D.O. (Doctor of Osteopathic Medicine), and/or M.B.B.S. (Bachelor's Medicine/Surgery) degrees.

Achieving ABAAM board certification is a two-step process, consisting of:

*Part I. Written Examination:* A three-hour, multiple choice written examination assesses proficiency in numerous areas of anti-aging clinical care, with a predominant focus on practical knowledge skills in diagnostic and therapeutic interventions, nutritional therapies, and pharmaceuticals, as well as sound textbook knowledge of endocrinology, neurophysiology, and cancer. Familiarity with key biomedical advancements and demographic trends relevant to life enhancement and life extension are also required. Those who pass Part I may refer to themselves as "Diplomates" of ABAAM.

*Part II. Chart Review & Oral Examination:* Upon receiving a passing grade in Part I, physicians submit eight (8) patient charts, evaluated by ABAAM to determine the candidate's skills in utilizing anti-aging diagnostic and treatment interventions in a safe and efficacious manner in their practices. At the A4M's USA conferences, the Oral Examination consists of a private exam interview conducted by two ABAAM oral examiners. Generally, the Oral Examination takes 45 to 60 minutes and consists of one or two mock cases and related clinical questions. Those who pass Part II may refer to themselves as "Board Certified" by ABAAM.

## A4M Official Academic Sanctioned Venues for ABAAM Anti-Aging Board Certifications, 2004

- Feb. 27-29, 2004 Bangkok, Thailand
- March 18-21, 2004 Paris, France
- June 24-27, 2004 Singapore
- Aug. 20-22, 2004 Chicago, Illinois USA*
- Sept. 11-12, 2004 Seoul, South Korea
- Oct. 8-11, 2004 Catania, Italy
- Oct. 22-24, 2004 Cancun, Mexico
- Dec. 2-5, 2004 Las Vegas, Nevada USA *
- Dec. 14-16, 2004 Dubai, United Arab Emirates

All venues above are scheduled to hold the ABAAM Written Examination (Part I). An asterisk (*) denotes venue at which the ABAAM Oral Examination (Part II) is scheduled to take place. Additional venues and dates in 2004 being added regularly. Visit www.a4minfo.net and click "Going Global" to stay apprised of the latest event schedule.

Inquire with Board Registrar at email: exam@worldhealth.net for exact examination date and time regarding your venue of interest.

## Requisites

- Membership in the A4M, current and in good standing.
- Attendance at two or more consecutive A4M-approved/sponsored conferences. (Attendance at future conferences may be used toward fulfilling this requirement.)
- An M.D., D.O., or M.B.B.S. degree from an accredited medical school
- An active medical license in the state, province, or nation where the applicant resides
- A minimum of five (5) years of clinical practice experience
- No significant disciplinary actions against the applicant (or a written appeal including full disclosure of all disciplinary actions accompanied by a full explanation of those actions accompanied by a request for a waiver of this requirement)
- Continuing Medical Education (CME) credits (or equivalent study) in their field of specialty during the past eight years, totalling 200 hours. In nations where CME is not offered, exception to this requisite may be granted on an individual basis, as determined by case-by-case review by the ABAAM Board.
- Submission of 5 multiple-choice examination questions, with correct answers supported by medical/scientific references
- Passing scores on Written (Part I) and then Oral (Part II) examination(s)
- Completion of the oral portion of the examination within 24 months of passing the written exam
- Payment of all mandatory board examination fees:
  - Credentials application & review: US$250
  - Written examination: US$ 1,470
  - Oral exam/Chart review: US$ 1,720
- Payment of annual ABAAM Credentialing/Certification/Documentation Fee: US$ 175 each year
- Purchase of Board Review Study Kit is recommended so candidate has access to relevant reference components for study.

*Qualifications and specifications for board examination may be subject to modification without notice by ABAAM at anytime.*

## About the Written Examination

| | |
|---|---|
| DURATION OF EXAMINATION: | 3 hours |
| OFFICIAL LANGUAGE OF EXAM: | English |

EXAM CONTENT:

| SUBJECT | APPROX % OF EXAM |
|---|---|
| **Foundation of understanding of importance/application of anti-aging medicine:** | 10% |
| Mechanisms of Aging | |
| Demographic / Sociological Aspects of Aging | |
| Biomedical and Biotechnological Advancements | |
| **Sound textbook knowledge of:** | |
| Endocrinology | 20% |
| Neurophysiology | 15% |
| Cancer | 10% |
| **Practical knowledge skills in:** | |
| Pharmaceuticals | 10% |
| Nutritional Therapies | 15% |
| Diagnostic and Therapeutic Interventions | 20% |

## BECOME A CANDIDATE FOR ANTI-AGING BOARD CERTIFICATION
Contact the Board Registrar at: email: exam@worldhealth.net ; tel: (773) 528-4333 ; fax (773) 528-5390

# American Board of Anti-Aging Medicine
## Board Certification Application for Physicians

### Certification and Credential Requirements

Medical Degree (Attach Copy of Degree/Diploma)   [ ] M.D.   [ ] D.O.   [ ] M.B.B.S.

Granting Institution _____   Date of Graduation _____

[ ] Attach copy of active medical license   [ ] Attach resume showing 5 years in clinical practice
[ ] Attach 250 word autobiography indicating primary areas   [ ] Attach copies of CME certificates/other evidence of current CME accrual of interest within anti-aging medicine

By signing this certification and credential request form, I hereby declare my intention to fulfill, prior to being granted final certification diploma, the following requirements:

1. Attendance at two (2) A4M-sponsored and/or supported conferences on anti-aging medicine and biotechnology*
2. Accrue two hundred (200) documented hours of Continuing Medical Education (CME) in related fields over the past eight (8) years*
3. Production of eight (8) clinical case studies in anti-aging medicine**
4. Pass both the written and oral sections of the board certification examination**

\* Requisite for Part I (Written Examination);   ** Requisite for Part II (Oral Examination).

### Contact Information (Home)

Name _____
Address _____
City, State, Zip _____
Country (if not United States of America) _____
Phone _____ Fax _____
E-mail _____

### Hospital/Practice Facility Information

Name of Practice/Facility _____
Address _____
City, State, Zip _____
Country (if not United States of America) _____
Phone _____ Fax _____
E-mail _____

### A4M Official Academic Sanctioned Venues for Continuing Medical Education Certifications in 2004: SELECT ONE Examination Venue:

[ ] Feb. 27-29, 2004 Bangkok, Thailand   Registration Deadline: Jan. 30, 2004
[ ] March 18-21, 2004 Paris, France   Registration Deadline: Feb. 25, 2004
[ ] June 24-27, 2004 Singapore   Registration Deadline: May 31, 2004
[ ] Aug. 20-22, 2004 Chicago, Illinois USA*   Registration Deadline: July 23, 2004   Specify: [ ] Part I (Written) [ ] Part II (Oral)

[ ] Sept. 11-12, 2004 Seoul, South Korea   Registration Deadline: Aug. 13, 2004
[ ] Oct. 8-11, 2004 Catania, Italy   Registration Deadline: Sept. 10, 2004
[ ] Oct. 22-24, 2004 Cancun, Mexico   Registration Deadline: Sept. 24, 2004
[ ] Dec. 2-5, 2004 Las Vegas, Nevada USA*   Registration Deadline: Nov. 5, 2004   Specify: [ ] Part I (Written) [ ] Part II (Oral)

[ ] Dec. 14-16, 2004 Dubai, United Arab Emirates   Registration Deadline: Nov. 19, 2004

Contact the ABAAM Board Registrar (email: exam@worldhealth.net) for exact sitting date and time. *Venues at which Oral Examination (Part II) will be offered (Board Registrar will confirm with Orals Candidates).

### Fees (Due With Application):

**PART I (Written Exam) CANDIDATES:**
US$ 250  Application Review Fee
US$ 1,470  Written Exam Fee

**PART II (Oral Exam) CANDIDATES:**
US$ 1,720  Chart Review & Examination

**ANNUAL Credentialing/Certification/Documentation:**
US$ 175 per year

### Method of Payment:

[ ] Check (payable to American Board of Anti-Aging Medicine)
[ ] Credit Card: [ ] Visa  [ ] Mastercard
Card # _____
Expiration Date: _____
Cardholder Name (print): _____
Cardholder Signature: _____

Application review fee is non-refundable. Should this application fail to meet board requirements, the written exam fee will be refunded. Cancellations for the written exam will be refunded if ABAAM is notified in writing thirty (30) days following Application receipt and prior to the stated Registration Deadline for the Sitting Date, minus a $200 processing fee. Cancellations beyond this date will be refunded minus a $300 processing fee. Books, review materials and/or courses beyond a syllabus and exam guide are not included in these fees. Qualifications and specifications for board examination may be subject to modification without notice by ABAAM at anytime.

I, the undersigned, hereby authorize the American Board of Anti-Aging Medicine to accept my application and fees and to review the enclosed materials. I certify that these materials are correct, complete, and true to the best of my knowledge. I have read and understand the provisions for refund of fees above. I certify with this signature that I will meet the ethical, academic, and professional standards set by the Board, and that I will have fulfilled all requirements for ABAAM certification by such time as such certification is awarded.

_____ Signature     _____ Date

*Speakers from the 2003 conference year have based their chapters in this book on lectures that they presented at A4M's scientific conferences. Cassettes and videos of the actual presentations are available from Insta-Tapes.*

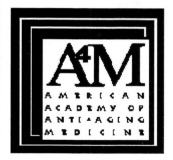

# American Academy of Anti-Aging Medicine

## Audio Cassette & Video Library by Insta-Tapes

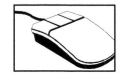

*"Tune In While You Drive"*

As a valued supporter of A4M since 1997, Insta-Tapes has been offering high quality audio and video productions of A4M's seminars.

To get the complete list via the internet go to:
**www.instatapes.com**

or EMAIL your request to:
**greg@instatapes.com**

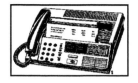

or FAX your request toll free to:
**(888) 346-8273**
Outside U.S.A. (208) 667-6834

*Cassettes • Audio CD's • VHS Videos • DVD's*

## Insta-Tapes
P.O. Box 908, Coeur d'Alene, ID 83816 U.S.A.